Endocrine Updates

Series Editor: *Shlomo Melmed, M.D.*

For further volumes:
http://www.springer.com/series/5917

Brooke Swearingen • Beverly M.K. Biller
Editors

Cushing's Disease

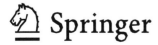 Springer

Editors
Brooke Swearingen, MD
Department of Neurosurgery
Massachusetts General Hospital
15 Parkman Street,
Boston, MA 02114, USA
BSwearingen@partners.org

Beverly M.K. Biller, MD
Neuroendocrine Unit
Massachusetts General Hospital
55 Fruit Street,
Boston, MA 02114, USA
BBiller@partners.org

ISSN 1566-0729
ISBN 978-1-4614-0010-3   e-ISBN 978-1-4614-0011-0
DOI 10.1007/978-1-4614-0011-0
Springer New York Dordrecht Heidelberg London

Library of Congress Control Number: 2011932355

© Springer Science+Business Media, LLC 2011
All rights reserved. This work may not be translated or copied in whole or in part without the written permission of the publisher (Springer Science+Business Media, LLC, 233 Spring Street, New York, NY 10013, USA), except for brief excerpts in connection with reviews or scholarly analysis. Use in connection with any form of information storage and retrieval, electronic adaptation, computer software, or by similar or dissimilar methodology now known or hereafter developed is forbidden.
The use in this publication of trade names, trademarks, service marks, and similar terms, even if they are not identified as such, is not to be taken as an expression of opinion as to whether or not they are subject to proprietary rights.
While the advice and information in this book are believed to be true and accurate at the date of going to press, neither the authors nor the editors nor the publisher can accept any legal responsibility for any errors or omissions that may be made. The publisher makes no warranty, express or implied, with respect to the material contained herein.

Printed on acid-free paper

Springer is part of Springer Science+Business Media (www.springer.com)

Preface

Investigations into the etiology and manifestations of Cushing's disease have served as a model for basic and clinical research in both endocrinology and neurosurgery since Cushing's original monograph in 1932. He worked from careful clinical observation back to underlying pathology; others, including Fuller Albright, elucidated the fundamental hormonal mechanisms. Even today, the complex interrelationships between cortisol dynamics and a wide spectrum of endocrine – e.g., the "metabolic syndrome" – and nonendocrine – e.g., depression – disorders continue to be described.

In this book, we review the pathogenesis, diagnostic algorithm, and treatment options for this complex disease, as presented by leading experts in the field. Dr. Aron discusses the fascinating history of Cushing's disease as well as its historical significance to both endocrinology and neurosurgery in Chap. 1. Dr. Melmed and colleagues present both their and others' work on the molecular pathogenesis of the disease in Chap. 2 while Drs. Cheunsuchon and Hedley-Whyte illustrate the anatomic pathology in Chap. 3. The diagnosis of Cushing's syndrome remains a major challenge; Dr. Nieman depicts the current diagnostic algorithm in Chap. 4 while Drs. Kaltsas and Chrousos review the differential of pseudo-Cushing's syndromes in Chap. 5. Cyclical hypercortisolemia can be extraordinarily difficult to diagnose; Drs. Tritos and Biller discuss its evaluation in Chap. 6. Dr. Findling and colleagues present their current approach to the differential diagnosis of Cushing's disease in Chap. 7. The source of the hypercortisolemia is localized by a combination of endocrine and radiographic techniques; Drs. Rapalino and Schaefer portray the imaging findings in Chap. 8.

The mainstay of treatment remains surgical removal of the corticotroph adenoma; current techniques and results are described by Drs. Tierney and Swearingen in Chap. 9. Dr. Vance reviews the postoperative management and assessment of remission in Chap. 10. If surgery is unsuccessful, adjunctive treatment is required. Dr. Loeffler and colleagues explain radiotherapeutic options in Chap. 11, and Dr. Petersenn describes recent exciting developments in medical therapy in Chap. 12. Even with initially successful surgical treatment, the disease will sometimes recur; the management of this difficult situation is reviewed by Dr. Kelly and colleagues in Chap. 13.

Although rare, Cushing's disease in the pediatric population is important to recognize, as its clinical manifestations and impact on growth can be severe; Dr. Savage and associates characterize its diagnosis and treatment in Chap. 14. Drs. Kaushal and Shalet review silent corticotroph adenomas as a distinct clinical entity in Chap. 15. The diagnosis and management of Cushing's disease during pregnancy can be especially difficult; this is highlighted in Chap. 16 by Drs. McCarroll and Lindsay. Although bilateral adrenalectomy is less frequently employed in treatment than several decades ago, postoperative progression of the underlying corticotroph tumor remains a potential complication of this approach, and is reviewed by Dr. Bertagna and associates in Chap. 17. Finally, the long-term psychological manifestations of hypercortisolemia can be significant even after disease remission; this important topic is discussed by Dr. Sonino in Chap. 18.

We would like to thank our colleagues for their excellent contributions, Ms. Ellen Green of Springer for her editorial assistance, and Dr. Shlomo Melmed, as senior editor of the series, for his initial invitation. All of us remain students of this fascinating disease.

Boston, MA, USA   Brooke Swearingen
                                                   Beverly M.K. Biller

Contents

1 Cushing's Disease: An Historical Perspective 1
   David C. Aron

2 Molecular Biology of Cushing's Disease 19
   Ning-Ai Liu, Anat Ben-Shlomo, and Shlomo Melmed

3 Pathology of Cushing's Disease 33
   Pornsuk Cheunsuchon and E.T. Hedley-Whyte

4 The Diagnosis of Cushing's Syndrome 45
   Lynnette K. Nieman

5 Pseudo-Cushing's Syndrome 57
   Gregory A. Kaltsas and George Chrousos

6 Cyclic Cushing's Disease 71
   Nicholas A. Tritos and Beverly M.K. Biller

7 Differential Diagnosis of Cushing's Syndrome 85
   Bradley R. Javorsky, Ty B. Carroll, and James W. Findling

8 Radiologic Imaging Techniques in Cushing's Disease 107
   Otto Rapalino and Pamela Schaefer

9 Surgical Treatment of Cushing's Disease 121
   Travis S. Tierney and Brooke Swearingen

10 Postoperative Management and Assessment of Cure 143
   Mary Lee Vance

11 Radiation Therapy in the Management
   of Cushing's Disease 151
   Kevin S. Oh, Helen A. Shih, and Jay S. Loeffler

12 Medical Management of Cushing's Disease 167
   Stephan Petersenn

13	**Recurrent Cushing's Disease**	183
	Nancy McLaughlin, Amin Kassam, Daniel Prevedello, and Daniel Kelly	
14	**Diagnosis and Treatment of Pediatric Cushing's Disease**	197
	Claire R. Hughes, Helen L. Storr, Ashley B. Grossman, and Martin O. Savage	
15	**Silent Corticotroph Adenomas**	211
	Kalpana Kaushal and Stephen M. Shalet	
16	**Cushing's Syndrome in Pregnancy**	223
	Frank McCarroll and John R. Lindsay	
17	**Nelson's Syndrome: Corticotroph Tumor Progression After Bilateral Adrenalectomy in Cushing's Disease**	237
	Guillaume Assie, Laurence Guignat, Jérôme Bertherat, and Xavier Bertagna	
18	**Psychosocial Aspects of Cushing's Disease**	247
	Nicoletta Sonino	
Index		259

Contributors

David C. Aron Division of Clinical and Molecular Endocrinology, Department of Medicine, Case Western Reserve University School of Medicine, Cleveland, OH, USA

VA Health Services Research and Development Center for Quality Improvement Research, Louis Stokes Cleveland VAMC, Cleveland, OH, USA

Education Office 14 (W), Louis Stokes Department of Veterans Affairs Medical Center, Cleveland, OH, USA

Guillaume Assie Department of Endocrinology, Faculté de Médecine Paris Descartes, Hôpital Cochin, Paris, France

Anat Ben-Shlomo Cedars-Sinai Medical Center, Los Angeles, CA, USA

Xavier Bertagna, Service des Maladies Endocriniennes et Métaboliques, Centre de Référence des Maladies, Rares de la Surrénale, INSERM U-567, Institut Cochin, Hôpital Cochin, Department of Endocrinology, Faculté de Médecine Paris Descartes, Paris, France

Jérôme Bertherat, Department of Endocrinology, Faculté de Médecine Paris Descartes, Hopital Cochin, Paris, France

Beverly M.K. Biller Neuroendocrine Unit, Massachusetts General Hospital, Harvard Medical School, Boston, MA, USA

Ty B. Carroll Department of Medicine, Endocrinology Center and Clinics, Medical College of Wisconsin, Milwaukee, WI, USA

Pornsuk Cheunsuchon Research Fellow in Neuropathology CS Kubik Laboratory for Neuropathology, Department of Pathology, Massachusetts General Hospital, Harvard Medical School, Boston, MA, USA

George Chrousos Department of Pediatrics, National University of Athens, Athens, Greece

James W. Findling Department of Medicine, Endocrinology Center and Clinics, Medical College of Wisconsin, Milwaukee, WI, USA

Ashley B. Grossman Department of Endocrinology, William Harvey Research Institute, Barts and the London School of Medicine and Dentistry, London, UK

Laurence Guignat Department of Endocrinology, Faculté de Médecine Paris Descartes, Hôpital Cochin, Paris, France

E. T. Hedley-Whyte CS Kubik Laboratory for Neuropathology, Department of Pathology, Massachusetts General Hospital, Harvard Medical School, Boston, MA, USA

Claire R. Hughes Department of Endocrinology, William Harvey Research Institute, Barts and the London School of Medicine and Dentistry, London, UK

Bradley R. Javorsky Department of Medicine, Endocrinology Center and Clinics, Medical College of Wisconsin, Milwaukee, WI, USA

Gregory A. Kaltsas Department of Pathophysiology, National University of Athens, Athens, Greece

Amin Kassam Department of Neurosurgery, The Ottawa Hospital, Ontario, Canada

Kalpana Kaushal Consultant Endocrinologist, Department of Endocrinology and Diabetes, Royal Preston Hospital, Preston, Lancashire, UK

Daniel Kelly Brain Tumor Center & Neuroscience Institute, John Wayne Cancer Institute at Saint John's Health Center, Santa Monica, CA, USA

John R. Lindsay Altnagelvin Area Hospital, Western Health & Social Care Trust, Londonderry, UK

Jay S. Loeffler Department of Radiation Oncology, Massachusetts General Hospital, Boston, MA, USA

Ning-Ai Liu Cedars-Sinai Medical Center, Los Angeles, CA, USA

Frank McCarroll Endocrinology & Diabetes Department, Altnagelvin Area Hospital, Londonderry, UK

Nancy McLaughlin Brain Tumor Center & Neurosciene Institute, John Wayne Cancer Institute at Saint John's Health Center, Santa Monica, CA, USA

Shlomo Melmed Cedars-Sinai Medical Center, Los Angeles, CA, USA

Lynnette K. Nieman Program on Reproductive and Adult Endocrinology, Eunice Kennedy Shriver National Institute of Child Health and Human Development, Bethesda, MD, USA

Kevin S. Oh Department of Radiation Oncology, Massachusetts General Hospital, Boston, MA, USA

Stephan Petersenn ENDOC Center for Endocrine Tumors, Hamburg, Germany
University of Duisburg-Essen, Essen, Germany

Daniel Prevedello Department of Neurosurgery, Ohio State University, Columbus, Ohio, CA, USA

Otto Rapalino Neuroradiology Division, Department of Radiology, Massachusetts General Hospital, Boston, MA, USA

Martin O. Savage Department of Endocrinology, William Harvey Research Institute, Barts and the London School of Medicine and Dentistry, London, UK

Pamela Schaefer Neuroradiology Division, Department of Radiology, Massachusetts General Hospital, Boston, MA, USA

Stephen M. Shalet Department of Endocrinology, Christie Hospital, Manchester, UK

Helen A. Shih Department of Radiation Oncology, Massachusetts General Hospital, Boston, MA, USA

Nicoletta Sonino Department of Statistical Sciences, University of Padova, Padova, Italy

Department of Mental Health, Padova City Hospital, Padova, Italy

Department of Psychiatry, State University of New York, Buffalo, NY, USA

Helen L. Storr Department of Endocrinology, William Harvey Research Institute, Barts and the London School of Medicine and Dentistry, London, UK

Brooke Swearingen Department of Neurosurgery, Massachusetts General Hospital and Harvard Medical School, Boston, MA, USA

Travis S. Tierney Department of Neurosurgery, Massachusetts General Hospital, Boston, MA, USA

Nicholas A. Tritos Neuroendocrine Unit, Massachusetts General Hospital, Boston, MA, USA

Mary Lee Vance Department of Medicine, University of Virginia Health System, Charlottesville, VA, USA

Chapter 1
Cushing's Disease: An Historical Perspective

David C. Aron

Abstract The history of Cushing's disease exemplifies one of the triumphs of clinical and experimental medicine, as well as some of their limitations. This history can be described in terms of the development of Cushing's disease as a clinical entity, which paralleled the history of medicine and the evolution of endocrinology as a discipline. Advances in endocrinology depended on clinical observations combined with laboratory studies – clinicians and chemists. The description of Cushing's disease and its elucidation depended upon these developments. Not only could treatment be effected by replacing a deficient hormone, but hormone excess could be treated by the removal of the pathologic hormone-secreting tumor, as demonstrated in Harvey Cushing's 1909 report of the successful treatment of acromegaly by the removal of a portion of the anterior lobe of the pituitary. The maturation of the field of endocrinology brought with it the recognition of the importance of feedback control and the development of the radioimmunoassay (among other scientific developments), as well as a shift in focus to hormone action, the rise of molecular biology, and the unification of endocrinology, immunology, and neuroscience into a single discipline.

This chapter is divided into three parts: (1) development of Cushing's disease as a clinical entity, a process that has moved from bedside to bench and back again, (2) further elucidation of the pathophysiology of Cushing's disease as the discipline of endocrinology moved from the organism to the organ to the cell, and (3) related developments that apply to issues in healthcare delivery.

D.C. Aron (✉)
Division of Clinical and Molecular Endocrinology, Department of Medicine,
Case Western Reserve University School of Medicine, Cleveland, OH, USA

VA Health Services Research and Development Center for Quality
Improvement Research, Louis Stokes Cleveland VAMC, Cleveland, OH, USA

Education Office 14 (W), Louis Stokes Department of Veterans Affairs
Medical Center, 10701 East Blvd., Cleveland, OH 44106, USA
e-mail: david.aron@va.gov

Keywords Endocrinology • Clinical medicine • Experimental medicine • Radio-immunoassay • Adenocorticotropic hormone • Hypercortisolism

Introduction

The history of Cushing's disease exemplifies one of the triumphs of clinical and experimental medicine, as well as some of their limitations. This history can be described in terms of the development of Cushing's disease as a clinical entity, which paralleled the history of medicine and the evolution of endocrinology as a discipline [1–4]. A discipline includes, among other elements, a paradigm, modes of inquiry, a community of scholars, an epistemology (requirements for what constitutes new knowledge), and a network for communication, e.g., learned journals and professional societies. This evolution has been described in part by Dr. Jean Wilson in his Plenary lecture at the 12th International Congress of Endocrinology [3]. He dates the birth of endocrinology to the presentation of a paper in 1889 to the Société de Biologie in Paris by Charles-Edouard Brown-Séquard, introducing the concept of chemical messengers secreted into the blood to exert systemic effects [5–8]. This is the essential paradigm. However, prior to this birth there was a long prenatal period during which many disorders now known to be endocrine in nature were described. For example, Thomas Addison described adrenal insufficiency in his book *On the Constitutional and Local Effects of Disease of the Supra-renal Capsules*, first published in London in 1855 [9]. At about the same time, Brown-Séquard's study of the effects of adrenalectomy indicated that the adrenals were necessary for life, though the reason remained unknown for many years. Endocrinology's adolescence was somewhat stormy; along with proof for the existence of multiple chemical messengers and astounding experiments involving administration of gland extracts, e.g., Murray's treatment of a case of myxedema and the discovery of insulin by Banting and Best; there were also extravagant claims for "organotherapy" [10–12]. However, the scientific approach to the generation of medical knowledge prevailed, and the importance of pathology in linking certain disorders to specific glands became evident. During this adolescence, the principles of hormone characterization were formulated by Doisy: (1) Identification of the tissue that produces a hormone; (2) Development of bioassay methods to identify the hormone; (3) Preparation of active extracts that can be purified, using the relevant bioassay; and (4) Isolation, identification of structure, and synthesis of the hormone [3, 13]. Advances in endocrinology depended on clinical observations combined with laboratory studies – clinicians and chemists. The description of Cushing's disease and its elucidation depended upon all of these developments. Not only could treatment be effected by replacing a deficient hormone, but hormone excess could be treated by the removal of the pathologic hormone-secreting tumor, as demonstrated in Harvey Cushing's 1909 report of the successful treatment of acromegaly by the removal of a portion of the anterior lobe of the pituitary [14].

The growing community of scholars' need for a professional society and journal was recognized with the founding in 1917 of The Association for the Study of

Internal Secretions (changing its name in 1952 to The Endocrine Society). The maturation of the field of endocrinology brought with it the recognition of the importance of feedback control and the development of the radioimmunoassay (among other scientific developments), as well as a shift in focus to hormone action, the rise of molecular biology, and the unification of endocrinology, immunology, and neuroscience into a single discipline. Paradigms were changing. Wilson stated: "The shift of focus to hormone action moved molecular endocrinology into the mainstream of cellular and developmental biology, and advances of several types have eroded the separations between endocrinology, neurobiology and immunology … There is probably no arena of medicine in which collaboration between the clinical and basic sciences has been more productive" [3]. In fact, the elucidation of the etiologies and pathophysiology of Cushing's disease has continued along with, and contributed to, these developments. Questions have been raised whether endocrinology is still a discipline or whether it has been reduced to molecular/cellular biology, but it is useful to view the development of Cushing's disease more broadly in context of health care delivery.

Although the emphasis in the current research paradigm as illustrated in the NIH Roadmap is conveniently described as being the linear progression of knowledge from bench to bedside to practice, the reality has always been far more complex [15]. The advance of medical practice depends on the interactions among the clinical practice, healthcare delivery, and biomedical research enterprises, all of which occur in a context with social, political, scientific, and philosophical aspects. For those interested in a detailed chronology of the events in the advance of knowledge of pituitary and adrenal anatomy, physiology, biochemistry, and pathophysiology, there are standard works and recent reviews [2, 3, 16–18]. This chapter is divided into three parts: (1) development of Cushing's disease as a clinical entity, a process that has moved from bedside to bench and back again, (2) further elucidation of the pathophysiology of Cushing's disease as the discipline of endocrinology moved from the organism to the organ to the cell, and (3) related developments that apply to issues in healthcare delivery.

Development of Cushing's Disease as a Clinical Entity

The description and elucidation of Cushing's disease has paralleled developments in medicine at large. Thomas Sydenham (1624–1689) became known as the English Hippocrates because of his idea that diseases were distinct and should be classified based on their clinical features and course. Critical to Sydenham's work (and the future of medicine) was his attention to accurate clinical observation and comparison of case with case and type with type. Thus, advancement in medicine proceeded following a clinical description, which consisted of a complex of signs and symptoms that were recognized as sufficiently different from other disease entities or syndromes to merit a new designation. The title of an essay from a book about the advancement of basic science is "By Their Diseases Ye Shall Know Them – The Endocrines" [19]. As knowledge accumulates, it helps us to understand the condition, how it came into being, how it relates to various other factors, various other

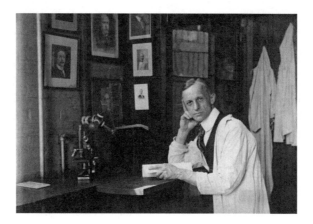

Fig. 1.1 Harvey Cushing http://webapps.jhu.edu/namedprofessorships/professorshipdetail.cfm?professorshipI D=125 accessed 11-28-04

states, i.e., it provides an "explanation" for a set of symptoms [20]. With time, it may prove valuable in the care of the patient and might also force us to modify the original concept of the clinical entity [20]. Although theories to explain the pattern (the science of medicine) may change through the ages, the clinical entity bridges the gap between theories, e.g., Cushing's disease due to hyperpituitarism versus hyperadrenalism. However, theories may broaden or narrow that clinical entity. For example, we now consider Cushing's disease to represent a spectrum from full blown Cushing's disease as it was initially described to a state of "sub-clinical" autonomous cortisol hypersecretion manifest solely by glucose intolerance or obesity [21]. The clinical entity is the persistent thread among the shifting theories and offers a way to examine the development of biomedical knowledge in ways that have implications for today. Following the clinical description of Cushing's disease some 300 years after Sydenham, the evolution of Cushing's disease as a clinical entity occurred in three periods: the description of the clinical syndrome, the explanation of the syndrome as hypercortisolism, and the delineation of three causes of hypercortisolism. In their 1969 article, Liddle and Shute recognized that this evolution was continuing to include the identification of atypical forms [1]. In the first two periods, the primary actors – Harvey Cushing (Fig. 1.1) and Fuller Albright (Fig. 1.2) combined clinical and experimental expertise. As consummate clinician–investigators, they were able to combine their knowledge and skills from each of these domains and the interactions were synergistic.

Harvey Cushing's Interest in the Pituitary and the Clinical Description of the Syndrome

Knowledge of the physiological role of both the adrenals and the pituitary began with recognition of clinical disorders. Bartolomeo Eustachius is the first person known to have described the adrenal glands, what in 1563 he termed the *"glandulae*

Fig. 1.2 Fuller Albright, from: Biographical Memoirs V.48 (1976) National Academy of Sciences, http://books.nap.edu/books/0309023491/html/2.html (NAS) accessed 11-28-04

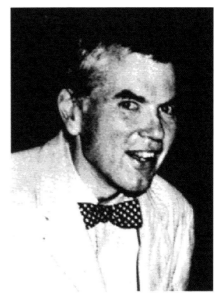

renibus incumbentes" and his drawing in the *Opuscula Anatomica* is the first known representation [2, 16, 18]. Virtually nothing was known about their function until the middle of the nineteenth century when Thomas Addison stated that "at the present moment, the function of the suprarenal capsules, and the influence they exercise in the general economy, are almost or altogether unknown" [9]. However, in this 1855 work, he described a series of patients with a variety of adrenal lesions – tuberculosis, metastases, and atrophy, some of whom clearly suffered from adrenal insufficiency. In fact, Addison's interest in the adrenals began with his observation of adrenal abnormalities in a form of fatal anemia (pernicious anemia). At around the same time, Brown-Séquard performed adrenalectomies and sham operations on dogs in the form of a controlled study and demonstrated that the adrenals were indispensable to life [2, 16, 18]. Tumors of the adrenal had been recognized at least since the eighteenth century and were associated with a variety of symptoms, particularly virilization [22, 23]. Individual cases, which fit the clinical picture of Cushing's disease, had also been described. However, the distinctness of the syndrome was not yet recognized.

The pituitary gland was identified earlier than the adrenals [24]. Galen, the court physician to the Roman Emperor Marcus Aurelius (third century CE), recognized the existence of the pituitary gland, and the conception of the pituitary as the source of phlegm was attributed to him; the pituitary was thus named (Latin *pituita*="phlegm"). Andreas Vesalius, the pioneering Flemish anatomist, named the structure *glandula pituitam cerebri excepiens* ("in the little phlegm acorn drawn out of the brain"). This was consistent with the Galenic concept of a structure necessary to eliminate waste products or residues generated in the brain. The English anatomist

Richard Lower suggested in his 1672 *Dissertatio de Origine Catarrhi* what might today be considered an endocrine function of the pituitary: "For whatever Serum is separated into the ventricles of the brain and tissues out of them through the Infundibulum to the Glandula pituitaria distills not upon the Palate but is poured again into the blood and mixed with it" [25]. By the turn of the twentieth century, apart from the clinical description of acromegaly and its association with a pituitary tumor, relatively little was known. In fact, in his classic monograph *The Pituitary Body and its Disorders,* Cushing contrasted the progress in investigation of the functions of the thyroid and adrenal glands: "The other glands have notably lagged behind, with the pituitary body at the tail of the procession. For though this structure was added to the group of so-called ductless glands by Liegeois some 50 years ago, its inaccessibility has been sufficient to discourage investigation even were there no other difficulties to be encountered" [26].

Harvey Cushing's interest in the pituitary gland may find its origin in a misdiagnosed case [27]. In 1901, Harvey Cushing returned to the USA from a European tour and began to develop his surgical career. Among his first cases was a sexually immature 14-year-old obese girl seeking treatment for progressive visual loss and headache. He was unable to localize the lesion clinically and rather than perform an exploratory craniotomy, he performed palliative decompressions. Although the headache improved, the girl's vision deteriorated. Cushing then explored the posterior fossa in the hopes of finding a cerebellar tumor, but to no avail and the girl died postoperatively of pneumonia. An autopsy revealed a pituitary cystic tumor. The misdiagnosis was made even worse because Cushing had recently spent time learning about brain tumor localization in the laboratory of one of the leading neurologists of the day, Charles Sherrington. Furthermore, several months after this case, Cushing earned of a similar case from someone who had studied with him in the same laboratory, Alfred Frohlich. Frohlich described a case of "adiposogenital dystrophy" in a boy with a pituitary tumor and sent a reprint to Cushing. Frohlich not only made the correct diagnosis, but also convinced a surgeon to operate. It may well have been wounded pride as well as intellectual interest in an intriguing case that set Cushing on the course to studying the functions and disorders of the pituitary gland. Cushing recognized the importance of clinical issues pointing the way in research. In his 1914 Weir Mitchell Lecture, Cushing emphasized the importance of tumors to the process of clarifying the function of an endocrine gland: "It may be recalled that much of our knowledge of pituitary disorders has revolved around the question of tumor-using the term *in* a comprehensive sense. It was the presence of a tumor which first led Marie, and subsequently Frohlich, to couple with this comparatively obscure gland the syndromes which bear their names. And for the most of us to-day manifestations of tumor continue to be a necessary guidepost, so that those who venture to predict pituitary disease in their absence do so with misgivings, and merely on the ground that similar constitutional symptoms have been known to arise in conjunction with a growth" [28].

Cushing's skill as neurosurgeon and his development of new techniques gave him an advantage over other experimental physiologists. When pituitary disorders were first being diagnosed, neurosurgery as a subspecialty had not yet come into being and the thought of surgical approaches to the deeply seated pituitary gland was a daunting prospect. This is illustrated in the words of a late twentieth century textbook: "Where the growth lies in contact with the base of the skull, that is, springs from the inferior surface of the brain, conservation would pronounce the word inaccessible. This warning, however, is quite unneeded by the genes audax omnia perpeti; for example, by such as announce that they think operations for the removal of tumors from the base *of* the brain are feasible; such daring characterized a specialist in cerebral surgery, whom the writer heard say that he believed it possible to so open the skull and lift up the brain as to catch a view of the foramen magnum. The reader may ask, Did he mean this of the living subject?" [29]. The first intracranial operation on the pituitary was performed only in 1889 by the British general surgeon Victor Horsley, who had an interest in the endocrine system and organotherapy and had already performed hypophysectomies and thyroidectomies in animals, but technical advancements occurred over the next two decades. Cushing's first approach to the pituitary via the extracranial (i.e., transsphenoidal) route took place in 1909, and an excellent surgical result was achieved. However, he remarked: "Surgeons, however, cannot afford to enter into this new field too precipitously, not simply by reason of the peculiar inaccessibility of the gland-for operative resources will overcome these difficulties – but principally on account of the present uncertainties in regard to its physiological properties" [14]. By 1912, Cushing had already achieved some excellent surgical outcomes, but he looked toward a different future: "It is conceivable that the day is not far distant when our present methods of dealing with hypophyseal enlargements, with scalpel, rongeur, and curette – new as these measures actually are and brilliant as the results may often be-will seem utterly crude and antiquated, for it is quite probable that surgery will, in the end, come to play a less, rather than a more important, role in ductless gland maladies. This Utopia, however, will be reached only when a sufficient understanding of the underlying aetiological agencies enables us to make more precocious diagnoses" [26].

Using his neurosurgical skills, Cushing was able to show in dogs that complete pituitary removal was lethal and concluded that the pituitary was essential to life. Although he was less successful in dissecting out the anterior and posterior lobes of the pituitary individually, he was able to show that partial destruction of the anterior pituitary was associated with the development of a Frohlich's syndrome. Although unable to prove it, Cushing, based on a clinical response to partial tumor resection in a patient with acromegaly, speculated that the acidophilic cells of the pituitary made a growth promoting factor that could account for the disordered growth. Though a researcher, Cushing was also a consummate clinician and sought to apply his knowledge in the clinic. Here is where he met Minnie G, one of his first patients with what Cushing called a polyglandular syndrome, but who in retrospect, clearly suffered from hypercortisolism (Fig. 1.3). Her case is described in his 1912 book, along with a group of cases exhibiting a polyglandular syndrome: "In brief, the term 'polyglandular syndrome' indicates merely that secondary functional alterations in members of the ductless gland series occur whenever the activity of one of the glands becomes primarily deranged. Further, the term as here employed is restricted to those cases in which it is difficult to tell which of the structures is primarily at

Fig. 1.3 Minnie G. Patient with Cushing's syndrome. From Cushing H. The pituitary body and its disorders. Philadelphia: J.B. Lippincott, 1912

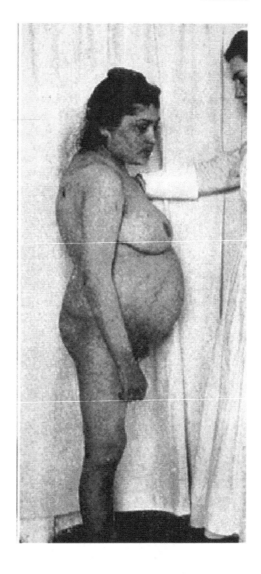

fault" [26]. Furthermore, her case description ends with the tantalizing statement: "An exploration of the adrenals is under consideration". However, this was never undertaken.

Cushing commented that in addition to skeletal undergrowth, adiposity and sexual dystrophy on the one hand, painful and tender adiposis with asthenia and psychic disturbances on the other, the case is an instance of the combination of intracranial pressure symptoms with amenorrhea, adiposity, and low physical stature. "A syndrome which might well be due to hypophyseal deficiency. But here, however, the similarity to the cases of hypopituitarism, which hasn't been heretofore discussed, ends ... A symptom-complex of this type has been described in association with certified *adrenal lesions,* which makes it appear that the adiposo-genital syndrome may occur with derangements of other of the ductless glands than the hypophysis itself ... It will thus be seen that we may perchance be on the way toward the recognition of the consequences of *hyperadrenalism*" [26]. He continued his clinical practice and laboratory investigation, accumulating a total of 12 cases that formed the basis of his classic 1932 paper [30]. Shortly thereafter, the syndrome was given the eponym Cushing's disease by Bishop and Close [31]. Although aware of the occurrence of adrenal hyperplasia in some cases, Cushing nevertheless held to the view that the pituitary was the primary problem, with the main factor being basophil adenomas of the pituitary gland which were found in two of the patients. He wrote: "While there is every reason to concede, therefore, that a disorder of somewhat similar aspect may occur in association with pineal, with gonadal, or with adrenal tumors, the fact that the peculiar polyglandular syndrome which pains have been taken herein conservatively to describe, may accompany a basophil adenoma in the absence of any apparent alteration in the adrenal cortex other than a possible secondary hyperplasia, will give pathologists reason in the future more carefully to scrutinize the anterior-pituitary for lesions of similar composition" [30]. He thought that hypersecretion of gonadotropin, along with growth hormone one of the two pituitary factors known, might be the factor responsible, but he was not able to produce this experimentally. Collip's discovery of adrenocorticotropic hormone (ACTH) would open the way to another path for investigation. Cushing's success owed to his keen powers of observation, skills as an experimentalist, as well as serendipity in his ability to relate disease syndromes to an overproduction or to an absence of secretory products of the pituitary; he set a very high standard for other clinician–investigators to follow [27]. Among those who met and probably exceeded this standard was Fuller Albright.

Fuller Albright and Hyperadrenocorticism

Fuller Albright (1900–1969) was considered to be the preeminent clinical and investigative endocrinologist of his day by many of his contemporaries and his 1944 address to the American Society for Clinical Investigation is considered a classic [32]. Schwartz noted that in a brief introductory note to his bibliography, Albright wrote, "In my opinion, my contributions divide themselves into two groups: (a) clinical descriptions and (b) elucidations of pathological physiology." In category (a), he, along with his students and associates, described de novo or made definitive contributions to the delineation of an astonishing 14 major syndromes over a 20-year-period [32]. In category (b), not only did he excel in the area of calcium metabolism for which he is best known, but also in the area of adrenal function (and others). I have elected to single out and describe in some detail his exploration of the workings of the adrenal cortex because his efforts in this area serve to illuminate the synergistic interactions between bedside medicine and basic science. At the same time, these studies provide elegant and instructive examples of how an astute clinical observer can unravel complex hormonal and metabolic interactions [32].

Interestingly, in Albright's diagram of the do's and don'ts of clinical investigation, a picture of a patient with Cushing's disease is prominently displayed [16]. This diagram was annotated by Felix Kolb, a member of the Metabolic Research Unit at University of California, San Francisco, which was led by Dr. Peter Forsham. This unit played an important role in describing a number of aspects of Cushing's disease and its management. In addition, among the most heavily cited life sciences papers between 1945 and 1954 was Albright's Harvey 1942–1943 Lectures on Cushing's syndrome [32, 33]. Here, Albright described the logical progression of his hypotheses and his moving from bench to bedside and back. His investigations stemmed from clinical observation. He wrote: "To be absolutely accurate, one should probably confine the term 'Cushing's Syndrome' to those individuals who present a certain striking clinical picture (vide infra) associated with a basophile tumor of the pituitary. However, the author will use the term to refer to patients with the clinical picture regardless of the etiology. From a clinical point of view, the syndrome is so striking that it seems almost certain that all individuals with it have some common denominator as regards the etiology" [32, 33].

His first attempt was to see whether this symptom complex could not be entirely explained on the basis of hypergluconeogenesis coupled with a resistance to glucose oxidation resulting from a hyperadrenocorticism. Since this hypothesis should lead not only to too much sugar, but also to too little protein, it might likewise explain the deficiency in tissues, notably the weakness of the muscles, osteoporosis, thin skin, and the easy bruisability. It might also explain the obesity. If the disorder does not involve a change in the total energy output but merely a change in the proportions of carbohydrates, fats, and proteins in the "metabolic mixture," one would expect the increased burning of protein to result in decreased burning and hence in storage of fats. However, Albright quickly saw problems with this hypothesis. He found it somewhat disconcerting that the patients with Cushing's disease studied in the clinic were never found to be in markedly negative nitrogen balance before therapy was instituted; indeed, most of them have been in slightly positive nitrogen balance. Moreover, patients with hypoinsulinemic diabetes, in whom the diabetes is not under control, do not develop a clinical picture like Cushing's disease in spite of the markedly increased conversion of proteins into sugars which occurs in that condition. This argument was stressed by Dr. Robert Loeb in a personal communication, who argued that the diabetes in Cushing's disease is the result of overproduction rather than the underconsumption of sugar. Finally, his hypothesis predicted that patients with Cushing's disease be resistant to ketosis. Abandoning that hypothesis, he tested another one, positing a fundamental disturbance in the ability to burn fat. However, a study in a single patient showed that not to be the case. Albright wrote: "When it came to looking around for a new hypothesis, the one certain fact from a clinical point of view was that the patients with Cushing's disease were suffering from deficiency of tissues. Since the evidence already presented made it quite clear that the disorder was not an excessive breakdown of tissue, the alternative thesis suggested itself, namely that there was a difficulty in synthesis of tissue. It seemed possible that the fundamental disorder was still a hyperadrenocorticism with respect to the 'S' hormone, but that this hormone, instead of converting proteins and hence tissues into sugar, inhibits the production of tissue" [32, 33]. In other words, as aptly put by Dr. E. C. Reifenstein, Jr., the hormone is anti-anabolic rather than catabolic. This hypothesis explained all the experimental results. He (Albright) wrote: "The author is aware of no data which do not harmonize with this new theory. However, he feels that such data will undoubtedly be forthcoming and that a new hypothesis or a further modification of the present one will be necessary" [32, 33]. The issue was not settled in the literature for several years, made more complicated by the different pathologic findings in different patients – basophilic adenomas of the pituitary, adrenal tumors, and adrenal hyperplasia. Ectopic ACTH syndrome was still to be recognized, although a case consistent with this diagnosis had been reported in 1928 [34]. For both Harvey Cushing and Fuller Albright, success was in large part a result of the combination of clinical and experimental expertise and the synergy of rigorous logic and knowledge-based intuition [32].

Further Elucidation of the Pathophysiology and Clinical Features of Cushing's Disease as the Discipline of Endocrinology Evolved

Following the periods of clinical description and identification of hypercortisolism as the underlying feature, in the third period, various causes of hypercortisolism were delineated: (1) autonomous secretion of cortisol by an adrenocortical neoplasm, (2) hypersecretion of cortisol in response to excessive secretion of ACTH by the pituitary gland and (3) hypersecretion of cortisol in response to "ectopic" ACTH. Other related conditions were described, e.g., Nelson's syndrome and the accelerated growth of an ACTH-secreting pituitary tumor following adrenalectomy for Cushing's disease [35]. However, when Grant Liddle described these three periods, the number of etiologies of Cushing's disease was relatively limited. In part, this reflected limitations in the technology of diagnosis [1]. However, during this time, advances in laboratory techniques and imaging facilitated more accurate diagnosis; tests were developed to distinguish among these types of hypercortisolism, e.g., dexamethasone suppression testing and ACTH measurements [36]. Developments in diagnosis and corresponding advances in imaging techniques and therapy continue to this day, e.g., inferior petrosal sinus sampling, salivary cortisol levels, CRH testing [37]. The identification of subclinical autonomous glucocorticoid hypersecretion which is a frequent finding in incidentally discovered adrenal masses reflects technological advances in radiologic imaging [38, 39].

As endocrinology narrowed its focus toward the inner workings of the cell, i.e., glucocorticoid receptors and genetic abnormalities, additional types of Cushing's disease were identified. Some cortisol-producing adrenal tumors or, more frequently, bilateral macronodular hyperplasias, are under the control of aberrant membrane hormone receptors, or altered activity of eutopic receptors. Food-dependent Cushing's disease was shown to be associated with ACTH-independent macronodular adrenal hyperplasia [40]. In this condition, cortisol secretion appears to be regulated by the aberrant expression of several G-protein-coupled receptors, specifically glucose-dependent insulinotropic polypeptide (GIP). In the adrenal tissue of affected individuals (both the adrenal nodules and the adjacent cortex), GIP and LH-receptor overexpression were found. Primary pigmented nodular adrenocortical disease (PPNAD) is a rare form of ACTH-independent Cushing's disease that may occur alone, but is found to be associated with the Carney complex (CNC) in 90% of the cases [41]. A form of multiple neoplasia syndrome, it is characterized by pigmented lesions on the skin; cardiac and cutaneous myxomas; multiple endocrinal tumors (adrenal, testicular or ovarian, thyroid, and hypophysis); and, less frequently psammomatous melanotic schwannoma, ductal adenoma of the breast, and rare bone tumors. It is an autosomally dominant inherited syndrome and somewhat fewer than half of the affected families have mutations in the gene *PRKAR1A*, which acts as a classical tumor suppressor. Additional developments in therapy have been based on molecular approaches, e.g., glucocorticoid receptor blockers [42]. However, notwithstanding the advances that have occurred in molecular biology and genetics, the endocrinologist practices in a context and developments outside the traditional discipline of endocrinology have also played a role in the way Cushing's disease is viewed, e.g., the elucidation of psychiatric manifestations of hypercortisolism [43]. Of note, Harvey Cushing himself was a pioneer in the psychosomatic approach to endocrine disease. This is reflected in his insistence on assessing every patient's mental status, in his insights into possible pathogenetic roles for stressful life events, in recognizing the occurrence of organic affective disorders ("the effects on the psyche and nervous system of chronic states of glandular overactivity or underactivity"), and in understanding the ailment of residual symptoms ("it is even more common for a physician or surgeon to eradicate or otherwise treat the obvious focus of disease, with more or less success, and to leave the mushroom of psychic deviation to vex and confuse the patient for long afterwards, if not actually imbalance him") [44]. The fact of residual symptoms implies long-term changes at the cellular/molecular level as a consequence of hypercortisolism.

Clinical Epidemiology and Healthcare Delivery (Health Services as They Apply)

As commonalities were found at the molecular level, there were developments in other areas, especially in health care delivery. The Institute of Medicine in 1995 offered the following definition of health services research: "Health services research is a multidisciplinary field of inquiry, both basic and applied, that examines the use, costs, quality, accessibility, delivery, organization, financing, and outcomes of health care services to increase knowledge and understanding of the structure, processes, and effects of health services for individuals and populations" [45]. This broad definition is explicitly concerned with several characteristics of health care and with the health of both individuals and populations. These concerns are especially relevant to the increasing interest in determining the value of health care and in managing the health of populations. Much of recent health services research has focused on medical outcomes defined as the health status of persons, groups, or communities that can be attributed to health care. Thus, outcomes research has been defined as the evaluation of medical practices integrating the best available information on safety, effectiveness, and outcomes as experienced by patients. Although outcomes research has a long history, its landmark application in the USA can be traced to a rivalry between two Harvard Medical School students: Ernest Codman and Harvey Cushing [46]. From 1894 to 1895, students were responsible for the administration of anesthesia at the Massachusetts General Hospital. After the death of Cushing's first patient, Cushing and Codman began a contest to obtain the lowest mortality rate. Although it is not clear who won, one result of the competition was the creation of anesthetic records. Codman became a surgeon in Boston and expanded upon his idea that the end results of treatment should be monitored and reported. In addition to keeping records of the patients' condition at discharge, he performed 1-year follow-up examinations and reported the results. His application of these ideas and their rejection by the medical establishment offers lessons for today. The development of measures of health care outcomes is critical to health services research. A wide variety of outcome measures have been developed and each has its problems. For example, mortality is easily defined but is usually such a rare event that the applicability of statistical analysis is limited. Although it is easier to establish criteria for an outcome measure in which data are collected prospectively, health services research frequently is performed retrospectively. Because outcomes may not be measurable for an extended period of time after the episode of care, conclusions about cause and effect are less certain. Measurement of health-related quality of life (HRQoL) is increasingly important in health services research, especially in evaluating the impact of chronic disease and the effectiveness of its treatment. Valid instruments are available to measure both comprehensive (generic) and disease-specific domains of function and well-being, and both are important in chronic illness. Chronic exposure to hypercortisolism has significant impact on patient's health and HRQoL, as demonstrated with generic questionnaires. Webb et al. developed a disease-specific questionnaire to evaluate HRQoL in patients with Cushing's disease (CushingQoL) [47]. Sonino et al. also developed a clinical index for rating severity in Cushing's disease to facilitate assessment of response to therapy [43].

Among the issues affecting the management of Cushing's is variation in practice. The Evidence-Based Medicine movement has reached endocrinology in general and Cushing's disease in particular. For example, systematic reviews of diagnostic tests have been conducted and evidence-based practice guidelines have been developed. An Endocrine Society Task Force developed a guideline for the diagnosis of Cushing's disease and Biller et al. reported on the development of a consensus approach to the treatment of patients with ACTH-dependent Cushing's disease [37, 48]. This process involved 32 leading endocrinologists, clinicians, and neurosurgeons with specific expertise in the management of ACTH-dependent Cushing's disease representing 9 countries. Another issue is that there is variation in outcomes across surgeons depending on experience, skill, and other factors. The consensus statement said: "The most important treatment recommendation that an endocrinologist makes to a patient with Cushing's disease is referral to a neurosurgeon with extensive experience in operating on patients with corticotroph microadenomas" [48]. Even under the best circumstances, remission rates after transsphenoidal pituitary microsurgery range from 42 to 86% [49]. Because Cushing's disease is rare, experience varies. An early example of practice variation is found in a letter to the New England Journal of Medicine which tabulated the number of cases and remission rates for transsphenoidal surgery for Cushing's disease [50]. Among 25 sites, the number of cases ranged from 2 to 15 per year and the remission rates ranged from 10 to 100% [50]. However, in a study of 958 neurosurgeons, Ciric et al. concluded that complication incidence is significantly higher in less-experienced surgeons in his study [51]. Cushing's disease treated by adrenalectomy presents similar issues. Moreover, Kissane and Cendan reported outcomes from laparoscopic adrenalectomy (LA) comparing patients with Cushing's disease with those with other adrenal pathology. LA in patients with Cushing's disease is associated with longer hospitalizations, more frequent major complications, and higher advanced care requirements, especially for patients undergoing bilateral adrenalectomy [52]. Thus, the history of Cushing's disease and its treatment continue to evolve.

Conclusion

The history of Cushing's disease has played out amid the background of developments in medicine and endocrinology. This history illustrates linkages between science and practice at multiple levels. Both Harvey Cushing and Fuller Albright played active roles to solidify the links. Each studied in the laboratory questions that arose at the bedside and contributed to the rise of endocrinology. Both served as Presidents of the Association for the Study of Internal Secretions (Cushing 1921–1922 and Allbright 1945–1946).

These efforts took place against a background of issues surprisingly relevant to contemporary issues. In a letter to Harvard Medical School Dean David Esall (7 March 1925), Cushing wrote: "If the pre-clinical departments succeed in driving the clinician out of the school entirely, instead of encouraging him to work there, it will be one more source of estrangement between those departments which deal with patients and those which do not" [53, 54]. Addressing the dedication of the William H. Welch Medical Library of the Johns Hopkins University School of Medicine in 1929, he commented upon the progressive decentralization of medical schools and the increasing specialization of both preclinical and clinical departments. He said: "More and more the preclinical chairs at most of our schools have come to be occupied by men whose scientific interests may be quite unrelated to anything that obviously has to do with Medicine, some of whom I, indeed, confess to a feeling that by engaging in problems that have an evident bearing on the healing art they lose caste among their fellows. They have come to have their own societies, separate journals of publication, a scientific lingo foreign to other ears, and are rarely seen in meetings of medical practitioners, with whom they have wholly lost contact" [55]. Similarly, Fuller Albright described the split personality of members of the American Society for Clinical Investigation. In his 1944 Presidential Address, he said that a member is "one trying to ride two horses – attempting to be an investigator and a clinician at one and the same time … this rider of two horses, however, must remember that there are two horses; he must avoid the danger on one side that he, as a clinician, be swamped with patients and the equal danger on the other side that he, an investigator, be segregated entirely from the bedside" [56].

Biomedical research is a complex network of processes and events. Much interest has been placed on distinctions between basic and clinical research or between basic and applied research. However, the dividing line between basic and applied biomedicine is at best elusive [27]. Similarly, there has been an emphasis on the process of going from bench to bedside rather than the other way around. The history of Cushing's disease illustrates the synergy between clinicians and researchers, particularly as personified by the same individual. This interplay, from bedside to bench and back in multiple iterations has brought us to the point where we can successfully treat the individuals afflicted with the group of disorders that bear the eponym "Cushing's disease." In fact, the advancement and expansion of endocrinology as a discipline has depended upon this iterative process. Only the continued interplay will allow us to make further progress and one wonders what the next phase in this process will bring.

References

1. Liddle GW, Shute AM. The evolution of Cushing's syndrome as a clinical entity. Adv Intern Med. 1969;15:155–75.
2. Lindholm J. Cushing's syndrome: historical aspects. Pituitary. 2000;3(2):97–104.
3. Wilson J. The evolution of endocrinologyPlenary lecture at the 12th International Congress of Endocrinology, Lisbon, Portugal, 31 August 2004. Clin Endocrinol. 2005;62:389–96.
4. Wilson LG. Internal secretions in disease: the historical relations of clinical medicine and scientific physiology. J Hist Med Allied Sci. 1984;39:263–302.
5. Brown-Sequard C. The effects produced in men by the injection of extracts of the testes of guinea pigs and dogs. Compte Rendu Societe de Biologie. 1899;1(Series 9):415–9.
6. Brown-Sequard C. The effects produced on man by subcutaneous injections of a liquid obtained from the testicules of animals. Lancet. 1899;2:105–7.
7. Olmsted J. Charles-Edouard Brown-Sequard: A Nineteenth Century Neurologist and Endocrinologist. Baltimore: The John Hopkins Press; 1946.
8. Wilson JD. Charles-Edouard Brown-Sequard and the centennial of endocrinology. J Clin Endocrinol Metab. 1990;71:1403–9.
9. Addison T. On the constitution and local effects of diseases of the suprarenal capsules. London: Samuel Highley; 1855.
10. Borell M. Brown-Sequard's organotherapy and its appearance in America at the endo of the nineteenth century. Bull Hist Med. 1976;50(1):309–20.
11. Borell M. Organotherapy, British physiology, and discovery of the internal secretions. J Hist Biol. 1976;9(2):235–68.
12. Hall DL. The critic and the advocate: contrasting British views on the state of endocrinology in the early 1920s. J Hist Biol. 1976;9(2):269–85.

13. Doisy E. Sex Hormones. Porter Lectures Delivered at the University of Kansas School of Medicine. Lawrence: University of Kansas Press; 1936.
14. Cushing H. Partial hypophysectomy for acromegly with remarks on the function of the hypophysis. Ann Surg. 1909;50:1002–17.
15. Green LW. From research to "best practices" in other settings and populations. Am J Health Behav. 2001;25:165–78.
16. Aron D. Cushing's syndrome from bedside to bench and back: a historical perspective. Endocrinol Metab Clin N Am. 2005;34(2):257–69.
17. Medvei V. A history of endocrinology. Lancaster, England: MTP; 1982.
18. Rolleston H. The Endocrine Organs in Health and Disease. London: Oxford University Press; 1936.
19. Means J. By their diseases ye shall know them the endocrines. In: Beecher HK, editor. Disease and the advancement of basic science. Cambridge, MA: Harvard University Press; 1960. p. 377–87.
20. King L. Medical Thinking. A Historical Preface. Princeton NJ: Princeton University Press; 1982.
21. Reincke M. Subclinical Cushing's syndrome. Endocrinol Metab Clin N Am. 2000;29:43–56.
22. Gabrilove J. The continuum of adrenocortical disease: a thesis and its lesson to medicine. Lancet. 1965;32:634–6.
23. Wilkins L. Adrenal disorders I: Cushing's syndrome and its puzzles. Arch Dis Child. 1962;37:1–8.
24. Aron DC. The path to the soul: Harvey Cushing and surgery on the pituitary and its environs in 1916. Perspect Biol Med. 1994;37:551–65.
25. Bell WB. The Pituitary: A Study of the Morphology, Physiology, Pathology, and Surgical Treatment of the Pituitary, Together with an Account of the Therapeutical Uses of the Extracts Made from this Organ. New York: William Wood & Co.; 1918.
26. Cushing H. The pituitary body and its disorders. Philadelphia: J.B. Lippincott; 1912.
27. Savitz S. Cushing's contributions to neuroscience, part 2: Cushing and several dwarfs. Neuroscientist. 2001;7(5):469–73.
28. Cushing H. The Weir Mitchell Lecture. Surgical experiences with pituitary disorders. JAMA. 1914;63:1515–25.
29. Johnson HC. Surgery of the hypophysis. In: Walker AE, editor. A History of Neurological Surgery. Baltimore: Williams & Wilkins; 1951.
30. Cushing H. The basophil adenomas of the pituitary body and their clinical manifestations (pituitary basophilism). Johns Hopkins Hosp Bull. 1932;50:137–95.
31. Bishop PMF, Close HG. A case of basophil adenoma of the anterior lobe of the pituitary: "Cushing's syndrome". Guys Hosp Rep. 1932;82:143–53.
32. Schwartz T. How to learn from patients: Fuller Albright's exploration of adrenal function. Ann Intern Med. 1995;123:225–9.
33. Albright F. Cushing's syndrome: its pathology and physiology, its relationship to the adreno-gential syndrome, and its connection with the problem of the reaction of the body to injurious agents. Harvey Lect. 1943;38:123–86.
34. Brown W. A case of pluriglandular syndrome: "diabetes of bearded women". Lancet. 1928;2:1022–3.
35. Hornyak M, Weiss MH, Nelson DH, Couldwell WT. Nelson syndrome: historical perspectives and current concepts. Neurosurg Focus. 2007;23(3):E12.
36. Liddle GW. Tests of pituitary-adrenal suppressibility in the diagnosis of Cushing's syndrome. J Clin Endocrinol Metab. 1960;20:1539–60.
37. Nieman L, Biller B, Findling J, Newell-Price J, et al. The diagnosis of Cushing's syndrome: an endocrine society clinical practice guideline. J Clin Endocrinol Metab. 2008;93:1526–40.
38. Chidiac RM, Aron DC. Incidentalomas: a disease of modern technology. Endocrinol Metab Clin N Am. 1997;26:233–53.
39. Ross NS, Aron DC. Hormonal evaluation of the patient with an incidentally discovered adrenal mass. N Engl J Med. 1990;323:1401–5.

40. Messidoro C, Elte J, Cabezas M, van Agteren M, et al. Food-dependent Cushing's syndrome. Neth Jounrnal Med. 2009;67(5):187–90.
41. Carney J. Discovery of the carney complex, a familial lentiginosis-multiple endocrine neoplasis syndrome: a medical odyssey. Endocrinologist. 2003;13(1):23–30.
42. Shomali MD, Hussain MA. Cushing's syndrome: from patients to proteins. Eur J Endocrinol. 2000;143:313–5.
43. Sonino N, Boscaro M, Fallo F, Fava G. A clinical index for rating severity in Cushing's syndrome. Psychother Psychosom. 2000;69(4):216–20.
44. Cushing H. Psychic disturbances associated with disorders of the ductless glands. Am J Insanity. 1913;69:965–90.
45. Field MJ, Tranquada RE, Feasley JC. Health Services Research: Work Force and Educational Issues. Washington, DC: Institute of Medicine-National Academy Press; 1995.
46. Beecher HK. The first anesthesia records (Codman, Cushing). Surg Gyn Obstet. 1940;71:689–93.
47. Webb S, Bandia X, Barahona M, et al. Evaluation of health-related quality of life in patients with Cushing's syndrome with new questionnaire. Eur J Endocrinol. 2008;158(5):623–30.
48. Biller B, Grossman A, Stewart P, et al. Treatment of adrenocorticotropin-dependant Cushing's syndrome: a consensus statement. J Clin Endocrinol Metab. 2008;93(7):2454–62.
49. Utz AL, Swearingen B, Biller BMK. Pituitary surgery and postoperative management in Cushing's disease. Endocrinol Metab Clin N Am. 2005;34:459–78.
50. Burch W. A survey of results with transsphenoidal surgery in Cushing's disease [letter]. N Engl J Med. 1983;308(2):216–20.
51. Ciric I et al. Complications of transsphenoidal surgery: results of a national survey, review of the literature, and personal experience. Neurosurgery. 1997;40(2):236–7.
52. Kissane N, Cendan J. Patients with Cushing's syndrome are care-intensive even in the era of laparoscopic adrenalectomy. Am Surg. 2008;75(4):279–83.
53. Tilney N. Harvey Cushing and the surgical research laboratory. Neurosurgery. 1980;151: 263–70.
54. Tilney N. Harvey Cushing and the evolution of a polymath. Surg Gyn Obstet. 1986;162:285–90.
55. Cushing H. The binding influence of a library on a subdiving profession in The Medical Career and Other Papers. Boston: Little Brown & Co.; 1940.
56. Albright F. Presidential Address to the American Society for Clinical Investigation, Atlantic City, New Jersey, 8 May 1944. Some of the "do's" and "do-not's" of clinical investigation. J Clin Invest. 1944;23:921–6.

Chapter 2
Molecular Biology of Cushing's Disease

Ning-Ai Liu, Anat Ben-Shlomo, and Shlomo Melmed

Abstract The proximal molecular pathogenesis of ACTH-secreting pituitary adenomas remains enigmatic. Several transgenic mice models have contributed important knowledge to understanding human pituitary disease; animal and cell models have provided novel insights into mechanisms underlying the pathogenesis of ACTH-secreting pituitary adenomas, mostly due to cell cycle disruption. Defective glucocorticoid feedback mechanisms also likely lead to enhanced POMC expression and corticotroph proliferation. Novel peptide therapies targeting somatostatin and/or dopamine (D2) receptors may also provide further insights into ACTH-secreting pituitary tumor pathogenesis. Studies investigating microRNA expression in pituitary corticotroph adenomas point to important functions of a unique class of gene regulators in the molecular biology of Cushing's disease. Continuing research advancement will lead to better understanding of Cushing's disease and development of novel therapeutic approaches.

Keywords Corticotroph cell • Proopiomelanocortin (POMC) • Transgenic mouse models • CRH • Adrenocorticotropic hormone (ACTH)

S. Melmed (✉)
Cedars-Sinai Medical Center, 8700 Beverly Blvd., Room 2015, Los Angeles, CA 90048, USA
e-mail: melmed@csmc.edu

Introduction

Despite advances leading to improved understanding of Cushing's disease, the pathogenesis of pituitary corticotroph adenomas remains enigmatic. We focus here on current knowledge and emphasize recent progress in identifying molecular and genetic mechanisms contributing to the development of pituitary corticotroph adenomas. Research progress on Cushing's disease pathogenesis is heavily dependent on animal studies largely due to the low disease incidence and small tumor size in humans.

Animal Models of Cushing's Disease and Related Tumors

Genetically manipulated mouse models have been used to recapitulate Cushing's disease, primarily because of striking homology in mammalian genomes as well as similar pituitary anatomy, cell biology, and physiology. Transgenic approaches have allowed overexpression of dominantly acting transgenes to phenocopy Cushing's disease pathology. Furthermore, specific allelic modification by homologous recombination gene ablation targeting endogenous cell cycle regulators have resulted in several mouse models with POMC-expressing tumors within the pituitary intermediate lobe.

Cushing's Disease Models with Transgenic Oncogene Overexpression

These models represent artificial phenomena generated using oncogenic viruses and, therefore, offer limited insight into corticotroph tumorigenesis. The first transgenic murine Cushing's disease model was produced by genetically introducing a hybrid gene consisting of the viral polyoma early region promoter linked to the polyoma large T antigen cDNA [1]. Transgenic mice developed pituitary microadenomas at 9 months of age, and large adenomas at 13–16 months of age, accompanied by features of Cushing's syndrome that progressed to wasting. The tumor latency period suggested the requirement for additional genetic or epigenetic alterations in pathogenesis of these tumors [1, 2]. Immunocompetent wild-type mice bearing transplants of PyLT transgenic pituitary tumors showed more pronounced effects of glucocorticoid excess than PyLT transgenic mice themselves. One of two PyLT transgenic lines developed pituitary tumors with 100% penetrance, suggesting that some viral oncogenes exhibit pituitary gland cell specificity.

Transgenic expression of the proopiomelanocortin (POMC) gene promoter (nucleotides −706 to +64) driving a simian virus (SV) 40 early gene encoding large T antigen induced large POMC-expressing pituitary tumors arising from the intermediate lobe [3]. Tumor cells expressed nuclear SV40 T antigen and POMC peptides, but not other pituitary hormones. Posttranslational pituitary

POMC processing was characterized by high proportions of acetylated and carboxyl-terminal shortened β-endorphins, as well as amino-terminal acetylated α-melanocyte-stimulating hormone, but virtually no ACTH(1–39), β-lipotropin or POMC. This pattern is indistinguishable from that of melanotrophs in the WT mouse intermediate lobe. In addition, tumor cells expressed abundant levels of mRNA for the prohormone convertase PC2 and undetectable levels of PC1, which is also similar to that of WT neurointermediate lobe, but distinct from the observed PC1 abundance in the anterior lobe.

Cushing's Disease Models with Transgenic Overexpression of Hormonal and Growth Factor Signals

Pituitary tumor growth appears to be promoted by hormones and growth factors implicated in normal pituitary function and development [6]. Mouse Cushing's disease models were developed by transgenic overexpression of hypothalamic stimulatory hormones or growth factors [4, 5]. Transgenic mice with metallothionein (mMT)-promoter-driven overexpression of CRH exhibited endocrine disruptions involving the hypothalamic-pituitary-adrenal (HPA) axis, manifesting as elevated plasma ACTH and glucocorticoid levels. These transgenic mice developed phenotypes similar to those seen in patients with Cushing's syndrome, such as excess fat accumulation, muscle atrophy, thin skin, and alopecia. However, there was no evidence of increased ACTH-expressing cells in the mMt-CRH transgenic pituitary, probably due to inhibitory feedback on pituitary corticotrophs by hypercortisolemia resulting from CRH stimulation [4].

Arginine-vasopressin is a potent ACTH-releasing hormone, which acts synergistically with CRH. Transgenic mice expressing the human V3 receptor under the control of rat POMC promoter sequences showed increased basal concentrations of corticosterone; however, no corticotroph tumors developed [7].

Leukemia inhibitory factor (LIF) is a pleiotropic cytokine that regulates the HPA axis and enhances POMC transcription as well as ACTH secretion by potently synergizing with CRH [8]. LIF also regulates corticotroph cell proliferation [9]. Transgenic LIF overexpression targeted by the pituitary glycoprotein hormone α-subunit (αGSU) promoter lead to corticotroph hyperplasia, truncal obesity, thin skin, and hypercortisolism, all characteristic phenotypes of Cushing's disease. αGSU-LIF transgenic mice also exhibited central hypogonadism, dwarfism, and mild hypothyroidism, with gonadotroph, somatotroph, lactotroph, and thyrotroph hypoplasia. In the mouse, pituitary organ commitment is initiated with expression of alpha-GSU [5]. In the transgenic pituitary, LIF overexpression diverts progenitor cell differentiation from Lhx3/Lim3-dependent cell lineages (gonadotroph, thyrotroph, somatotroph, and lactotroph) to an Lhx3/Lim3-independent cell lineage, i.e., corticotrophs. Pituitary LIF signaling is further potentiated by glucocorticoids [10], therefore suggesting that neuro-immune-endocrine interfacing molecules act as important players in pituitary corticotroph homeostasis and tumor formation.

Table 2.1 Disrupted cell cycle regulators in mouse and human Cushing's disease and related tumors

Gene	Tumor-associated change	Tumor type	References
pRb	Mouse: heterozygous null mutation	IL tumors	[13]
p27	Mouse: null mutation	IL tumors in mouse	[15, 17]
	Human: reduced expression level a 19-bp duplication in exon 1	Corticotroph tumor and pituitary carcinoma	[44]
		MEN1-like syndrome including corticotroph tumor	[55, 56]
p18	Mouse: null mutation	IL and pituitary tumors	[20]
	Human: reduced expression level	Corticotroph adenomas	[48]
Cyclin E	Human: overexpression	Corticotroph adenomas	[47]
Pttg	Human: overexpression	All types of pituitary tumors including corticotroph adenomas	[42]

Genetic Knockout of Cell Cycle Regulators in Pituitary POMC-Cell Tumors

Multiple targeted gene knockout models have implicated cell cycle regulators in the pathogenesis of pituitary POMC-expressing tumors [11–13]. These gene knockout animals exhibit a high incidence of pituitary intermediate lobe POMC cell tumors, which are an otherwise rare tumor type in WT mice (Table 2.1). A classical example indicating the association of cell cycle regulators and pituitary tumorigenesis is derived from the heterozygous Rb mice [11–13]. The Rb gene encodes a tumor suppressor that controls the G1/S checkpoint. Rb phosphorylation by cyclin dependent kinases (Cdk) releases E2F, enabling S phase progression. Ink4-type inhibitors (p16, p15, p18, p19) and Cip/Kip-type (p21, p27, p57) suppress Cdk actions. Sequential activation and inactivation of protein kinase complexes regulate cell-cycle progression [14]. $Rb^{+/-}$ mice develop pituitary intermediate lobe POMC cell tumors at 12 months with 100% penetrance. p27 (Kip1) deletion, like deletion of the Rb gene, also leads to neoplastic growth within the intermediate lobe. However, intermediate lobe adenomas due to p27 deletion are less prominent than the POMC-expressing adenocarcinomas arising in $Rb^{+/-}$ animals [15–17]. Deletion of p27 or p21 in $Rb^{+/-}$ animals enhances intermediate lobe tumorigenesis and shortens the murine lifespan [18, 19]. Additionally, p18 deletion leads to intermediate lobe hyperplasia, which is further enhanced by compound loss of p27 or p21 [20, 21]. Overall, tumor incidence and phenotype are highly dependent on the mouse strain suggesting involvement of additional genetic factors in tumorigenesis [22]. Increased tumor incidence in $Rb^{+/-}$ mice is partially rescued by mutations of Rb effectors such as E2f1 or E2f4 [23, 24], as well as by pituitary tumor transforming gene (PTTG) [25]. PTTG is a securin that regulates sister-chromatid separation by binding to separase in the APC complex, and plays multiple roles in cell cycle regulation at different stages [26]. PTTG deletion decreased pituitary tumor incidence in $Rb^{+/-}$ mice by triggering p53/p21-dependent senescence [27, 28]. Therefore, multiple cell cycle regulatory pathways are involved in initiating and maintaining pituitary corticotroph tumorigenesis.

Spontaneous Cushing's Disease in Large Animals

Spontaneous disorders mimicking human Cushing's disease have been described in dogs, horses, and less commonly cats [29–32]. Equine Cushing's disease usually results from intermediate lobe tumors, and rarely from those of the anterior lobe [29, 30]. Canine Cushing's disease has an estimated incidence of 1–2 cases/1,000 dogs/year [31, 32] and represents one of the most common endocrine disorders in dogs. Approximately 30% of canine Cushing's disease results from intermediate lobe tumors. In addition to typical melanotrophs, the canine pituitary intermediate lobe contains a substantial percentage of a second cell type that stains intensely for ACTH, but not for MSH [33]. Although molecular, cellular, and genetic makeup of canine corticotroph adenomas are yet to be identified, the high natural incidence and many clinical phenotypes similar to human Cushing's disease render canine Cushing's disease a potentially important system for both in vitro and in vivo studies to understand Cushing's disease pathogenesis, as well as to develop and test new therapeutic strategies.

Molecular Pathogenesis of Human Cushing's Disease

It remains unresolved whether corticotroph tumors arise from a primary defect in the hypothalamus or the pituitary [34]. However, currently, most evidence supports the primary pituitary origin of these tumors. Hypothalamic dysfunction was supported by the fact that many Cushing's disease associated endocrinopathies manifested as inhibition of growth, hypogonadotropic hypogonadism, and hypothyroidism. Moreover, in many cases the pituitary adenoma is not identified at surgery and these tumors often recur after apparently complete resection, while some pituitary glands harboring corticotroph adenomas exhibit corticotroph hyperplasia [35, 36]. However, corticotroph hyperplasia is difficult to detect as differences from normal corticotroph cells are subtle [37]. The evidence for a primary pituitary origin is more compelling. High cure rates with reversal of major abnormalities associated with Cushing's disease are observed after complete tumor resection and cortisol level normalization. Pituitary hyper-responsiveness to CRH before corticotroph adenoma removal reverses to hyporesponsiveness 1 week after resection [38]. Most corticotroph adenomas do not exhibit surrounding hyperplastic corticotrophs [37]. Moreover, pituitary tumors were proven to be monoclonal in origin [39, 40].

Biochemically and histologically, corticotroph tumor cells show relative and subtle abnormalities compared with normal ACTH-secreting cells, suggesting that tumorigenesis is likely associated with mutations or derangements of normal corticotroph-specific regulatory pathways. The initial event of corticotroph transformation likely involves multifactorial etiologies such as genetic and epigenetic silencing of tumor suppressors, as well as hormonal and growth factor dysregulation, all of which may further promote tumor cell proliferation and expansion.

Tumor Suppressor Genes and Other Cell Cycle Regulators

Pituitary cells are rarely affected by oncogene activation or loss of tumor suppressor genes. Most protooncogene and tumor suppressor gene mutations implicated in nonpituitary cancers have not been identified in corticotroph adenomas. These include RAS, c-ERB2/neu, c-MYC, PKC, RET, c-MYB, c-FOS, Gα subunit of the G-protein, p53, Rb1, p16, and p18 [41].

As a cell cycle regulator and global transcription factor modulating G1/S and G2/M phase transition, human PTTG1 is overexpressed in more than 90% of all type of pituitary tumors, including corticotroph adenomas [42]. PTTG1 is regulated by CDK1-mediated phosphorylation [43], suggesting a link between cell cycle control by CDKs and PTTG1 function and implicating cell cycle deregulation in pituitary tumorigenesis. The p27 tumor suppressor regulates cell cycle progression by interacting with and inhibiting cyclin/Cdk complexes. Although early studies detected no p27 genomic mutations or consistent change in p27 messenger RNA expression in human sporadic pituitary tumors, downregulation of p27 protein expression is often observed in corticotroph adenomas and pituitary carcinomas suggesting underlying mechanisms involving posttranslational dysregulation [44]. Degradation of p27 is a critical event for the G1/S transition and occurs through ubiquitination by SCF(Skp2) and subsequent degradation by the 26S-proteasome [45]. In a study of 59 human pituitary samples (seven normal pituitary glands, 52 adenomas including 12 ACTH-secreting tumors), no significant difference of Skp2 mRNA or nuclear protein expression was detected between the normal pituitary and tumor tissue; therefore, it is not yet clear whether SKP2 is the relevant F-box protein for degradation of p27Kip1 in corticotropinomas [46]. In addition, increased cyclin E protein expression is frequently observed in corticotroph tumors, probably in relation to the low p27 protein expression levels [47]. Using Affymetrix GeneChip microarray analysis combined with RT-PCR analysis for gene expression profile of major pituitary adenoma subtypes, ACTH-secreting adenomas ($n=13$) were shown to exhibit significantly underexpressed p18, in which murine gene deletion has been shown to produce pituitary ACTH cell hyperplasia and adenomas [48]. Both p27 and p18 are directly regulated by MEN1 (multiple endocrine neoplasia type 1), and loss of MEN1 function results in downregulation of these two inhibitors with subsequent deregulation in cell proliferation [49, 50]. The multiple endocrine neoplasia syndrome is characterized by predisposition to pituitary adenomas, parathyroid hyperplasia, and pancreatic endocrine tumors. Pituitary adenomas affect between 25 and 30% of MEN-1 patients [51]. According to the France–Belgium MEN1 multicenter study, 6 of 136 cases of MEN1 with pituitary adenomas harbored

ACTH-secreting corticotroph adenomas [52]. However, expression of MEN1 mRNA is normal in sporadic pituitary corticotroph adenomas [53, 54]. Recently, the CDKN1B/p27^{Kip1} gene has been identified as a new susceptibility gene for a MEN1-like syndrome that is MEN1-gene mutation negative (now designated MEN4), in one family segregating endocrine neoplasia (pituitary adenoma, acromegaly, and primary hyperparathyroidism) [55]. Subsequently, a second germ-line CDKN1B/p27^{Kip1} mutation was identified in 1 of 36 (2.8%) Dutch patients clinically suspected for MEN1, however, tested negative for *MEN1* gene mutation [56]. A 19-bp duplication within CDKN1B/p27^{Kip1} exon 1 changes the amino-acid sequence after 26 residues and leads to a premature stop codon 69 amino acids earlier than the wild type. The patient was diagnosed with small-cell neuroendocrine cervical carcinoma, ACTH-secreting pituitary adenoma, and hyperparathyroidism, all lesions compatible with MEN1 [56]. Overall, somatic CDKN1B/p27^{Kip1} mutations are uncommon in suspected MEN1 cases and sporadic pituitary adenoma patients [56–58] (Table 2.1).

Neuroendocrine Hormones and Regulatory Factors

Corticotroph proliferation and ACTH secretion are controlled by stimulatory factors, such as CRH, vasopressin, leukemia inhibitory factor (LIF), and inhibitory factors, such as glucocorticoid and somatostatin (SRIF), as well as their specific receptors. Genes encoding proteins involved in corticotroph regulatory pathways are potential candidates as tumorigenic mutations in Cushing's disease. However, studies investigating classic corticotroph regulatory factors are yet to provide clear evidence of a common genetic defect in these tumors.

CRH is the main hypothalamic stimulator of corticotroph proliferation and ACTH secretion. In humans with CRH-secreting tumors, excess CRH induces corticotroph hyperplasia and hypercortisolism but no corticotroph tumor formation [59, 60]. In a study of 43 corticotroph adenomas, CRH mRNA levels were significantly higher in tumor tissues vs. normal pituitary and also in macroadenoma and locally invasive adenomas vs. microadenomas. CRH expression correlated with Ki-67 expression, suggesting CRH autocrine/paracrine functions in corticotroph adenomas [61]. Some corticotroph adenoma cells exhibit increased CRH receptor type 1 mRNA levels; however, mutations of CRH receptor coding sequence have not been found [62]. Vasopressin type 3 receptor (V$_3$R) stimulation enhances ACTH secretion and mRNA expression is increased in ACTH-secreting tumors, probably as a consequence of chronic glucocorticoid exposure. However, no mutation in the V$_3$R gene has been found in corticotroph adenomas [63]. While the pathophysiological significance of V$_3$R and CRH/CRH-R overexpression in Cushing's disease remains to be determined, they may be associated with proproliferative effects sustaining corticotroph tumor growth.

One of the hallmarks of corticotroph adenomas is partial resistance to corticosteroid feedback, which may represent an early event of corticotroph tumorigenesis.

Corticotroph tumors likely develop from cells with genetic mutations rendering partial resistance to the physiological negative feedback [64], therefore leading to a set-point defect and inappropriately high ACTH levels. Peritumoral normal corticotrophs would likely exhibit growth suppression in response to the supraphysiological level of cortisol, thus providing the mutant clone with a further growth advantage. ACTH may suppress its own secretion from corticotrophs via an ultrashort paracrine/autocrine loop. Indeed, ACTH receptor and melanocortin 2 receptor (MC2) mRNAs were absent in 16 of 22 pituitary corticotroph adenomas, but were detectable in normal human pituitary. Plasma ACTH levels were significantly higher with tumors that did not express the receptor compared to those that did [65]. Loss of normal ACTH receptor expression and/or function in corticotroph adenomas may contribute to partial corticosteroid resistance, although no mutations of ACTH and MC2 receptors were found in corticotroph tumors that still exhibit receptor expression. Glucocorticoid exerts feedback on corticotrophs via the glucocorticoid receptor (GR), and GR disruption may contribute to pituitary-specific glucocorticoid resistance seen in corticotroph adenomas. The human GR exhibits two isoforms resulting from alternative transcript splicing [66]. GR-β differs from GR-α at the carboxyl terminus, which prevents corticosteroid binding and transcriptional activation [66]. A nonsense mutation leading to a truncated GR was discovered in a patient with Nelson's syndrome; however, no similar defect was identified in a series of 19 ACTH-secreting tumors, including two cases of Nelson's syndrome, three ectopic secretors, and one malignant corticotropinoma [67]. While a GR gene mutation does not appear to be a common defect contributing to glucocorticoid resistance in corticotroph adenomas, it remains to be determined whether GR LOH, or altered levels of GR-α and GR-β isoform expression are associated with Cushing's disease pathogenesis.

Investigation of mechanisms underlying glucocorticoid resistance has led to identification of two essential proteins for repression of proopiomelanocortin (POMC), a precursor of ACTH. Corticosteroids repress POMC transcription through protein–protein interactions of GR with NGFI-B to form a transrepression complex at the POMC promoter. The ATPase subunit of the chromatin remodeling Swi/Snf complex Brg1 is essential to stabilize GR and NGFI-B interactions, and critical for recruitment of the histone deacetylase HDAC2 to the complex [68]. In a series of 36 human corticotroph adenomas obtained at surgery, 50% of tumors were deficient in nuclear Brg1 or HDAC2. Brg1 was delocalized to the cytoplasm in a subset of tumors, while it was detected in nuclei of surrounding peritumoral corticotroph cells. This observation was apparent in both human and canine pituitary corticotroph adenoma cells [68, 69]. The relative high frequency of Brg1 and/or HDAC2 misexpression in corticotroph adenomas supports their importance in pituitary corticosteroid resistance associated with Cushing's disease.

Pituitary Nelson's tumors arise in patients with Cushing's disease who have undergone bilateral adrenalectomy. The cause for growth of Nelson's tumor is yet unknown, and recent studies suggest that tumors do not appear de novo, but rather grow from a persistent pituitary corticotroph microadenoma [70]. Potential causes of

Nelson's tumors may include restored CRH and AVP tone, elimination of the suppressive growth effect of endogenous cortisol and insufficient levels of exogenous cortisone [71]. Although usually slow growing, some tumors can grow rapidly to a large size [72]. Crooke hyalinization is usually absent in nontumorous corticotroph cells derived from pituitary glands harboring Nelson's tumors.

Corticotrophs are also negatively regulated by somatostatin (SRIF) signaling pathways. Somatostatin actions are mediated through five different membrane-bound receptors (SSTR 1–5). SSTRs are members of the G protein-coupled receptor family. SSTR signaling leads to inhibition of hormone secretion and cell proliferation, or may induce apoptosis. Human corticotroph adenomas exhibit abundant SSTR5, in addition to SSTR1, -2, and -3, mRNA and protein levels. Pasireotide (SOM230), a synthetic SRIF analog, inhibits ACTH secretion from ACTH-secreting adenomas not responsive to octreotide in vitro and is more effective than octreotide to inhibit CRH-induced rat ACTH and cortisol secretion. In a proof-of-concept, open-label, 15-day phase II trial, 76% of patients with Cushing's disease receiving pasireotide exhibited lowered urinary free cortisol levels [73]. Enhanced pasireotide action in corticotrophs is determined by SST5 dominance that maximally stimulates short- and long-term corticotroph responses to SRIF analogs [74].

In addition to the aforementioned hormonal and regulatory factors, other cytokines, growth and developmental factors have been investigated for potential roles in corticotroph tumor formation, including epidermal growth factor (EGF) and receptor (EGFR), PTX family members and Tpit/Tbx19 [41, 69], none of which has been found to play a major role in corticotroph tumorigenesis. These factors may regulate a preexisting tumor clone or promote establishment of an oncogenic background, therefore contributing to tumor formation and/or expansion. A mutation in the DAX1 gene that controls HPA axis development was found in a 33-year-old patient with X-linked adrenal hypoplasia congenita and pituitary corticotroph adenoma [75]. Recently, pituitary corticotroph microadenomas have been reported in two patients with tuberous sclerosis complex, an autosomal dominant neurocutaneous disorder characterized by benign tumors (hamartomas), epilepsy, and mental retardation. This complex is a result of mutation in the *TSC1* and *TSC2* genes that encode the proteins hamartin and tuberin, respectively. Mechanisms promoting corticotroph adenoma growth in this disorder are unknown [76].

MicroRNA Expression in Corticotroph Adenomas

MicroRNAs (miRNAs) are noncoding, single-stranded RNAs constituting a novel class of gene regulators. MicroRNAs control diverse biological processes including cell growth, differentiation and apoptosis by posttranscriptional regulation of target gene expression [77]. More than 50% of identified human microRNAs are located in the fragile sites of genome areas [78]. miRNA mutations or misexpression correlate with several human cancers suggesting that miRNAs can function as tumor suppressors [79]. In a recent study of 11 ACTH-secreting pituitary adenomas and seven normal pituitaries, real-time PCR analysis revealed downregulation of several miRNAs in corticotroph adenomas compared with normal pituitary, including miR-15a, miR-16, and Let-7a among others [80]. Reduced miR-15a and miR-16 expression was also discovered in GH- or PRL-secreting pituitary adenomas, and levels of reduction correlated inversely with tumor diameter [81, 82]. Interestingly, miR-15a and miR-16 genes are colocalized with the Rb tumor suppressor on chromosome region 13q14, which is frequently deleted in pituitary adenomas including corticotropinomas [83, 84]. There has been evidence that additional putative tumor-suppressor gene(s) at the 13q14 locus are closely linked to, but distinct from, Rb1 and might be important in pituitary tumorigenesis [85]. Let-7 microRNA negatively regulates high-mobility group A2 (HMGA2), an embryonic and oncogenic protein that is highly expressed in many tumors including pituitary adenomas [86–88]. In a series of 55 postsurgical pituitary adenomas, decreased let-7 expression was present in 23 of 55 (42%) adenomas, including 12 of 18 (67%) corticotroph adenomas, and correlated with high-grade tumors ($P<0.05$). An inverse correlation between let-7 and high-mobility group A2 expression was evident ($R=-0.33$, $P<0.05$) [89]. These findings support a causal link between let-7 and HMGA2 whereby loss of let-7 expression induces HMGA2, contributing to pituitary tumorigenesis and progression.

Conclusion

In summary, human corticotroph tumor studies are difficult to undertake as the disease is rare. Moreover, these tumors are small, and in many cases the tumor specimen is accompanied by surrounding normal pituitary tissue. In addition, direct comparison of tumorous to normal corticotroph cell function is challenging in most cases, as normal pituitary tissue from the same patient is usually unavailable, and even if available, the degree of "normalcy" is questionable. Recently, Roussel-Gervais et al showed that overexpression of cyclin E in murine pituitary POMC cells leads to abnormal reentry into cell cycle of differentiated POMC cells and to centrosome instability. These alterations are consistent with the intermediate lobe hyperplasia and anterior lobe adenomas observed in these pituitaries [90]. As this chapter was in press, we published a germline transgenic zebrafish overexpressing PTTG targeting the pituitary POMC lineage, which recapitulated features pathognomonic of corticotroph adenomas including corticotroph expansion, partial glucocorticoid resistance, and pituitary cyclin E up-regulation, as well as metabolic disturbances mimicking hypercortisolism due to Cushing's disease [91]. Selective CDK inhibitors effectively targeted zebrafish and murine corticotroph tumor growth and hormone secretion [91]. A better understanding of the specific genetic and epigenetic alterations in human Cushing's disease will be necessary for selecting the appropriate combination of current treatments and/or developing new therapeutic approaches.

References

1. Helseth A, Siegal GP, Haug E, Bautch VL. Transgenic mice that develop pituitary tumors. A model for Cushing's disease. Am J Pathol. 1992;140:1071–80.
2. Bautch VL, Toda S, Hassell JA, Hanahan D. Endothelial cell tumors develop in transgenic mice carrying polyoma virus middle T oncogene. Cell. 1987;51:529–37.
3. Low MJ, Liu B, Hammer GD, Rubinstein M, Allen RG. Post-translational processing of proopiomelanocortin (POMC) in mouse pituitary melanotroph tumors induced by a POMC-simian virus 40 large T antigen transgene. J Biol Chem. 1993;268:24967–75.
4. Stenzel-Poore MP, Cameron VA, Vaughan J, Sawchenko PE, Vale W. Development of Cushing's syndrome in corticotropin-releasing factor transgenic mice. Endocrinology. 1992;130:3378–86.
5. Yano H, Readhead C, Nakashima M, Ren SG, Melmed S. Pituitary-directed leukemia inhibitory factor transgene causes Cushing's syndrome: neuro-immune-endocrine modulation of pituitary development. Mol Endocrinol. 1998;12:1708–20.
6. Melmed S. Mechanisms for pituitary tumorigenesis: the plastic pituitary. J Clin Invest. 2003;112:1603–18.
7. Rene P et al. Overexpression of the V3 vasopressin receptor in transgenic mice corticotropes leads to increased basal corticosterone. J Neuroendocrinol. 2002;14:737–44.
8. Auernhammer CJ, Melmed S. Leukemia-inhibitory factor-neuroimmune modulator of endocrine function. Endocr Rev. 2000;21:313–45.
9. Stefana B, Ray DW, Melmed S. Leukemia inhibitory factor induces differentiation of pituitary corticotroph function: an immuno-neuroendocrine phenotypic switch. Proc Natl Acad Sci USA. 1996;93:12502–6.
10. Langlais D, Couture C, Balsalobre A, Drouin J. Regulatory network analyses reveal genome-wide potentiation of LIF signaling by glucocorticoids and define an innate cell defense response. PLoS Genet. 2008;4:e1000224.
11. Lee EY et al. Mice deficient for Rb are nonviable and show defects in neurogenesis and haematopoiesis. Nature. 1992;359:288–94.
12. Clarke AR et al. Requirement for a functional Rb-1 gene in murine development. Nature. 1992;359:328–30.
13. Jacks T et al. Effects of an Rb mutation in the mouse. Nature. 1992;359:295–300.
14. Quereda V, Malumbres M. Cell cycle control of pituitary development and disease. J Mol Endocrinol. 2009;42:75–86.
15. Nakayama K et al. Mice lacking p27(Kip1) display increased body size, multiple organ hyperplasia, retinal dysplasia, and pituitary tumors. Cell. 1996;85:707–20.
16. Fero ML et al. A syndrome of multiorgan hyperplasia with features of gigantism, tumorigenesis, and female sterility in p27(Kip1)-deficient mice. Cell. 1996;85:733–44.
17. Kiyokawa H et al. Enhanced growth of mice lacking the cyclin-dependent kinase inhibitor function of p27(Kip1). Cell. 1996;85:721–32.
18. Brugarolas J, Bronson RT, Jacks T. p21 is a critical CDK2 regulator essential for proliferation control in Rb-deficient cells. J Cell Biol. 1998;141:503–14.
19. Park MS et al. p27 and Rb are on overlapping pathways suppressing tumorigenesis in mice. Proc Natl Acad Sci USA. 1999;96:6382–7.
20. Franklin DS et al. CDK inhibitors p18(INK4c) and p27(Kip1) mediate two separate pathways to collaboratively suppress pituitary tumorigenesis. Genes Dev. 1998;12:2899–911.
21. Franklin DS, Godfrey VL, O'Brien DA, Deng C, Xiong Y. Functional collaboration between different cyclin-dependent kinase inhibitors suppresses tumor growth with distinct tissue specificity. Mol Cell Biol. 2000;20:6147–58.
22. Leung SW et al. A dynamic switch in $Rb^{+/-}$ mediated neuroendocrine tumorigenesis. Oncogene. 2004;23:3296–307.
23. Yamasaki L et al. Loss of E2F-1 reduces tumorigenesis and extends the lifespan of Rb1(+/−) mice. Nat Genet. 1998;18:360–4.

24. Lee EY et al. E2F4 loss suppresses tumorigenesis in Rb mutant mice. Cancer Cell. 2002;2: 463–72.
25. Chesnokova V, Kovacs K, Castro AV, Zonis S, Melmed S. Pituitary hypoplasia in Pttg$^{-/-}$ mice is protective for Rb$^{+/-}$ pituitary tumorigenesis. Mol Endocrinol. 2005;19:2371–9.
26. Vlotides G, Eigler T, Melmed S. Pituitary tumor-transforming gene: physiology and implications for tumorigenesis. Endocr Rev. 2007;28:165–86.
27. Chesnokova V et al. p21(Cip1) restrains pituitary tumor growth. Proc Natl Acad Sci USA. 2008;105:17498–503.
28. Chesnokova V et al. Senescence mediates pituitary hypoplasia and restrains pituitary tumor growth. Cancer Res. 2007;67:10564–72.
29. Orth DN et al. Equine Cushing's disease: plasma immunoreactive proopiolipomelanocortin peptide and cortisol levels basally and in response to diagnostic tests. Endocrinology. 1982;110:1430–41.
30. Wilson MG et al. Proopiolipomelanocortin peptides in normal pituitary, pituitary tumor, and plasma of normal and Cushing's horses. Endocrinology. 1982;110:941–54.
31. de Bruin C et al. Cushing's disease in dogs and humans. Horm Res. 2009;71 Suppl 1:140–3.
32. Willeberg PPW. Epidemiological aspects of clinical hyperadrenocorticism in dogs (canine Cushing's syndrome). J Am Anim Hosp Assoc. 1982;18:717–24.
33. Halmi NS, Peterson ME, Colurso GJ, Liotta AS, Krieger DT. Pituitary intermediate lobe in dog: two cell types and high bioactive adrenocorticotropin content. Science. 1981;211:72–4.
34. Burch WM. Cushing's disease. A review. Arch Intern Med. 1985;145:1106–11.
35. Lamberts SW et al. The mechanism of the suppressive action of bromocriptine on adrenocorticotropin secretion in patients with Cushing's disease and Nelson's syndrome. J Clin Endocrinol Metab. 1980;51:307–11.
36. Lamberts SW et al. Failure of clinical remission after transsphenoidal removal of a microadenoma in a patient with Cushing's disease: multiple hyperplastic and adenomatous cell nets in surrounding pituitary tissue. J Clin Endocrinol Metab. 1980;50:793–5.
37. Kovacs K. The pathology of Cushing's disease. J Steroid Biochem Mol Biol. 1993;45:179–82.
38. Orth DN et al. Pituitary microadenomas causing Cushing's disease respond to corticotropin-releasing factor. J Clin Endocrinol Metab. 1982;55:1017–9.
39. Alexander JM et al. Clinically nonfunctioning pituitary tumors are monoclonal in origin. J Clin Invest. 1990;86:336–40.
40. Herman V, Fagin J, Gonsky R, Kovacs K, Melmed S. Clonal origin of pituitary adenomas. J Clin Endocrinol Metab. 1990;71:1427–33.
41. Dahia PL, Grossman AB. The molecular pathogenesis of corticotroph tumors. Endocr Rev. 1999;20:136–55.
42. Zhang X et al. Pituitary tumor transforming gene (PTTG) expression in pituitary adenomas. J Clin Endocrinol Metab. 1999;84:761–7.
43. Holt LJ, Krutchinsky AN, Morgan DO. Positive feedback sharpens the anaphase switch. Nature. 2008;454:353–7.
44. Lidhar K et al. Low expression of the cell cycle inhibitor p27Kip1 in normal corticotroph cells, corticotroph tumors, and malignant pituitary tumors. J Clin Endocrinol Metab. 1999;84: 3823–30.
45. Frescas D, Pagano M. Deregulated proteolysis by the F-box proteins SKP2 and beta-TrCP: tipping the scales of cancer. Nat Rev Cancer. 2008;8:438–49.
46. Musat M et al. The expression of the F-box protein Skp2 is negatively associated with p27 expression in human pituitary tumors. Pituitary. 2002;5:235–42.
47. Jordan S, Lidhar K, Korbonits M, Lowe DG, Grossman AB. Cyclin D and cyclin E expression in normal and adenomatous pituitary. Eur J Endocrinol. 2000;143:R1–6.
48. Morris DG et al. Differential gene expression in pituitary adenomas by oligonucleotide array analysis. Eur J Endocrinol. 2005;153:143–51.
49. Karnik SK et al. Menin regulates pancreatic islet growth by promoting histone methylation and expression of genes encoding p27Kip1 and p18INK4c. Proc Natl Acad Sci USA. 2005;102:14659–64.

50. Milne TA et al. Menin and MLL cooperatively regulate expression of cyclin-dependent kinase inhibitors. Proc Natl Acad Sci USA. 2005;102:749–54.
51. Burgess JR, Greenaway TM, Shepherd JJ. Expression of the MEN-1 gene in a large kindred with multiple endocrine neoplasia type 1. J Intern Med. 1998;243:465–70.
52. Verges B et al. Pituitary disease in MEN type 1 (MEN1): data from the France-Belgium MEN1 multicenter study. J Clin Endocrinol Metab. 2002;87:457–65.
53. Asa SL, Somers K, Ezzat S. The MEN-1 gene is rarely down-regulated in pituitary adenomas. J Clin Endocrinol Metab. 1998;83:3210–2.
54. Satta MA et al. Expression of menin gene mRNA in pituitary tumours. Eur J Endocrinol. 1999;140:358–61.
55. Pellegata NS et al. Germ-line mutations in p27Kip1 cause a multiple endocrine neoplasia syndrome in rats and humans. Proc Natl Acad Sci USA. 2006;103:15558–63.
56. Georgitsi M et al. Germline CDKN1B/p27Kip1 mutation in multiple endocrine neoplasia. J Clin Endocrinol Metab. 2007;92:3321–5.
57. Igreja S et al. Assessment of p27 (cyclin-dependent kinase inhibitor 1B) and aryl hydrocarbon receptor-interacting protein (AIP) genes in multiple endocrine neoplasia (MEN1) syndrome patients without any detectable MEN1 gene mutations. Clin Endocrinol (Oxf). 2009;70:259–64.
58. Ozawa A et al. The parathyroid/pituitary variant of multiple endocrine neoplasia type 1 usually has causes other than p27Kip1 mutations. J Clin Endocrinol Metab. 2007;92:1948–51.
59. Carey RM et al. Ectopic secretion of corticotropin-releasing factor as a cause of Cushing's syndrome. A clinical, morphologic, and biochemical study. N Engl J Med. 1984;311:13–20.
60. Schteingart DE et al. Cushing's syndrome secondary to ectopic corticotropin-releasing hormone-adrenocorticotropin secretion. J Clin Endocrinol Metab. 1986;63:770–5.
61. Xu B, Sano T, Yamada S, Li CC, Hirokawa M. Expression of corticotropin-releasing hormone messenger ribonucleic acid in human pituitary corticotroph adenomas associated with proliferative potential. J Clin Endocrinol Metab. 2000;85:1220–5.
62. Dieterich KD, Gundelfinger ED, Ludecke DK, Lehnert H. Mutation and expression analysis of corticotropin-releasing factor 1 receptor in adrenocorticotropin-secreting pituitary adenomas. J Clin Endocrinol Metab. 1998;83:3327–31.
63. Dahia PL et al. Vasopressin receptor expression and mutation analysis in corticotropin-secreting tumors. J Clin Endocrinol Metab. 1996;81:1768–71.
64. Wolfsen AR, Odell WD. The dose-response relationship of ACTH and cortisol in Cushing's disease. Clin Endocrinol (Oxf). 1980;12:557–68.
65. Morris DG et al. Identification of adrenocorticotropin receptor messenger ribonucleic acid in the human pituitary and its loss of expression in pituitary adenomas. J Clin Endocrinol Metab. 2003;88:6080–7.
66. Bamberger CM, Schulte HM, Chrousos GP. Molecular determinants of glucocorticoid receptor function and tissue sensitivity to glucocorticoids. Endocr Rev. 1996;17:245–61.
67. Dahia PL et al. Expression of glucocorticoid receptor gene isoforms in corticotropin-secreting tumors. J Clin Endocrinol Metab. 1997;82:1088–93.
68. Bilodeau S et al. Role of Brg1 and HDAC2 in GR trans-repression of the pituitary POMC gene and misexpression in Cushing disease. Genes Dev. 2006;20:2871–86.
69. Drouin J, Bilodeau S, Vallette S. Of old and new diseases: genetics of pituitary ACTH excess (Cushing) and deficiency. Clin Genet. 2007;72:175–82.
70. Assie G et al. Corticotroph tumor progression after adrenalectomy in Cushing's Disease: a reappraisal of Nelson's Syndrome. J Clin Endocrinol Metab. 2007;92:172–9.
71. Assie G et al. The Nelson's syndrome (revisited). Pituitary. 2004;7:209–15.
72. Challa VR, Marshall RB, Hopkins 3rd MB, Kelly Jr DL, Civantos F. Pathobiologic study of pituitary tumors: report of 62 cases with a review of the recent literature. Hum Pathol. 1985;16:873–84.
73. Boscaro M et al. Treatment of pituitary-dependent Cushing's disease with the multireceptor ligand somatostatin analog pasireotide (SOM230): a multicenter, phase II trial. J Clin Endocrinol Metab. 2009;94:115–22.

74. Ben-Shlomo A et al. Differential ligand-mediated pituitary somatostatin receptor subtype signaling: implications for corticotroph tumor therapy. J Clin Endocrinol Metab. 2009;94: 4342–50.
75. De Menis E et al. Corticotroph adenoma of the pituitary in a patient with X-linked adrenal hypoplasia congenita due to a novel mutation of the DAX-1 gene. Eur J Endocrinol. 2005;153: 211–5.
76. Dworakowska D, Grossman AB. Are neuroendocrine tumours a feature of tuberous sclerosis? A systematic review. Endocr Relat Cancer. 2009;16:45–58.
77. He L, Hannon GJ. MicroRNAs: small RNAs with a big role in gene regulation. Nat Rev Genet. 2004;5:522–31.
78. Calin GA et al. Human microRNA genes are frequently located at fragile sites and genomic regions involved in cancers. Proc Natl Acad Sci USA. 2004;101:2999–3004.
79. Esquela-Kerscher A, Slack FJ. Oncomirs – microRNAs with a role in cancer. Nat Rev Cancer. 2006;6:259–69.
80. Amaral FC et al. MicroRNAs differentially expressed in ACTH-secreting pituitary tumors. J Clin Endocrinol Metab. 2009;94:320–3.
81. Bottoni A et al. miR-15a and miR-16-1 down-regulation in pituitary adenomas. J Cell Physiol. 2005;204:280–5.
82. Bottoni A et al. Identification of differentially expressed microRNAs by microarray: a possible role for microRNA genes in pituitary adenomas. J Cell Physiol. 2007;210:370–7.
83. Bates AS et al. Allelic deletion in pituitary adenomas reflects aggressive biological activity and has potential value as a prognostic marker. J Clin Endocrinol Metab. 1997;82:818–24.
84. Fan X et al. Gain of chromosome 3 and loss of 13q are frequent alterations in pituitary adenomas. Cancer Genet Cytogenet. 2001;128:97–103.
85. Pei L et al. Frequent loss of heterozygosity at the retinoblastoma susceptibility gene (RB) locus in aggressive pituitary tumors: evidence for a chromosome 13 tumor suppressor gene other than RB. Cancer Res. 1995;55:1613–6.
86. Lee YS, Dutta A. The tumor suppressor microRNA let-7 represses the HMGA2 oncogene. Genes Dev. 2007;21:1025–30.
87. Mayr C, Hemann MT, Bartel DP. Disrupting the pairing between let-7 and Hmga2 enhances oncogenic transformation. Science. 2007;315:1576–9.
88. Yu F et al. let-7 regulates self renewal and tumorigenicity of breast cancer cells. Cell. 2007;131: 1109–23.
89. Qian ZR et al. Overexpression of HMGA2 relates to reduction of the let-7 and its relationship to clinicopathological features in pituitary adenomas. Mod Pathol. 2009;22:431–41.
90. Roussel-Gervais A et al. Cooperation between cyclin E and p27(Kip1) in pituitary tumorigenesis. Mol Endocrinol. 2010;9:1835–45.
91. Liu et al. Targeting zebrafish and murine pituitary corticotroph tumors with a cyclin-dependent kinase (CDK) inhibitor. Proc Natl Acad Sci USA. 2011;108(20):8414–9.

Chapter 3
Pathology of Cushing's Disease

Pornsuk Cheunsuchon and E.T. Hedley-Whyte

Abstract Adrenocorticotropin (ACTH)-producing pituitary adenomas are derived from corticotroph cells in the anterior pituitary gland. Most of them secrete excess ACTH leading to cortisol overproduction or Cushing's disease. However, ACTH-producing pituitary tumors are heterogeneous and differ in histologic, immunohistochemical, and ultrastructural findings as well as in clinical presentations and prognosis. In this chapter, the histopathology of ACTH-producing adenomas and their clinicopathologic correlations are described.

Keywords ACTH-secreting pituitary adenoma • Pathology • Nelson's syndrome

Introduction

The pituitary gland is a part of the hypothalamic–pituitary–endocrine axis and plays an important role in regulating endocrine organs. It is situated in the sella turcica and consists of anterior and posterior lobes. The anterior lobe can be further divided into a central part (mucoid wedge) and two lateral wings. Major cell types in the anterior pituitary are hormone-secreting cells including somatotrophs, lactotrophs, corticotrophs, gonadotrophs, and thyrotrophs which produce growth hormone, prolactin, adrenocorticotropin (ACTH), gonadotropins, and thyrotropin, respectively. These cells are unequally distributed within the anterior pituitary, and the various types of cells are packed in nests or acini surrounded by an interlacing capillary network. On classical hematoxylin and eosin (H&E) staining, they have different staining affinities and can be classified into three groups as basophils, acidophils,

---

E.T. Hedley-Whyte (✉)
CS Kubik Laboratory for Neuropathology, Department of Pathology,
Massachusetts General Hospital, Harvard Medical School,
55 Fruit Street, Boston, MA 02114, USA
e-mail: ehedleywhyte@partners.org

and chromophobes. However, this classification does not correlate well with the types of hormones they produce. Immunohistochemistry is now the most commonly used method to detect the hormone produced by each cell type.

Corticotrophs or ACTH-producing cells constitute about 10–20% of all cells and are most numerous in the middle and posterior portions of the mucoid wedge. They are basophilic on H&E stain and strongly positive for periodic acid schiff (PAS) stain because they contain the ACTH precursor, pro-opiomelanocortin (POMC) [1]. In the anterior pituitary, POMC is synthesized and cleaved in corticotrophs to generate ACTH and β-lipotropin (LPH) as the major end products [2]. Immunostaining for both ACTH and β-LPH can be used to distinguish corticotrophs from other cell types but ACTH immunostaining is most commonly used in neuropathology practice.

Pathology of ACTH-Producing Pituitary Tumors

ACTH-producing pituitary tumors are derived from corticotroph cells in the anterior pituitary gland. Most of them are benign adenomas. Pituitary carcinomas are rare. Benign ACTH-producing adenomas associated with ACTH hypersecretion cause the clinical syndrome of glucocorticoid overproduction known as Cushing's disease. However, some of them, called silent corticotroph adenomas, produce ACTH as seen by immunohistochemical study but do not secrete ACTH into the systemic circulation. These patients usually present with symptoms of clinically nonfunctioning adenomas, such as headache or visual disturbance, instead of Cushing's disease. In addition to functional status, pituitary adenomas can also be classified by their growth patterns seen radiologically, grossly, or microscopically as noninvasive or invasive tumors. The latter tumors involve adjacent structures in the sellar region such as the cavernous sinus or sphenoid sinus. ACTH-producing pituitary tumors are also classified by their histologic, immunohistochemical, and ultrastructural features.

ACTH-Producing Pituitary Adenomas

Functional ACTH-Producing Adenomas

These corticotroph adenomas produce and secrete ACTH as evidenced by clinical symptoms and biochemical study. They are associated with two clinical syndromes.

Adenomas of Cushing's Disease

ACTH-producing adenomas in the setting of Cushing's disease account for about 10–15% of all pituitary adenomas and typically are microadenomas. The peak incidence is the third and fourth decades and they are more common in women [3]. Most are associated with ACTH hypersecretion. Grossly, the tumors are usually small, softer and paler than the nontumorous pituitary but sometimes it is difficult to distinguish one from the other. Microscopically, tumor cells are monomorphic, round, and basophilic or amphophilic on H&E stain. The cytoplasm is densely granulated and PAS-positive. Some degree of pleomorphism can be observed but mitoses are infrequent. The tumor cells show ACTH immunoreactivity in which the intensity varies (Fig. 3.1a–c). Other peptides derived from POMC can be detected as well. Production of gonadotropic hormones such as luteinizing hormones (LH) or the α-subunit of the glycoprotein hormones can also be seen but infrequently (Table 3.1).

Although classical ACTH adenomas are small and noninvasive, about 15% are macroadenomas and frequently invade adjacent structures such as bone, dura, and nerve [4]. These patients usually have less florid hormone excess [5]. Macroadenomas are more often chromophobic, sparsely granulated, less PAS-positive, and have weaker ACTH immunoreactivity and are more likely to behave aggressively. Another variant of ACTH-producing adenomas are Crooke's cell adenomas which are usually invasive macroadenomas [6]. The cells in Crooke's adenomas resemble the cells with Crooke's hyaline change seen in normal corticotrophs as a response to excess glucocorticoids from exogenous or endogenous sources. Crooke's cells are large with eosinophilic hyaline cytoplasm due to an accumulation of low molecular weight cytokeratin pushing cellular organelles and secretory granules to the periphery of the cells (Fig. 3.1d–f).

Ultrastructurally, most functioning corticotroph adenoma cells resemble normal corticotroph cells. The cells have an oval to polygonal shape with eccentric large, polygonal to ovoid nuclei. The cytoplasm contains moderately developed Golgi and rough endoplasmic reticulum (RER). Perinuclear bundles of intermediate filaments of cytokeratin are characteristic. The secretory granules are usually abundant and vary in electron density, shape, and size, ranging from 150 to 450 nm. The secretory granules tend to accumulate under the cell membrane. In Crooke's cell adenomas and cells with Crooke's hyaline change, perinuclear accumulation of cytokeratin filaments is abundant and secretory granules are trapped inside them (Fig. 3.1f).

Adenomas of Nelson's Syndrome

This type of adenoma is found in the patients who have undergone bilateral adrenalectomy in order to control refractory glucocorticoid overproduction. It is hypothesized that lack of glucocorticoid negative feedback following bilateral adrenalectomy is associated with the progression of a pre-existing corticotroph adenoma [7]. Most of the adenomas in Nelson's syndrome are macroadenomas and invasive. The tumors have similar histologic appearances and identical molecular features to those seen in macroadenomas of Cushing's disease [8]. However, some ultrastructural features are different, and the intermediate cytokeratin filaments and Crooke's hyaline change are absent [5, 7]. Unlike Cushing's disease, adenomas of Nelson's syndrome have a high proliferative activity, more aggressive behavior, and a higher recurrence rate [7].

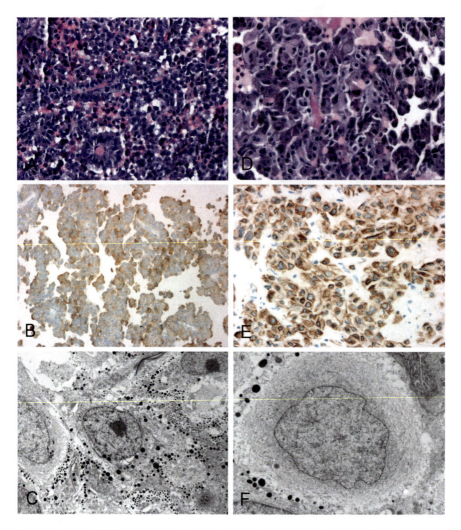

Fig. 3.1 (**a–c**) ACTH-producing pituitary adenoma. (**a**) Adenoma has a variety of histologic growth patterns. Diffuse, trabecular, and papillary growth patterns are seen. The tumor cells are basophilic and densely granulated (H&E, 20×). (**b**) Immunohistochemical study demonstrates ACTH immunoreactivity with varying intensity (ACTH immunoperoxidase, 20×). (**c**) Electron micrograph showing numerous secretory granules with varying size and electron density (3,400× magnification). (**d–f**) Crooke's cell adenoma. (**d**) The cells show homogenous cytoplasmic pink hyaline change around the nuclei (H&E, 40×). (**e**) Accumulations of intermediate filaments in Crooke's hyaline change are positive for cytokeratin immunohistochemical staining (pan-cytokeratin immunoperoxidase, 40×). (**f**) Electron micrograph, the perinuclear accumulation of cytokeratin pushes cytoplasmic organelles to the periphery of the cell next to the cell membrane and traps the secretory granules inside (7,100× magnification)

3 Pathology of Cushing's Disease

Table 3.1 Summary of characteristics of ACTH-producing pituitary adenomas

Type	Size	Histology	Immunohistochemistry	Functional status
Adenomas of Cushing's disease	Microadenoma (85%)	Basophilic to amphophilic Densely granulated Strong PAS	ACTH, β-LPH LH, α-subunit	Functioning adenomas
	Macroadenoma (15%)	Chromophobic Sparsely granulated Weak PAS	Weaker ACTH	Can also occur in Nelson's syndrome
Crooke's cell adenomas	Macroadenoma	Crooke's hyaline change	ACTH Low molecular weight cytokeratin (perinuclear pattern)	Functioning adenomas
Silent corticotroph adenomas subtype 1	Macroadenoma	Basophilic Densely granulated	ACTH	Nonfunctioning adenomas
Silent corticotroph adenomas subtype 2	Macroadenoma	Chromophobic Sparsely granulated	Weaker ACTH	Nonfunctioning adenomas

ACTH adrenocorticotropic hormone, *LH* luteinizing hormone, *LPH* lipotropic hormone

Silent ACTH-Producing Adenomas

Silent ACTH-producing adenomas are uncommon. They account for 1–6% of all pituitary adenomas and approximately 10–15% of all corticotroph adenomas [9]. They produce ACTH as seen in immunohistochemical staining but have no clinical or biological evidence of excess ACTH secretion. Most are macroadenomas and frequently invasive. Clinically, patients present with clinically nonfunctioning adenomas and symptoms due to mass effect are common manifestations. There are two subtypes of silent corticotroph adenomas, subtype 1 and 2, which display different levels of differentiation. Silent subtype 1 adenomas are more differentiated and have similar histologic, immunohistochemical, and ultrastructural features to functional corticotroph adenomas. Those features are a basophilic, densely granulated cytoplasm with strong PAS and ACTH positivity while the subtype 2 adenomas are chromophobic, sparsely granulated with weak PAS and ACTH immunoreactivity (Table 3.1).

Ultrastructurally, silent corticotroph adenomas have two different subtypes. Silent subtype 1 adenomas resemble those of functional corticotroph adenomas, while silent type 2 adenomas have less differentiated ultrastructural features. The cells of subtype 2 are smaller in size and have a polyhedral shape with centrally placed nuclei. The Golgi complex and RER are poorly developed. The secretory granules are sparse, drop-shaped, and range from 150 to 300 nm in diameter. Perinuclear intermediate cytokeratin filaments are absent.

It is unclear why silent corticotroph adenomas are unable to secrete bioactive ACTH. In functional corticotroph adenomas, transcription of the POMC gene and the processing of its products are similar to those that occur in normal corticotrophs [2]. In comparing silent corticotroph adenomas to functional adenomas, the expression profile of the POMC gene, POMC transcription factors, and genes related to processing and secretion of POMC products are different and might partially explain the pathogenesis of silent corticotroph adenomas [10, 11]. Among those genes that are differentially expressed in silent corticotroph adenomas, expression of prohormone convertase (PC) 1/3, an enzyme that cleaves POMC to ACTH in anterior pituitary, is lower in silent adenomas than in functional tumors. Absence of PC1/3 immunoreactivity in silent corticotroph adenomas has been reported and may be useful as a marker to distinguish these two entities [12, 13].

Prognosis and Predictive Factors

Most ACTH-producing adenomas are surgically treated and have a remission rate of 70–98% after surgery [14, 15]. The major factors contributing to long-term remission are tumor size and invasiveness. Microadenomas of Cushing's disease have a higher remission rate than macroadenomas and invasive adenomas [14, 15]. The recurrence rate of adenomas of Cushing's disease varies from 3% to 25% depending on the centers [14, 15] and late recurrence can occur [14, 15]. Some histologic types of ACTH-producing adenomas, e.g., Crooke's cell adenomas, adenomas of Nelson's syndrome, and silent corticotroph adenomas, are more likely to recur, possibly related to the large tumor size and invasiveness [15].

Histologic markers predicting progression or recurrence specific for corticotroph adenomas are not well established. In general, independent predictive markers for pituitary adenomas are still inconclusive. The Ki-67 labeling index (LI), assessed by MIB-1 antibody to detect the Ki-67 protein which is expressed in non-G0 cell cycle phase, is variable and has no clear-cut predictive threshold. In one study, a Ki-67 LI more than 3% and an extensive nuclear staining of p53 were found to be correlated with invasiveness [3]. In other studies, this Ki-67 threshold was shown to be lower at about 2% [16, 17]. Staining for proliferative cell nuclear antigen (PCNA) gave a similar result to Ki-67 [18]. However, combinations of markers may have greater predictive value. Features that may help indicate aggressive behavior are elevated mitotic index, Ki-67 LI more than 3%, and an extensive nuclear staining of p53 immunoreactivity [3].

ACTH-Producing Pituitary Carcinomas

Pituitary carcinomas are rare neoplasms accounting for only 0.1–0.2% of all pituitary tumors [3, 19]. The definition requires the presence of craniospinal metastasis and/or distant extracranial spread where lymph nodes, liver, and bone are common sites. Pituitary carcinomas are often endocrinologically active with prolactin- and corticotropin-producing lesions being the most common [3]. Interestingly, ACTH-producing pituitary carcinomas account for approximately 40% of all pituitary carcinomas and have a higher prevalence in patients with Nelson's syndrome [20]. Grossly, pituitary carcinomas are indistinguishable from invasive adenomas. Craniospinal spread, if present, may manifest as single or multiple discontinuous nodules in the subarachnoid space, dura, and brain or spinal cord parenchyma. Extracranial metastatic lesions are grossly similar to metastatic carcinomas from other organs.

As with other endocrine neoplasms, clear-cut criteria and predictive markers for malignant behavior of pituitary tumors are still problematic because their histologic appearances do not correlate well with their behavior. Most of the carcinomas have a well differentiated histology but they can range from no or mild atypia to frank malignancy, and mitoses can vary from few to abundant. Although brisk mitotic activity is not an indicator for malignancy and a particular threshold does not exist, it is associated with invasive growth and malignant potential [19]. On electron microscopy, pituitary carcinomas show less differentiation than their benign counterparts. The features of an endocrine neoplasm are usually confirmed but cannot be used for further classification or behavioral prediction [3, 4].

Prognosis and Predictive Factors

Because the diagnosis of pituitary carcinoma requires the presence of metastasis, early diagnosis cannot be made on the initial pathological specimen, thus contributing to the poor prognosis of this tumor. Efforts to identify predictive markers have been made but have been inconclusive. Among those predictive factors, Ki-67 LI is higher in malignant and invasive tumors than benign adenomas (about 12, 4.5, and 1%, respectively) [21, 22]. However, one should be aware that there is a considerable case-to-case variability of Ki-67 LI (0–22%) in pituitary carcinomas and also a great overlap between carcinomas and adenomas [3, 19]. Although assessment of Ki-67 LI does not allow one to diagnose pituitary carcinoma, a high LI greater than 10% should raise a suspicion about the malignant potential of the tumor [19].

Overexpression of p53 protein has been detected in both pituitary adenomas and carcinomas but the frequency varies. Immunohistochemical staining is the most widely used method to assess p53 overexpression. The mutations of the p53 gene lead to conformation change of p53 protein and make it more stable, and thus it can be detected by immunohistochemical techniques. However, there is a discrepancy between p53 immunopositivity and the mutation status of p53 tumor suppressor gene. In pituitary tumors, the p53 gene mutation is not a common genetic event, thus the mechanisms of p53 protein overexpression in pituitary tumors are still elusive [23]. Although p53 overexpression may not reflect p53 gene inactivation in pituitary tumors, extensive p53 nuclear staining has been found to be correlated with their invasiveness and aggressive behaviors. However, p53 expression alone is not a predictor for malignancy, and some pituitary carcinomas are p53-negative. Therefore, combinations of p53 expression and high Ki-67 LI may have a greater predictive value than either method alone [19].

Role of Intraoperative Consultation in Cushing's Disease

Since most of the adenomas in Cushing's disease are microadenomas, there can be problems identifying the tumors either by imaging study or during surgery. To ensure that the adenomas are removed, intraoperative consultation for frozen section diagnosis is usually performed. In routine intraoperative consultation, part of the tissue is divided for a smear preparation and the remainder is frozen and sections are stained with H&E. Specimens of adenomas of Cushing's disease are often very small and there may not be enough tissue to make both a smear and a frozen section. Moreover, the tumor may be only a small part of a specimen and hard to distinguish from non-tumor pituitary tissue, which can make pathologic diagnosis very difficult. In this case, the cytologic smears may be the best choice. The cytologic smears can be performed either by a neurosurgeon intraoperatively or by a pathologist in the frozen lab. The cytologic preparation can be made by smear, touch, or squash techniques. They are immediately fixed in 95% ethanol and then stained with rapid H&E. In our institution, the cytologic smears are often made intraoperatively by the neurosurgeon, fixed in ethanol, and sent to the frozen lab for staining and interpretation. In this way, the region most likely to be a tumor is selected during tumor removal and is confirmed by frozen section examination.

One should keep in mind that both normal pituitary tissue and adenomas are susceptible to crush artifact during specimen handling, although this is generally

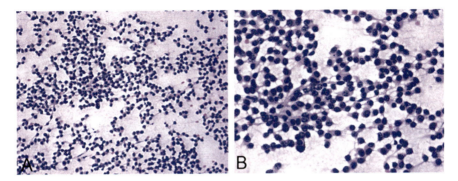

Fig. 3.2 Cytologic preparation of an ACTH-producing pituitary adenoma. (**a**) Intraoperative smear of the adenoma shows a monotonous population of cells. Discohesive fragments and single-cell spread are characteristic of pituitary adenoma smear (H&E, 20×). (**b**) The cells have relatively uniform and regular nuclei, inconspicuous nucleoli, and fine granular chromatin. The cytoplasm is scant and poorly defined (H&E, 40×)

less of a problem with adenomatous tissue. Proper handling of tissue should be practiced by both surgeons and pathologists. Generally, pituitary tissue is soft and a significant amount can be lost while handling on the cutting board, paper towels, or gauze pad. The specimens should be handled gently and placed on a nonadhesive material or container. During the gross examination in the frozen lab, handling the tissue on a glass slide or nonadhesive surface will help prevent tissue loss. Freezing artifacts during frozen section can cause distortion of morphology and make the H&E section hard to interpret. Morphological and architectural appearances are the most important features for making the diagnosis of pituitary adenomas and distinguishing between normal anterior pituitary gland and adenoma, especially in small biopsy specimens. In this latter circumstance, a good cytologic smear may have an advantage over frozen sections due to better preserved cytology and lack of freezing artifact. The nuclear features of an endocrine neoplasm (finely stippled or salt and pepper chromatin) and a monotonous population of cells are the usually recognized characteristics of pituitary adenomas (Fig. 3.2). The smears can be used for subsequent immunohistochemical staining. The smears are destained and then standard immunohistochemical methods are applied. It is preferable to have two separate smears so that in addition to ACTH another hormone such as prolactin can be used as a control, both for the immunohistochemical technique and either confirming or refuting that only ACTH is present.

Summary

In summary, ACTH-producing pituitary adenomas that are derived from corticotrophs have different clinical, biochemical, and pathological features. Most of them present as functioning microadenomas causing a characteristic clinical picture, Cushing's disease. However, functioning macroadenomas and silent corticotroph tumors also occur and have their own histopathology and clinical courses. Pathologic assessment, including standard histological and immunostaining techniques used to classify subtypes of ACTH adenomas, can provide additional information regarding their behavior.

References

1. Lopes MBS, Pernicone PJ, Scheithauer BW, Horvath E, Kovacs K. Pituitary and sellar region. In: Mills SE, editor. Histology for pathologists. 3rd ed. Philadelphia, PA: Lippincott Williams and Wilkins; 2007. p. 321–44.
2. Raffin-Sanson ML, de Keyzer Y, Bertagna X. Proopiomelanocortin, a polypeptide precursor with multiple functions: from physiology to pathological conditions. Eur J Endocrinol. 2003;149(2):79–90.
3. Lloyd RV, Kovacs K, Young Jr WF, et al. Tumours of the pituitary. In: DeLellis RA, Lloyd RV, Heitz PU, Eng C, editors. World health organization classification of tumours. Pathology and genetics of tumours of endocrine organs. Lyon: IARC; 2004. p. 9–39.
4. Burger PC, Scheithauer BW, Vogel FS. Region of the sella turcica. In: Burger PC, Scheithauer BW, Vogel FS, editors. Surgical pathology of the nervous system and its coverings. 4th ed. Philadelphia, PA: Churchill Livingstone; 2002. p. 437–97.
5. Asa SL. Pituitary and suprasellar tumours. In: Love S, Louis DN, Ellison DW, editors. Greenfield's neuropathology. 8th ed. London: Hodder Arnold; 2008. p. 2088–107.
6. George DH, Scheithauer BW, Kovacs K, et al. Crooke's cell adenoma of the pituitary: an aggressive variant of corticotroph adenoma. Am J Surg Pathol. 2003;27(10):1330–6.
7. Banasiak MJ, Malek AR. Nelson syndrome: comprehensive review of pathophysiology, diagnosis, and management. Neurosurg Focus. 2007;23(3):E13.
8. Assie G, Bahurel H, Bertherat J, Kujas M, Legmann P, Bertagna X. The Nelson's syndrome… revisited. Pituitary. 2004;7(4):209–15.
9. Karavitaki N, Ansorge O, Wass JA. Silent corticotroph adenomas. Arq Bras Endocrinol Metabol. 2007;51(8):1314–8.
10. Stefaneanu L, Kovacs K, Horvath E, Lloyd RV. In situ hybridization study of pro-opiomelanocortin (POMC) gene expression in human pituitary corticotrophs and their adenomas. Virchows Arch A Pathol Anat Histopathol. 1991;419(2):107–13.
11. Tateno T, Izumiyama H, Doi M, et al. Differential gene expression in ACTH-secreting and non-functioning pituitary tumors. Eur J Endocrinol. 2007;157(6):717–24.
12. Ohta S, Nishizawa S, Oki Y, Yokoyama T, Namba H. Significance of absent prohormone convertase 1/3 in inducing clinically silent corticotroph pituitary adenoma of subtype I–immunohistochemical study. Pituitary. 2002;5(4):221–3.
13. Tateno T, Izumiyama H, Doi M, Akashi T, Ohno K, Hirata Y. Defective expression of prohormone convertase 1/3 in silent corticotroph adenoma. Endocr J. 2007;54(5):777–82.
14. Utz AL, Swearingen B, Biller BM. Pituitary surgery and postoperative management in Cushing's disease. Endocrinol Metab Clin North Am. 2005;34(2):459–78. xi.
15. Kelly DF. Transsphenoidal surgery for Cushing's disease: a review of success rates, remission predictors, management of failed surgery, and Nelson's Syndrome. Neurosurg Focus. 2007;23(3):E5.
16. Gejman R, Swearingen B, Hedley-Whyte ET. Role of Ki-67 proliferation index and p53 expression in predicting progression of pituitary adenomas. Hum Pathol. 2008;39(5):758–66.
17. Saeger W, Ludecke B, Ludecke DK. Clinical tumor growth and comparison with proliferation markers in non-functioning (inactive) pituitary adenomas. Exp Clin Endocrinol Diabetes. 2008;116(2):80–5.

18. Hsu DW, Hakim F, Biller BM, et al. Significance of proliferating cell nuclear antigen index in predicting pituitary adenoma recurrence. J Neurosurg. 1993;78(5):753–61.
19. Kaltsas GA, Nomikos P, Kontogeorgos G, Buchfelder M, Grossman AB. Clinical review: diagnosis and management of pituitary carcinomas. J Clin Endocrinol Metab. 2005;90(5):3089–99.
20. van der Klaauw AA, Kienitz T, Strasburger CJ, Smit JW, Romijn JA. Malignant pituitary corticotroph adenomas: report of two cases and a comprehensive review of the literature. Pituitary. 2009;12(1):57–69.
21. Thapar K, Kovacs K, Scheithauer BW, et al. Proliferative activity and invasiveness among pituitary adenomas and carcinomas: an analysis using the MIB-1 antibody. Neurosurgery. 1996;38(1):99–107.
22. Hosaka N, Kitajiri S, Hiraumi H, et al. Ectopic pituitary adenoma with malignant transformation. Am J Surg Pathol. 2002;26(8):1078–82.
23. Tanizaki Y, Jin L, Scheithauer BW, Kovacs K, Roncaroli F, Lloyd RV. P53 gene mutations in pituitary carcinomas. Endocr Pathol. 2007;18(4):217–22.

Chapter 4
The Diagnosis of Cushing's Syndrome

Lynnette K. Nieman

Abstract Cushing's syndrome is characterized by exposure to excess glucocorticoid. It can be caused by exogenous administration of these compounds, usually in supraphysiologic treatment doses. Endogenous Cushing's syndrome is caused either by excessive ACTH production from a pituitary or other tumor, or by autonomous adrenal cortisol production. Clinical features suggestive of the disorder should prompt biochemical screening. Case detection of this rare disorder is justified by the high standardized mortality rate, which is normalized after successful treatment.

Keywords Glucocorticoids • Adrenocorticotropic hormone • Cortisol • Biochemical screening

Introduction

Cushing's syndrome is a rare symptom complex that reflects excessive tissue exposure to glucocorticoid(s). Endogenous Cushing's syndrome is caused by excessive autonomous adrenal production of cortisol, or by increased ACTH secretion from a pituitary or other tumor, which in turn stimulates cortisol production. The syndrome complex also develops with chronic administration of supra-pharmacologic doses of agents with glucocorticoid action. In general, Cushing's syndrome is diagnosed only if there are both clinical features and biochemical abnormalities. Thus, clinical features consistent with the syndrome provoke biochemical screening. The rationale for such case detection is that the syndrome is progressive and carries an

L.K. Nieman (✉)
Program on Reproductive and Adult Endocrinology, Eunice Kennedy Shriver
National Institute of Child Health and Human Development,
Building 10, CRC, 1 East, Room 1-3140, 10 Center Drive, MSC 1109,
Bethesda, MD 20892-1109, USA
e-mail: NiemanL@nih.gov

increased risk of death: the standardized mortality rate for untreated patients has been estimated to increase 3.8- to 5.0-fold compared with the general population [1, 2]. By contrast, successfully treated patients have a standardized mortality rate similar to that of an age- and gender-matched United States population (0.98) [3].

Clinical Features

Table 4.1 illustrates the incidence of clinical features of Cushing's syndrome as described in 1952 [4]. These symptoms reflect the amount and duration of exposure to excess cortisol in this group, which had moderate-to-severe hypercortisolism. A 2007 study compared 32 patients with Cushing's syndrome and 23 patients with "pseudo-Cushing's," who had clinical features of Cushing's syndrome but proved not to have the disorder [5]. The Cushing's syndrome group included patients with relatively mild hypercortisolism. There was a higher prevalence of obesity in the pseudo-Cushing's group (74 vs. 31%), and similar rates of hypertension, diabetes mellitus, menstrual disorders, hirsutism, and acne in both groups. Only osteoporosis and easy bruising were more common in Cushing's syndrome. Two important points derive from these data. First, compared to 50 years ago, Cushing's syndrome is

Table 4.1 The frequency of clinical signs and symptoms of Cushing's syndrome [4]

Sign/symptom	% of 70
Decreased libido	100
Obesity or weight gain	97
Plethora	94
Round face	88
Menstrual changes	84
Hirsutism	81
Hypertension	74
Ecchymoses	62
Lethargy, depression	62
Striae	56
Weakness	56
EKG changes or atherosclerosis	55
Dorsal fat pad	54
Edema	50
Abnormal glucose tolerance	50
Osteopenia or fracture	50
Headache	47
Backache	43
Recurrent infections	25
Abdominal pain	21
Acne	21
Female balding	13

currently considered and diagnosed in patients with less severe hypercortisolism. As a result, there are fewer symptoms in the group overall. Second, there is a great overlap in the "snapshot" of symptoms in the current Cushing's syndrome and pseudo-Cushing's groups. Thus, not all patients have all clinical features, and patients with mild or intermittent cortisol excess have fewer signs and symptoms than those with very high glucocorticoid production.

Since many clinical features of Cushing's syndrome are common in the general population, and patients with mild hypercortisolism have less impressive features, the question arises, who should be screened for Cushing's syndrome? The Endocrine Society recently considered this question and published guidelines on the diagnosis of Cushing's syndrome in 2008 after an evidence-based review [6]. This chapter reviews those recommendations.

Biochemical Testing

Before proceeding to biochemical testing, it is essential to question a Cushingoid patient about current or previous medications to exclude exposure to glucocorticoids via any route of administration. It is important to ask specifically if any injections were given for joint or other pain, as often patients do not know that an injection contained a glucocorticoid. Prolonged release, particularly of a potent glucocorticoid, from a depot into the circulation can be equivalent to giving a supra-physiologic dose over many weeks, causing a Cushingoid appearance and suppression of the hypothalamic–pituitary–adrenal axis. It is important to inquire about agents used for non-glucocorticoid reasons, such as megestrol acetate, which have glucocorticoid activity. Finally, herbal preparations, "tonics," and skin bleaching creams (all of which may contain glucocorticoids) should be specifically sought, as the patient may not mention them.

The Endocrine Society guidelines recommend testing in patients most likely to have Cushing's syndrome: those with unusual features for age (e.g., osteoporosis, hypertension in a young patient), those with multiple and progressive features, children with decreasing height percentile and increasing weight, and patients with an adrenal incidentaloma compatible with adenoma [6]. It was not felt to be cost-effective to screen patients with other single features of Cushing's syndrome, such as diabetes mellitus, unless additional features develop. The panel recognized that testing carries a probability of a falsely positive result, leading to further testing and anxiety. Limiting testing to individuals with a higher likelihood of having the disorder diminishes the chance of a falsely abnormal result.

A thorough history, with attention to the timeframe and tempo of the progression of signs and symptoms, is an essential part of the decision regarding screening. Comparison of the current facies or body habitus with old photographs may help establish progression. Cognitive and psychiatric symptoms may not be mentioned spontaneously: decreased short-term memory, irritability and emotional liability, an exaggeration of "baseline" personality (e.g., mild depression becoming severe) or new psychiatric disorder are common in Cushing's syndrome [7, 8]. Disordered sleep is common, as manifest by insomnia and vivid dreams. However, each of these features may occur outside of Cushing's syndrome. It is the number, type, and increasing tempo of signs and symptoms that provoke screening.

Biochemical Screening Tests for Cushing's Syndrome

There are two inter-related biochemical characteristics of Cushing's syndrome: glucocorticoid production is increased, but does not provide adequate negative feedback to normalize cortisol production. Three tests were recommended to evaluate these possibilities (Fig. 4.1). Urine cortisol excretion over 24 h (UFC) reflects the integrated cortisol production during that time. A late-night salivary cortisol is normally quite low; patients with Cushing's syndrome have a blunted circadian rhythm so that values at this time are elevated. Finally, dexamethasone suppression testing (DST) assesses the integrity of negative feedback. It is recommended that one test should be obtained; if it is abnormal, or if there is a strong

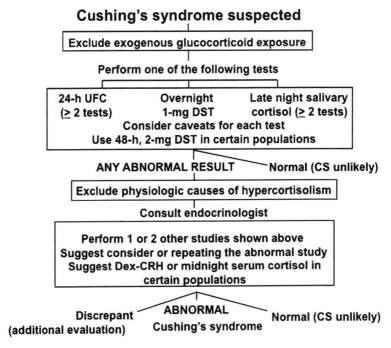

Fig. 4.1 Guidelines for evaluation for the diagnosis of Cushing's syndrome (reprinted with permission from ref. [6])

clinical suspicion, another should be done. Both must be abnormal to make the diagnosis [6]. Since each of the tests has caveats or situations when it is more likely to give inaccurate results, these three choices allow for individualized testing that is tailored to each patient.

There are some general concerns to keep in mind when choosing a screening test. A major concern is to understand the performance of the assay, be it to measure urine, serum, or salivary cortisol. Because assays vary in their accuracy and precision, results that are close to the diagnostic criterion should be viewed with skepticism. This is particularly a problem for the salivary and serum cortisol assays, as the expected normal result is very low and may be close to the functional limit of detection of the assay. Also, the reference ranges differ amongst assays, depending on whether the assay uses an antibody or structurally based detection method. Finally, each test must be performed properly for the results to be accepted. At least two measurements of UFC or salivary cortisol should be obtained, because of possible variability in hypercortisolism.

Urine Cortisol Excretion

Urine cortisol reflects the increased production of cortisol in Cushing's syndrome. It represents the free fraction in blood that is filtered and excreted. This unbound fraction increases in Cushing's syndrome because the levels of serum cortisol exceed the binding capacity of corticosteroid-binding globulin (CBG), so that the circulating free fraction increases. It is important to collect a full 24-h specimen and measure volume and creatinine to evaluate the completeness of the collection.

False-negative UFC results may occur in a renal failure patient who has decreased filtration and urine output, in a patient who finds the process inconvenient and under-collects the specimen, and in a patient who has cyclic or intermittent Cushing's syndrome and collects urine during an inactive period. Conversely, results may be falsely abnormal (using the upper reference range as a cut-off point) in the so-called pseudo-Cushing states and other physiologic states that increase cortisol (e.g., pregnancy), when the urine volume is very high (>5 L), or if there is more than a 24-h collection (Table 4.2).

Pseudo-Cushing states, characterized by mild over-activation of the hypothalamic–pituitary–adrenal axis without true Cushing's syndrome, include certain psychiatric disorders (depression, anxiety disorder, obsessive-compulsive disorder), morbid obesity, poorly controlled diabetes mellitus, and alcoholism. In these disorders, UFC may be only mildly elevated or may be increased up to fourfold the upper normal limit; values greater than this nearly always indicate Cushing's syndrome [9]. If values are lower but still abnormal, physiologic hypercortisolism should be sought. If identified, one approach is to treat the condition and see if the UFC normalizes, which would exclude Cushing's syndrome.

Table 4.2 Conditions associated with hypercortisolism in the absence of Cushing's syndrome[a]

Some clinical features of Cushing's syndrome may be present
Pregnancy
Depression and other psychiatric conditions
Alcohol dependence
Glucocorticoid resistance
Morbid obesity
Poorly controlled diabetes mellitus
Unlikely to have any clinical features of Cushing's syndrome
Physical stress (hospitalization, surgery, pain)
Malnutrition, anorexia nervosa
Intense chronic exercise
Hypothalamic amenorrhea
CBG excess (increased serum but not urine cortisol)

[a]Whereas Cushing's syndrome is unlikely in these conditions, it may rarely be present. If there is a high clinical index of suspicion, the patient should undergo testing, particularly those within the first group

Salivary Cortisol Assays

Like UFC, late-night pre-bedtime measurement of salivary cortisol also reflects the free fraction in blood. The nadir in salivary cortisol that occurs around the time of sleep in healthy individuals is lost in Cushing's syndrome. As a result, just as UFC is elevated, late-night salivary cortisol levels are increased in Cushing's syndrome. The morning values of salivary cortisol in healthy and hypercortisolemic people overlap so that measurement at this time is not useful for diagnosis [10]. One advantage of saliva over urine collections is that saliva can be collected at home by passive drooling or chewing on a pledget. Salivary cortisol is stable at room temperature and can be mailed to the laboratory.

Because various studies propose different diagnostic cut-off points, salivary cortisol assays may need local validation unless previously characterized assays are used. These different criteria may reflect differences in assay performance. For example, in one study of split samples, tandem mass spectrometry gave fewer false-positive results than radioimmunoassay [11]. Using ELISA and mass spectrometry, values between 2300 and 2400 h are usually less than 145 ng/dL (4 nmol/L).

Most reference ranges for salivary cortisol are based on a relatively small sample, comprised mostly of younger individuals. By contrast, recent publications show that late-night salivary cortisol values exceed the reference range in elderly, hypertensive, and diabetic men and in current smokers [12, 13]. Because of this, the test may not be a good choice in such patients, unless smokers can abstain for the day of collection. The question of whether age and co-morbidities increase the normal upper reference limit is important and deserves further study.

4 The Diagnosis of Cushing's Syndrome   51

Additionally, because the circadian rhythm is blunted in shift workers and is shifted in time when bedtime is much later than midnight, late-night salivary cortisol measurements potentially may give a false result [14]. The environment theoretically could influence results – if a collection were done at a stressful time, the result might be falsely increased. Despite these concerns, in a study of healthy volunteers sampled 1 h after watching an exciting football game, only 1 of 15 had an elevated value at 2300 h [10].

Dexamethasone Suppression Test

In healthy individuals, dexamethasone negative feedback decreases ACTH. As a result serum cortisol levels fall. This response is lost in Cushing's syndrome, so that cortisol levels remain elevated above 1.8 μg/dL (50 nmol/L). In the United States, the DST usually is performed using a 1 mg dose given orally between 2300 and 2400 h, with measurement of serum cortisol between 0800 h and 0900 h the following day. In the United Kingdom and elsewhere, a 2-day 2 mg DST (also known as the low dose dexamethasone suppression test, LDDST) often is used instead. This test involves taking dexamethasone, 500 μg, orally every 6 h for eight doses and measuring serum cortisol 2 or 6 h after the last dose, using a test-specific cortisol criterion (1.4 or 1.8 μg/dL; 39 or 50 nmol/L) [9, 15]. This version of the test requires greater patient compliance than the 1 mg test.

The DST is susceptible to error if dexamethasone is metabolized more quickly than usual, resulting in a less biologically effective dose, or if cortisol values are perturbed by changes in CBG. A variety of medications induce CYP3A4 enzymes and accelerate dexamethasone clearance [16]. Conversely, other medications and hepatic and renal failure may prolong dexamethasone clearance, leading to a falsely normal result. Recent data indicate that patients taking multiple medications (not all of which are known to interact with CYP3A4) are more likely to have a falsely abnormal result with the LDDST [17].

The plasma dexamethasone concentration can be measured at the time of cortisol measurement to assess the possibility of abnormal metabolism. If an adequate level (>5.6 nmol/L [0.22 μg/dL]) is present, a falsely abnormal test is unlikely [18]. If an inadequate level is found, the dose can be increased. Unfortunately, this measurement is not widely available outside of the United States.

Estrogen-induced increases in CBG (from oral contraceptives or pregnancy) or decreases caused by critical illness or nephrotic syndrome, also can affect the validity of the DST by increasing or decreasing the total blood cortisol level [19, 20].

There is up to a 30% false-positive rate for the DST in chronic illness, obesity, psychiatric disorders, and even normal individuals [21], and a rate of 50% in women taking oral contraceptive pill [22]. Conversely, an inappropriately normal serum cortisol result was found in 8% of patients with Cushing's disease after the 1 mg test, and in 17% after the LDDST when urine endpoints were used [23]. (Thus, serum cortisol must be used as an endpoint.)

Second Line Tests

The guidelines recommended a midnight serum cortisol and the dexamethasone-CRH stimulation test as possible second line tests [6]. The serum cortisol test excludes Cushing's syndrome if it is low. Just as with salivary cortisol, nadir serum cortisol values occur at this time. A variety of cut-off points have been proposed to enhance diagnostic accuracy but no single criterion has worked well in all studies [5].

The Dexamethasone-CRH stimulation test is generally reserved for subsequent analysis, particularly in patients considered to have physiologic hypercortisolism. The test has had mixed reviews in terms of its ability to distinguish patients with pseudo-Cushing's syndrome from those with Cushing's syndrome [17]. The variables underlying these differences are not clear, but may relate to medication-induced enhanced dexamethasone metabolism [17]. Unfortunately, dexamethasone levels were not measured in most series with less encouraging results.

The guidelines also recommend case detection for patients with an adrenal incidentaloma compatible with an adenoma on imaging. UFC may be less sensitive in this setting, in part because the hypercortisolism may be intermittent or mild, while an abnormal response to dexamethasone is common in patients with a functioning adenoma. Often these patients have symptoms that are compatible with Cushing's syndrome, such as hypertension or diabetes, and it is uncertain whether these are caused or exacerbated by mild hypercortisolism. Ultimately, a decision for resection should be chosen based on this judgment [24]. In this setting only, documentation of a suppressed plasma ACTH or dehydroepiandrosterone concentration is helpful, as it suggests the presence of hypercortisolism sufficient to suppress the corticotrope.

Apart from patients with adrenal masses, tests used for the differential diagnosis of Cushing's syndrome (e.g. plasma ACTH level, CRH stimulation test) should not be used to make the initial diagnosis. This includes magnetic resonance imaging of the pituitary gland. Since 10% of healthy volunteers have an apparent microadenoma using 1.5 T machine, abnormal imaging cannot be used to establish the diagnosis of Cushing's disease in the absence of biochemical data [25].

In many cases the chance of a false-positive result for any of the screening tests is greater than the chance of a truly positive result. Because of this, when the results are abnormal, one should review again the choice of tests with a view of ignoring the results if the tests were suboptimal. As examples, a salivary sample obtained at midnight after a car accident may be abnormal, but the effect of a stress response could not be excluded; an abnormal DST result potentially may be explained by a medication that the patient had not disclosed previously; an abnormal UFC may be discarded if the creatinine excretion was 4.0 g. Conversely, a normal response in a context that might be problematic can generally be accepted. As examples, a normal salivary cortisol after a car accident, a normal response to DST while taking oral contraceptives, and a normal UFC with a creatinine of 4 g can be considered normal.

Having correctly performed appropriate screening tests, it is next critical to assess the results in light of the pretest probability of Cushing's syndrome based on clinical judgment [26]. If the pretest probability is low, and two screening tests are minimally abnormal, the patient probably does not have Cushing's syndrome. A third test could be done, or the patient could be asked to return for additional testing if new symptoms appear. Conversely, if the pretest probability is very high and the test results are normal, it is reasonable to continue to screen with UFC and/or salivary cortisol based on a potential diagnosis of cyclic Cushing's syndrome. In this setting, it is sometimes helpful to instruct the patient to collect samples on days when they feel worst.

The Differential Diagnosis of Cushing's Syndrome

Once the diagnosis of Cushing's syndrome is established, its cause must be determined. Individual tests for this purpose are reviewed elsewhere in this book and the differential diagnosis is discussed in detail in Chap. 7, but a few general observations may be helpful.

All biochemical tests for the differential diagnosis of Cushing's syndrome require suppression of the normal corticotrope cells. Patients with mild or cyclic Cushing's syndrome whose normal corticotropes can respond to dexamethasone or CRH will have a normal response – the ACTH and cortisol levels will increase after CRH administration and decrease after dexamethasone administration. Corticotrope tumors have the same responses. As a result, Cushing's syndrome patients without a corticotrope tumor may be falsely diagnosed as having Cushing's disease if tested when they have not been hypercortisolemic.

Because of corticotrope suppression, patients with autonomous adrenal cortisol production have very low or undetectable plasma ACTH levels. This forms the basis for the first diagnostic step. Imaging of the adrenal gland in these patients is done next to identify whether the lesions are unilateral or bilateral. An unresolved issue is how to interpret single bilateral masses – is this an unusual presentation of macronodular adrenal disease, or an adenoma with a contralateral nonfunctioning mass? Another question is how to interpret an intermediate ACTH level (10–20 pg/mL), which might be seen in both adrenal and nonadrenal causes. In a young person, measurement of dehydroepiandrosterone might be useful if it is low, indicating functional corticotrope suppression. This author would evaluate for mild or cyclic hypercortisolism and image the adrenal gland to exclude primary adrenal disease with inadequate corticotrope suppression. If this evaluation is negative, in such a patient, it is reasonable to proceed to investigate ACTH-dependent causes.

Two Strategies for the Differential Diagnosis

In most centers, a pituitary MRI is obtained first after a primary adrenal cause has been excluded, as an obvious large mass may influence subsequent testing choices. When there is no obvious tumor, or a mass is ≤6 mm, other testing is needed.

Since inferior petrosal sinus sampling (IPSS) has the best diagnostic accuracy, it can be done as the sole procedure [27]. However, reliable results require performance by an experienced radiologist and correct catheter placement. If there is a step-up in the petrosal sinus ACTH samples compared to peripheral values (more than 2:1 before or 3:1 after CRH administration), and the corticotropes are suppressed, the patient has Cushing's disease (or very rarely, ectopic CRH secretion). If there is no central gradient the patient is most likely to have ectopic ACTH secretion, although false-negative IPSS results have been reported in Cushing's disease patients with anomalous or hypoplastic petrosal sinuses [28].

When access to IPSS is limited, both the 8 mg DST and the CRH test may be useful. If both are positive, Cushing's disease is very likely [29]. However, if results are discordant or both negative, either ectopic ACTH secretion or Cushing's disease is possible.

References

1. Etxabe J, Vazquez JA. Morbidity and mortality in Cushing's disease: an epidemiological approach. Clin Endocrinol (Oxf). 1994;40(4):479–84.
2. Lindholm J, Juul S, Jorgensen JO, et al. Incidence and late prognosis of Cushing's syndrome: a population-based study. J Clin Endocrinol Metab. 2001;86(1):117–23.
3. Swearingen B, Biller BM, Barker 2nd FG, et al. Long-term mortality after transsphenoidal surgery for Cushing disease. Ann Intern Med. 1999;130(10):821–4.
4. Plotz CM, Knowlton AI, Ragan C. The natural history of Cushing's syndrome. Am J Med. 1952;13(5):597–614.
5. Pecori Giraldi F, Pivonello R, Ambrogio AG, et al. The dexamethasone-suppressed corticotropin-releasing hormone stimulation test and the desmopressin test to distinguish Cushing's syndrome from pseudo-Cushing's states. Clin Endocrinol (Oxf). 2007;66(2):251–7.
6. Nieman LK, Biller BM, Findling JW, et al. The diagnosis of Cushing's syndrome: an Endocrine Society Clinical Practice Guideline. J Clin Endocrinol Metab. 2008;93(5):1526–40.
7. Sonino N, Fava GA. Psychiatric disorders associated with Cushing's syndrome. Epidemiology, pathophysiology and treatment. CNS Drugs. 2001;15(5):361–73.
8. Starkman MN, Schteingart DE, Schork MA. Correlation of bedside cognitive and neuropsychological tests in patients with Cushing's syndrome. Psychosomatics. 1986;27(7):508–11.
9. Yanovski JA, Cutler Jr GB, Chrousos GP, Nieman LK. Corticotropin-releasing hormone stimulation following low-dose dexamethasone administration. A new test to distinguish Cushing's syndrome from pseudo-Cushing's states. JAMA. 1993;269(17):2232–8.
10. Raff H, Raff JL, Findling JW. Late-night salivary cortisol as a screening test for Cushing's syndrome. J Clin Endocrinol Metab. 1998;83(8):2681–6.
11. Baid SK, Sinaii N, Wade M, Rubino D, Nieman LK. Radioimmunassay and tandem mass spectrometry measurement of bedtime salivary cortisol levels: a comparison of assays to establish hypercortisolism. J Clin Endocrinol Metab. 2007;92:3102–7.
12. Badrick E, Kirschbaum C, Kumari M. The relationship between smoking status and cortisol secretion. J Clin Endocrinol Metab. 2007;92(3):819–24.
13. Liu H, Bravata DM, Cabaccan J, Raff H, Ryzen E. Elevated late-night salivary cortisol levels in elderly male type 2 diabetic veterans. Clin Endocrinol (Oxf). 2005;63(6):642–9.
14. Touitou Y, Motohashi Y, Reinberg A, et al. Effect of shift work on the night-time secretory patterns of melatonin, prolactin, cortisol and testosterone. Eur J Appl Physiol Occup Physiol. 1990;60(4):288–92.

15. Newell-Price J, Trainer P, Besser M, Grossman A. The diagnosis and differential diagnosis of Cushing's syndrome and pseudo-Cushing's states. Endocr Rev. 1998;19(5):647–72.
16. Luo G, Cunningham M, Kim S, et al. CYP3A4 induction by drugs: correlation between a pregnane X receptor reporter gene assay and CYP3A4 expression in human hepatocytes. Drug Metab Dispos. 2002;30(7):795–804.
17. Valassi E, Swearingen B, Lee H, et al. Concomitant medication use can confound interpretation of the combined dexamethasone-corticotropin releasing hormone test in Cushing's syndrome. J Clin Endocrinol Metab. 2009;94(12):4851–9.
18. Meikle AW. Dexamethasone suppression tests: usefulness of simultaneous measurement of plasma cortisol and dexamethasone. Clin Endocrinol (Oxf). 1982;16(4):401–8.
19. Klose M, Lange M, Rasmussen AK, et al. Factors influencing the adrenocorticotropin test: role of contemporary cortisol assays, body composition, and oral contraceptive agents. J Clin Endocrinol Metab. 2007;92(4):1326–33.
20. Hamrahian AH, Oseni TS, Arafah BM. Measurements of serum free cortisol in critically ill patients. N Engl J Med. 2004;350(16):1629–38.
21. Kaye TB, Crapo L. The Cushing syndrome: an update on diagnostic tests. Ann Intern Med. 1990;112(6):434–44.
22. Nickelsen T, Lissner W, Schoffling K. The dexamethasone suppression test and long-term contraceptive treatment: measurement of ACTH or salivary cortisol does not improve the reliability of the test. Exp Clin Endocrinol. 1989;94(3):275–80.
23. Findling JW, Raff H, Aron DC. The low-dose dexamethasone suppression test: a reevaluation in patients with Cushing's syndrome. J Clin Endocrinol Metab. 2004;89(3):1222–6.
24. Chiodini I, Morelli V, Salcuni AS, et al. Beneficial metabolic effects of prompt surgical treatment in patients with an adrenal incidentaloma causing biochemical hypercortisolism. J Clin Endocrinol Metab. 2010;95:2736–45.
25. Hall WA, Luciano MG, Doppman JL, Patronas NJ, Oldfield EH. Pituitary magnetic resonance imaging in normal human volunteers: occult adenomas in the general population. Ann Intern Med. 1994;120(10):817–20.
26. Elamin MB, Murad MH, Mullan R, et al. Accuracy of diagnostic tests for Cushing's syndrome: a systematic review and metaanalyses. J Clin Endocrinol Metab. 2008;93(5):1553–62.
27. Findling JW, Raff H. Cushing's Syndrome: important issues in diagnosis and management. J Clin Endocrinol Metab. 2006;91(10):3746–53.
28. Doppman JL, Chang R, Oldfield EH, Chrousos G, Stratakis CA, Nieman LK. The hypoplastic inferior petrosal sinus: a potential source of false-negative results in petrosal sampling for Cushing's disease. J Clin Endocrinol Metab. 1999;84(2):533–40.
29. Nieman LK, Chrousos GP, Oldfield EH, Avgerinos PC, Cutler Jr GB, Loriaux DL. The ovine corticotropin-releasing hormone stimulation test and the dexamethasone suppression test in the differential diagnosis of Cushing's syndrome. Ann Intern Med. 1986;105(6):862–7.

Chapter 5
Pseudo-Cushing's Syndrome

Gregory A. Kaltsas and George Chrousos

Abstract Pseudo-Cushing's syndromes (PCS) are defined as states associated with increased cortisol production with all or some of the clinical features of Cushing's syndrome (CS), combined with biochemical evidence of hypercortisolism, but without evidence for a neoplastic etiology. These states include conditions such as severe physical or emotional stress, alcoholism or alcohol withdrawal, and chronic medical and psychiatric diseases such as depression and various psychoses. Although resolution of the primary condition usually leads to disappearance of the Cushingoid features and hypercortisolism, the underlying mechanisms remain unclear. Most evidence suggests that central stimulation of corticotropin-releasing hormone (CRH), either at the hypothalamic or suprahypothalamic level, is responsible. This leads to characteristic alterations in endocrine testing aimed at differentiating PCS from true states of excessive cortisol production. Distinguishing PCS from CS is clinically relevant, because a patient with a PCS who is misdiagnosed as CS may undergo needless testing and potentially harmful treatments, while missing the diagnosis of CS can lead to increased morbidity and mortality risk from the underlying disease.

Keywords Cushing's syndrome • Hypercortisolism • Corticotropin-releasing hormone • Endocrine testing

G.A. Kaltsas (✉)
Department of Pathophysiology, National University of Athens,
Mikras Asias 75, Athens 11527, Greece
e-mail: gkaltsas@endo.gr

Introduction

Endogenous Cushing's syndrome (CS) is a relatively rare disorder that presents with hallmark signs such as proximal myopathy, thin skin and easy bruisability, and may affect multiple organ systems [1]. As glucocorticoids exert a wide range of actions and modulate metabolism, electrolytes, and energy expenditure, a number of common but less specific symptoms/signs such as hypertension, abnormalities in glucose metabolism, central obesity, and osteoporosis are often present [1, 2]. Following the introduction of more sensitive endocrine testing and the widespread application of imaging modalities, particularly abdominal computerized tomography (CT), increasing numbers of patients are being recognized with mild CS. They may exhibit a constellation of symptoms/signs, including weight gain, menstrual irregularity, hirsutism, emotional instability, and hypertension, that may overlap with those observed in other relatively common disorders not associated with the increased morbidity and mortality seen in true endogenous CS [3]. In order to detect patients with CS, particularly those with milder forms, accurate tests are required that can discriminate patients with and without sustained hypercortisolism [4].

Patients with a number of other medical conditions may also manifest some of the symptoms/signs seen in patients with CS, without actually having the disease [1, 2]. This is particularly relevant as the aging population and the obesity epidemic are making some of the features of CS, such as central obesity, hypertension, hyperglycemia, and bone fragility, more common [4]. Furthermore, a number of conditions may lead to increased cortisol production with or without the physical phenotype found in patients with CS [2]. Such conditions are defined as pseudo-Cushing's states (PCS) and include severe physical and mental stress, alcoholism or alcohol withdrawal, extreme nutritional alterations, and mental disorders, especially depression [1, 2]. Patients with PCS exhibit increased cortisol production (documented by increased urinary free cortisol (UFC) measurement) that is usually moderate and not sufficiently sustained to produce the full hallmarks of CS [2]. Furthermore, resolution of the underlying condition is usually associated with disappearance of the clinical and biochemical abnormalities [2]. Therefore, it is important to determine whether a patient has PCS, since if this is misdiagnosed as CS the patient may undergo costly and invasive testing and/or potentially harmful therapies. Conversely, if CS is missed, a potentially curable condition associated with considerable morbidity and mortality may remain untreated. In order to reach the appropriate diagnosis, it is important to understand the clinical and laboratory features of the conditions that may be associated with PCS in order to evaluate patients with suspected CS in a safe and cost-effective manner.

Diseases/Conditions Associated with PCS

A number of physical and mental stresses can lead to elevated cortisol production and development of some of the symptoms/signs of hypercortisolism. (Table 5.1) Physical conditions include surgery, trauma and severe illness, extreme caloric

5 Pseudo-Cushing's Syndrome

Table 5.1 Symptoms/signs encountered in patients with CS and PCS

Symptoms	Signs	Other condition
Features that when present exert a high sensitivity and specificity		
	Easy bruising	Factitious glucocorticoid intake [23]
	Proximal myopathy	
	Thin skin	
	Combination of weight gain and decrease in growth velocity in children	
Features that when present exert a high sensitivity but relatively low specificity		
	Facial plethora	Obesity
	Striae (reddish purple and >1 cm in diameter)	
	Dorsocervical fat pad ("buffalo hump")	
	Supraclavicular fullness	
Features of CS that are also found in other common disorders		
Weight gain/abdominal adiposity	Hypertension	Metabolic syndrome
Fatigue	Obesity	Diabetes mellitus Type 2
Emotional liability – decline intellectual performance		PCOS
Menstrual abnormality – Hirsutism		Adrenal incidentaloma
Backpain		Hypopituitarism, GH, and/or gonadotrophin deficiency
		Osteoporosis

alterations, starvation, morbid obesity, and intensive exercise, whereas mental conditions include everyday emotional stresses and losses [2, 5, 6]. Psychiatric disorders and alcoholism are important states associated with PCS; the psychiatric disorders that are most commonly confused with CS include depression and anxiety states [5, 6]. Although these conditions are associated with the activation of the hypothalamo–pituitary–adrenal (HPA) axis, not all patients develop the characteristic symptoms/signs of CS. Nonetheless, they can be associated with alterations of cortisol secretion manifested as either hypercortisolism and/or alterations of cortisol dynamics, i.e., loss of cortisol diurnal rhythm of secretion and/or inability of adequate suppression to dexamethasone administration.

Physical Stresses (Aerobic Exercise)

Strenuous and/or prolonged physical activity leads to muscle and other tissue damage and induces an inflammatory response characterized by secretion of proinflammatory cytokines, chemokines, and other mediators of inflammation, in addition to cortisol secretion [7]. It is well established that several cytokines, especially interleukin-6 (IL-6), exert a stimulatory effect on HPA axis [8]. Strenuous exercise is associated with dramatic increases of IL-6, and although cortisol levels were not directly measured, they would also be expected to substantially increase [7].

Emotional Stress

Stressful events are environmental reactions perceived to threaten homeostatic status that, when accompanied with feelings of defeat or helplessness, are associated with activation of the HPA axis. Subsequent inhibition of gonadal and growth axes predisposes to the development of central obesity [9]. Stress-related cortisol hypersecretion is associated with lack of cortisol diurnal rhythm, hypertension, hyperlipidemia, and insulin resistance along with failure of dexamethasone suppression, all features of CS [9].

Depression

Patients with depression develop many laboratory features suggestive of CS, including hypercortisolemia and altered cortisol dynamics. They may be unable to achieve adequate cortisol suppression following dexamethasone administration. Depression is likely to represent a state of relative corticotrophin (CRH) excess, in contrast to CS which is a state of CRH deficiency, occurring as a result of hypothalamic suppression from the autonomous glucocorticoid production. This hypothesis that depression increases CRH is further supported by the finding that the adrenal glands hypertrophy follows CRH hypersecretion, leading to increased cortisol response to adrenocorticotrophin (ACTH) hypersecretion [10–12]. Cortisol feedback to corticotrophs remains relatively intact (although at a higher level compared to controls) so that exogenous CRH induces a blunted ACTH but normal cortisol response [10–12].

Severe and Chronic Diseases

Patients with severe illnesses and chronic diseases can develop some of the biochemical features of CS, although their symptoms/signs are not usually those of hypercortisolism but rather of the underlying disease. The degree of HPA-axis suppression depends on the severity and duration of the underlying disease.

Severe Illnesses

Life-threatening conditions, surgical procedures, and severe illnesses activate the HPA axis, leading to excessive cortisol production that is initially appropriate for the intensity of the insult. Perpetuation of this event may lead to sustainable hypercortisolism and abnormalities in cortisol secretory dynamics.

Chronic Diseases

Abnormalities of HPA function, as observed in PCS, are common in diabetic patients, even in the absence of ketoacidosis [13]. These include higher plasma cortisol levels than in non-diabetics [14] and increases in counter-regulatory hormone secretion [15]. Diabetic subjects with abdominal obesity, particularly women, may also have slightly increased activity of the HPA axis together with blunted cortisol circadian variability [16], increased nocturnal cortisol secretion [17], and higher ACTH and cortisol concentration after HPA stimulation [18]. In addition, the depression that commonly accompanies diabetes [19] may also contribute to the functional activation of the HPA axis [13]. Patients with renal failure may also show biochemical features of CS and abnormalities in laboratory tests of autonomous cortisol secretion, but maintain normal cortisol secretory rhythm [20].

Nutrition (Morbid Obesity, Anorexia)

Obesity and malnutrition have opposing effects in normal physiology and are associated with changes in hormonal secretion. Some of the changes are adaptive but may create diagnostic problems with primary states of hormonal excess [21]. Circulating cortisol concentrations are usually normal (or slightly reduced) in obesity, but morbid obesity is associated with raised UFC levels [22]. Higher brain centers stimulate CRH release and subsequent activation of the HPA axis that is, however, under relative negative feedback restraining the resulting hypercortisolemia [5, 6]. Due the presence of relative feedback inhibition, UFC excretion is limited to values less than three to fourfold normal [2]. Based initially on studies performed in animal models [23], it was later confirmed that human subjects with abdominal obesity exhibit a hyperactivity of the HPA axis [24]. These subjects have increased UFC excretion and increased cortisol responsiveness both to ACTH stimulation and to physical and mental stresses [24]. In a comparative study of women with abdominal and gluteofemoral obesity, the former had significantly higher absolute and percentage increases in ACTH and cortisol levels following CRH stimulation, and higher UFC and cortisol metabolite excretion [18]. However, these patients maintain a normal cortisol circadian rhythm and the majority obtain adequate cortisol suppression to dexamethasone administration [22].

Patients with anorexia nervosa develop biochemical evidence of hypercortisolism, but the increased cortisol levels have been associated with normal ACTH levels [25]. This state of hypercortisolism is thought to develop due to a combination of a relative increase in cortisol secretion and a decrease in cortisol clearance [21].

Increased cortisol secretion develops as a result of central activation of the stress axis, as documented by the increased CRH levels in the cerebrospinal fluid of underweight patients [26]. In addition, there is decreased feedback sensitivity, as shown by an abnormal suppressibility with dexamethasone postulating intact pituitary but impaired hypothalamic feedback [26]. The distinction from CS can be made by the absence of clinical stigmata of CS and the preservation of cortisol circadian rhythm [26].

Factitious Glucocorticoid Administration

Factitious intake of glucocorticoids may be difficult to distinguish from CS as it leads to the same phenotypic features [27]. When hydrocortisone is ingested, UFC and serum cortisol levels are increased, whereas intake of synthetic glucocorticoids is associated with low or high levels depending on the cross-reactivity of these compounds with the cortisol assay [2]. In all such cases ACTH levels are low and imaging of the adrenal glands shows absence of adrenal pathology.

Metabolic Syndrome, Polycystic Ovary Syndrome, Hypopituitarism: Growth Hormone Deficiency

The central obesity that accompanies the metabolic syndrome may be associated with mildly elevated cortisol production and inability to adequately suppress cortisol levels following dexamethasone administration, without any of the classical symptoms/signs suggestive of hypercortisolemia [24, 28]. Women with polycystic ovary syndrome (PCOS) may also exhibit many nonspecific symptoms/signs similar to those encountered in CS; however, such patients do not exhibit any of the signs considered specific for CS [29]. Patients with hypopituitarism, and particularly adult growth hormone deficiency (AGHD), may present with symptoms similar to those with CS, including weight gain and central obesity, low energy and fatigue, reduced muscle strength, altered lipid composition, and impaired sense of well-being [30]. Although patients with AGHD are usually eucortisolemic, in the presence of concomitant ACTH deficiency particular attention should be paid to symptoms/signs of glucocorticoid deficiency, because initiation of GH replacement can induce increased cortisol to cortisone metabolism due to modulation of 11β-hydroxysteroid dehydrogenase (HSD) type 1 [31].

Drug Induced

Human immunodeficiency virus-1 (HIV-1) positive patients, particularly those treated with retroviral protease inhibitors, may develop some of the stigmata of patients with CS, including new onset central obesity, dorsocervical fat accumulation, hyperlipidemia, and abnormal glucose homeostasis [32]. Acromegalic patients receiving the GH-antagonist, pegvisomant, may also develop central obesity [33]. Drugs that interfere with some of the analytical methods used for the laboratory confirmation of hypercortisolism may also cause diagnostic confusion. The interference with UFC by fenofibrate and anticonvulsants could lead to a false diagnosis of CS [34, 35]. In addition, alterations in cortisol binding globulin (CBG), either as a constitutive increase or from drug effect, and alterations in dexamethasone metabolism could account for biochemical abnormalities that mimic CS [2].

Alcohol Intake

Excessive alcohol intake can produce typical clinical and laboratory features similar to those of patients with CS [26]. Twenty-four-hour UFC levels are usually twofold higher in alcoholics compared to controls, and alcoholics also fail to achieve adequate cortisol suppression following dexamethasone administration [26]. Although a subset of alcoholics demonstrate enhanced basal production of cortisol, most alcoholics have a blunted response to acute intervening stresses, including CRH, low dose ACTH-(1–24), and metyrapone blockade. These data suggest that alcoholics have ethanol-induced HPA-axis injury, resulting in an inappropriately reduced response to nonethanol-induced stress [26]. It is very difficult to differentiate such patients from those with CS, and the diagnosis is established either by demonstrating increased alcohol levels or by repeating the investigations after a period of alcohol abstinence when HPA-axis dynamics have returned to normal [26, 36]. Adrenocorticoid hyposensitivity persists after oCRH infusion for at least 1 month after cessation of drinking, whereas hyporesponsiveness of the pituitary corticotrophs to CRH seems to resolve with continued abstinence [37].

Peripheral Cortisol Metabolism (11β-HSD)

Glucocorticoid action at the pre-receptor level is regulated mostly by 11β-hydroxysteroid dehydrogenase (11β-HSD), an enzyme that interconverts bioactive cortisol into bioinactive cortisone [31]. The low affinity type 1 isoform of the enzyme is mainly found in omental fat cells and converts cortisone to cortisol, while the high affinity type 2 isoform is found in the kidney and inactivates cortisol, thus protecting the mineralocorticoid receptor from cortisol excess [38]. Increased activity of 11β-HSD1 could lead to the characteristic stigmata of CS with relatively normal cortisol levels [31].

Glucocorticoid Receptor Abnormalities

The possibility of increased sensitivity of the glucocorticoid receptor (GR) to circulating cortisol levels has been raised as a potential cause of PCS, after the description of a patient with symptoms of hypercortisolemia and low cortisol levels [39, 40]. A specific polymorphism of the GR, found in 6% of normal Dutch men, was associated with cortisol hyperresponsivity, as manifested by greater cortisol suppression by dexamethasone, higher body mass index, and lower bone mineral density in these men as compared to non-carriers. It is therefore possible that such patients may have evaded conventional diagnostic testing, as screening tests would fail to reveal any evidence of hypercortisolism [40]. Resistance to GR is far better characterized and, although many biochemical features resemble those of CS, the maintenance of normal cortisol rhythm and the absence of stigmata related to the disease distinguishes it from CS [41].

Laboratory Confirmation and Tests Used to Distinguish CS from PCS

Initial Tests to Confirm Hypercortisolism

Careful medical history and clinical examination can help identify patients with CS, especially those with florid disease. Particular attention should be paid to the time course of symptom development and the presence of the characteristic clinical stigmata of the disease [2]. The diagnosis can then be substantiated with the establishment of excessive cortisol secretion and/or failure to obtain adequate cortisol suppression to dexamethasone administration [1, 2] However, the optimal laboratory test for establishing the diagnosis and distinguishing patients with CS from normals and from those with PCS has not yet been established [42]. Elevated UFC levels are found at least once following several measurements in 95% of patients with CS [2]. After three normal UFC measurements, it is unlikely that the patient has CS, whereas the diagnosis of CS is highly likely if a UFC value of 3.5 times more than the upper normal limit is found [2]. For all intermediate values more sophisticated tests are needed to distinguish patents with CS from PCS.

Tests Used for Distinguishing CS from PCS

Morning serum total and free cortisol levels among patients with CS, PCS, and normal subjects overlap, making this test unsuitable for the diagnosis of CS and/or PCS [2, 43]. Similarly, the absence of diurnal serum cortisol rhythm fails to discriminate patients with PCS from patients with CS [44]. Twenty-four-hour UFC levels can be mildly elevated in patients with PCS, but can also be normal in approximately 10–20% of patients with CS [43]. Both the 1 mg overnight and the formal 2-day low-dose dexamethasone suppression tests (LDDST) are highly sensitive but have a low specificity, as inadequate cortisol suppression has been documented in patients with obesity, severe illness, alcoholism, depression, and other psychiatric disorders [8, 22]. In a recent study including patients with both CS and PCS, the specificity of the above tests in correctly identifying patients with CS was 18% for abnormal cortisol rhythm, 44% for UFC, 58% for the 1 mg DST, and 74% for the LDDST, respectively [44].

Midnight Serum or Salivary Cortisol

The loss of normal cortisol circadian rhythm combined with the absence of a late-night cortisol nadir is consistent with the abnormal cortisol dynamics seen in patients with CS. Midnight serum cortisol (MSC) levels have been used to distinguish patients with CS from those with PCS. In a study that included 240 patients with CS and 23 patients with PCS, an MSC value greater than 7.5 μg/dl correctly identified 96% patients with CS, while a value less then this threshold was found in all patients with PCS (96% sensitivity and 100% specificity) [8]. In a more recent study using an MSC threshold of 9.3 μg/dl, the test achieved 100% sensitivity and specificity in distinguishing patients with CS from PCS [42]. The midnight cortisol measurement requires inpatient admission for a period of 48 h or longer to avoid false-positive responses due to the stress of hospitalization. The blood sample must be drawn within 5–10 min after waking the patient, or through an indwelling line, to avoid false-positive results. Recently, measurement of salivary cortisol (SC) has also been used as it is in equilibrium with serum free cortisol and independent of saliva production [45]. In a study that included 151 subjects, a threshold SC value of 3.6 nmol/L (0.13 μg/dl) at 11 P.M. achieved a sensitivity and specificity of 92% and 96%, respectively [46]. In a more recent study of 122 patients with CS and 21 patients with PCS, a 93% sensitivity and 100% specificity was obtained using a 15.2 nmol/L (0.55 μg/dl) SC value as a cut-off [47]. Several factors that can affect SC measurement should be considered when evaluating the results. Patients are advised to refrain from smoking or liquorice consumption on the day of the test, as both contain the 11β-HSD type 2 inhibitor, glycyrrhizic acid, and may lead to false elevated results [48].

Dexamethasone-CRH Test

The dexamethasone-CRH test, which combines the LDDST and the CRH tests, has been proposed to distinguish between mild CD and PCS. Two hours after the last dexamethasone dose of the LDDST, 1 μg/kg of ovine CRH is administered intravenously and serum cortisol is measured 15 min later. In theory, dexamethasone suppresses serum cortisol levels in individuals without CS as well as in a small number of those with CD, but following CRH administration only those patients with CD respond with an increase in ACTH and cortisol secretion. In a study that included 39 patients with mild CD and UFC values that overlapped with those of 19 patients with PCS, a serum cortisol measured 15 min after CRH of greater than 1.4 μg/dl (38 nmol/L) correctly identified all patients with CD, while all patients with PCS had values less than 1.4 μg/dl (100% sensitivity and specificity) [22]. In the same study, the CRH test without dexamethasone pre-treatment exhibited 100% specificity and 64% sensitivity. However, subsequent studies did not confirm these findings and revealed a lower diagnostic accuracy of the dexamethasone-CRH Test (sensitivity 100% and specificity 50–62.5%) [42, 44]. By increasing the threshold to 4 μg/dl, sensitivity was maintained at 100% and specificity was improved to 86% [42]. The reasons for the differences in the responses to the combined test are not clear. In part, they may be attributed to conditions that alter the metabolic clearance of dexamethasone or differences in the performance of cortisol assays used. Furthermore, a recent study has suggested that concomitant medication can affect the performance of the test, as its sensitivity and specificity were found to be higher in the group of patients who were not receiving any other medication while being investigated [49].

Desmopressin Test

The vasopressin analog desmopressin (1-deamino-8-D-arginine vasopressin, DDAVP) stimulates ACTH release in patients with CD but not in the majority of normal, obese, and depressed subjects. It has also been used to distinguish patients with PCS from those with CD. In a study that included 20 patients with CD and 30 patients with PCS, a peak absolute ACTH increase of 6 pmol/L (27.2 pg/mL) within 30 min after DDAVP infusion exhibited a sensitivity of 90% and a specificity of 96.7% [44]. In a similar study including 29 patients with CD and 23 patients with PCS, using the same peak ACTH cut-off, the sensitivity and specificity were 81.5% and 90%, respectively [50].

Other Less Commonly Used Tests

The insulin tolerance test (ITT) measures corticotroph secretion of ACTH after adequate hypoglycemia (glucose levels less than 40 mg/dl) following insulin (0.15 U/kg) administration. Patients with CS fail to obtain an adequate cortisol or ACTH response (a more than twofold increment compared to baseline), whereas the majority of patients with PCS respond; however, the discriminative ability of this test is only 75% [43]. The opiate antagonist loperamide has also been used, as it is expected to reduce ACTH secretion differentially in PCS and CS patients

Table 5.2 Tests used to distinguish Cushing's syndrome from Pseudo-Cushing's states and their respective sensitivity and specificity

Test used	Diagnostic cut-off	Sensitivity (%)	Specificity (%)	Reference
Midnight serum cortisol	7.5 μg/dl	96	100	8
	9.3 μg/dl	100	100	40
Midnight salivary cortisol	3.6 nmol/L	92	96	43
	15.2 nmol/L	93	100	44
Dexamethasone-CRH test (serum cortisol 15 min after CRH administration)	1.4 μg/dl	100	100	4
	1.4 μg/dl	100	50	42
	1.4 μg/dl	100	62.5	40
	4 μg/dl	100	86	40
Desmopressin test (peak absolute ACTH increase within 30 min after DDAVP)	6 pmol/L	90	96.7	42
	6 pmol/L	81.5	90	46

[51]. However, the test has not been extensively evaluated and is rarely used [51]. Although IL-6 administration has been proposed as a method to distinguish patients with CS from those with PCS, it has not been extensively studied and its use is restricted by the unavailability of the compound [52]. The rationale of this test relies on the ability of IL-6 to stimulate cortisol and ACTH secretion by enhancing CRH activity at the hypothalamus, which should be present in patients with PCS but not in those with CS [52].

Despite numerous tests available, the distinction between CS and PCS still represents a considerable challenge, as no single test provides 100% diagnostic accuracy (Table 5.2), and further studies are necessary.

Treatment and Follow-Up

Treatment of the PCS state is based on therapy of the underlying cause, while CS needs directed treatment according to its etiology. Occasionally, it is very difficult to reach an accurate diagnosis, as many cases of true CS can be mild and occasionally periodic, where states of eucortisolism follow that of excessive cortisol secretion. In contrast, cases of PCS may resolve when their underlying cause remits and may reappear with exacerbation of the underlying disease. It is therefore appropriate to continue evaluation of such patients until a definite diagnosis is established.

References

1. Newell-Price J, Trainer P, Besser M, Grossman A. The diagnosis and differential diagnosis of Cushing's syndrome and pseudo-Cushing's states. Endocr Rev. 1998;19(5):647–72.
2. Nieman LK, Biller BM, Findling JW, et al. The diagnosis of Cushing's syndrome: an Endocrine Society Clinical Practice Guideline. J Clin Endocrinol Metab. 2008;93(5):1526–40.

3. Tsagarakis S, Vassiliadi D, Thalassinos N. Endogenous subclinical hypercortisolism: diagnostic uncertainties and clinical implications. J Endocrinol Invest. 2006;29(5):471–82.
4. Elamin MB, Murad MH, Mullan R, et al. Accuracy of diagnostic tests for Cushing's syndrome: a systematic review and metaanalyses. J Clin Endocrinol Metab. 2008;93(5):1553–62.
5. Gold PW, Goodwin FK, Chrousos GP. Clinical and biochemical manifestations of depression. Relation to the neurobiology of stress (2). N Engl J Med. 1988;319(7):413–20.
6. Gold PW, Goodwin FK, Chrousos GP. Clinical and biochemical manifestations of depression. Relation to the neurobiology of stress (1). N Engl J Med. 1988;319(6):348–53.
7. Margeli A, Skenderi K, Tsironi M, et al. Dramatic elevations of interleukin-6 and acute-phase reactants in athletes participating in the ultradistance foot race spartathlon: severe systemic inflammation and lipid and lipoprotein changes in protracted exercise. J Clin Endocrinol Metab. 2005;90(7):3914–8.
8. Papanicolaou DA, Yanovski JA, Cutler Jr GB, Chrousos GP, Nieman LK. A single midnight serum cortisol measurement distinguishes Cushing's syndrome from pseudo-Cushing states. J Clin Endocrinol Metab. 1998;83(4):1163–7.
9. Rosmond R, Bjorntorp P. The interactions between hypothalamic-pituitary-adrenal axis activity, testosterone, insulin-like growth factor I and abdominal obesity with metabolism and blood pressure in men. Int J Obes Relat Metab Disord. 1998;22(12):1184–96.
10. Arana GW, Mossman D. The dexamethasone suppression test and depression. Approaches to the use of a laboratory test in psychiatry. Neurol Clin. 1988;6(1):21–39.
11. Carroll BJ, Curtis GC, Davies BM, Mendels J, Sugerman AA. Urinary free cortisol excretion in depression. Psychol Med. 1976;6(1):43–50.
12. Carroll BJ. Use of the dexamethasone suppression test in depression. J Clin Psychiatry. 1982;43(11 Pt 2):44–50.
13. Catargi B, Rigalleau V, Poussin A, et al. Occult Cushing's syndrome in type-2 diabetes. J Clin Endocrinol Metab. 2003;88(12):5808–13.
14. Cameron OG, Thomas B, Tiongco D, Hariharan M, Greden JF. Hypercortisolism in diabetes mellitus. Diabetes Care. 1987;10(5):662–4.
15. Spyer G, Hattersley AT, MacDonald IA, Amiel S, MacLeod KM. Hypoglycaemic counter-regulation at normal blood glucose concentrations in patients with well controlled type-2 diabetes. Lancet. 2000;356(9246):1970–4.
16. Bjorntorp P, Holm G, Rosmond R. Hypothalamic arousal, insulin resistance and type 2 diabetes mellitus. Diabet Med. 1999;16(5):373–83.
17. Duclos M, Gatta B, Corcuff JB, Rashedi M, Pehourcq F, Roger P. Fat distribution in obese women is associated with subtle alterations of the hypothalamic-pituitary-adrenal axis activity and sensitivity to glucocorticoids. Clin Endocrinol (Oxf). 2001;55(4):447–54.
18. Pasquali R, Cantobelli S, Casimirri F, et al. The hypothalamic-pituitary-adrenal axis in obese women with different patterns of body fat distribution. J Clin Endocrinol Metab. 1993;77(2):341–6.
19. Anderson RJ, Freedland KE, Clouse RE, Lustman PJ. The prevalence of comorbid depression in adults with diabetes: a meta-analysis. Diabetes Care. 2001;24(6):1069–78.
20. Sharp NA, Devlin JT, Rimmer JM. Renal failure obfuscates the diagnosis of Cushing's disease. JAMA. 1986;256(18):2564–5.
21. Douyon L, Schteingart DE. Effect of obesity and starvation on thyroid hormone, growth hormone, and cortisol secretion. Endocrinol Metab Clin North Am. 2002;31(1):173–89.
22. Yanovski JA, Cutler Jr GB, Chrousos GP, Nieman LK. Corticotropin-releasing hormone stimulation following low-dose dexamethasone administration. A new test to distinguish Cushing's syndrome from pseudo-Cushing's states. JAMA. 1993;269(17):2232–8.
23. Jeanrenaud B, Halimi S, van de Werve G. Neuro-endocrine disorders seen as triggers of the triad: obesity–insulin resistance–abnormal glucose tolerance. Diabetes Metab Rev. 1985;1(3):261–91.
24. Marin P, Darin N, Amemiya T, Andersson B, Jern S, Bjorntorp P. Cortisol secretion in relation to body fat distribution in obese premenopausal women. Metabolism. 1992;41(8):882–6.

25. Licinio J, Wong ML, Gold PW. The hypothalamic-pituitary-adrenal axis in anorexia nervosa. Psychiatry Res. 1996;62(1):75–83.
26. Duclos M, Corcuff JB, Roger P, Tabarin A. The dexamethasone-suppressed corticotrophin-releasing hormone stimulation test in anorexia nervosa. Clin Endocrinol (Oxf). 1999;51(6): 725–31.
27. Cizza G, Nieman LK, Doppman JL, et al. Factitious Cushing syndrome. J Clin Endocrinol Metab. 1996;81(10):3573–7.
28. Peeke PM, Chrousos GP. Hypercortisolism and obesity. Ann NY Acad Sci. 1995;771:665–76.
29. Kaltsas GA, Isidori AM, Besser GM, Grossman AB. Secondary forms of polycystic ovary syndrome. Trends Endocrinol Metab. 2004;15(5):204–10.
30. Gibney J, Wallace JD, Spinks T, et al. The effects of 10 years of recombinant human growth hormone (GH) in adult GH-deficient patients. J Clin Endocrinol Metab. 1999;84(8): 2596–602.
31. Stewart PM. 11 beta-Hydroxysteroid dehydrogenase: implications for clinical medicine. Clin Endocrinol (Oxf). 1996;44(5):493–9.
32. Ho TT, Chan KC, Wong KH, Lee SS. Abnormal fat distribution and use of protease inhibitors. Lancet. 1998;351(9117):1736–7.
33. Plockinger U, Reuter T. Pegvisomant increases intra-abdominal fat in patients with acromegaly: a pilot study. Eur J Endocrinol. 2008;158(4):467–71.
34. Putignano P, Kaltsas GA, Satta MA, Grossman AB. The effects of anti-convulsant drugs on adrenal function. Horm Metab Res. 1998;30(6–7):389–97.
35. Meikle AW, Findling J, Kushnir MM, Rockwood AL, Nelson GJ, Terry AH. Pseudo-Cushing syndrome caused by fenofibrate interference with urinary cortisol assayed by high-performance liquid chromatography. J Clin Endocrinol Metab. 2003;88(8):3521–4.
36. Junghanns K, Horbach R, Ehrenthal D, Blank S, Backhaus J. Cortisol awakening response in abstinent alcohol-dependent patients as a marker of HPA-axis dysfunction. Psychoneuroendocrinology. 2007;32(8–10):1133–7.
37. Adinoff B, Junghanns K, Kiefer F, Krishnan-Sarin S. Suppression of the HPA axis stress-response: implications for relapse. Alcohol Clin Exp Res. 2005;29(7):1351–5.
38. Stewart PM, Boulton A, Kumar S, Clark PM, Shackleton CH. Cortisol metabolism in human obesity: impaired cortisone cortisol conversion in subjects with central adiposity. J Clin Endocrinol Metab. 1999;84(3):1022–7.
39. Fujii H, Iida S, Gomi M, Tsugawa M, Kitani T, Moriwaki K. Augmented induction by dexamethasone of metallothionein IIa messenger ribonucleic acid in fibroblasts from a patient with cortisol hyperreactive syndrome. J Clin Endocrinol Metab. 1993;76(2):445–9.
40. Huizenga NA, Koper JW, De LP, et al. A polymorphism in the glucocorticoid receptor gene may be associated with and increased sensitivity to glucocorticoids in vivo. J Clin Endocrinol Metab. 1998;83(1):144–51.
41. Charmandari E, Kino T, Ichijo T, Chrousos GP. Generalized glucocorticoid resistance: clinical aspects, molecular mechanisms, and implications of a rare genetic disorder. J Clin Endocrinol Metab. 2008;93(5):1563–72.
42. Gatta B, Chabre O, Cortet C, et al. Reevaluation of the combined dexamethasone suppression-corticotropin-releasing hormone test for differentiation of mild cushing's disease from pseudo-Cushing's syndrome. J Clin Endocrinol Metab. 2007;92(11):4290–3.
43. Nieman LK. Diagnostic tests for Cushing's syndrome. Ann NY Acad Sci. 2002;970:112–8.
44. Pecori GF, Pivonello R, Ambrogio AG, et al. The dexamethasone-suppressed corticotropin-releasing hormone stimulation test and the desmopressin test to distinguish Cushing's syndrome from pseudo-Cushing's states. Clin Endocrinol (Oxf). 2007;66(2):251–7.
45. Dorn LD, Lucke JF, Loucks TL, Berga SL. Salivary cortisol reflects serum cortisol: analysis of circadian profiles. Ann Clin Biochem. 2007;44(Pt 3):281–4.
46. Raff H, Raff JL, Findling JW. Late-night salivary cortisol as a screening test for Cushing's syndrome. J Clin Endocrinol Metab. 1998;83(8):2681–6.

47. Papanicolaou DA, Mullen N, Kyrou I, Nieman LK. Nighttime salivary cortisol: a useful test for the diagnosis of Cushing's syndrome. J Clin Endocrinol Metab. 2002;87(10):4515–21.
48. Badrick E, Bobak M, Britton A, Kirschbaum C, Marmot M, Kumari M. The relationship between alcohol consumption and cortisol secretion in an aging cohort. J Clin Endocrinol Metab. 2008;93(3):750–7.
49. Valassi E, Swearingen B, Lee H, et al. Concomitant medication use can confound interpretation of the combined dexamethasone-corticotropin releasing hormone test in Cushing's syndrome. J Clin Endocrinol Metab. 2009;94(12):4851–9.
50. Moro M, Putignano P, Losa M, Invitti C, Maraschini C, Cavagnini F. The desmopressin test in the differential diagnosis between Cushing's disease and pseudo-Cushing states. J Clin Endocrinol Metab. 2000;85(10):3569–74.
51. Ambrosi B, Bochicchio D, Colombo P, Fadin C, Faglia G. Loperamide to diagnose Cushing's syndrome. JAMA. 1993;270(19):2301–2.
52. Tsigos C, Papanicolaou DA, Defensor R, Mitsiadis CS, Kyrou I, Chrousos GP. Dose effects of recombinant human interleukin-6 on pituitary hormone secretion and energy expenditure. Neuroendocrinology. 1997;66(1):54–62.

Chapter 6
Cyclic Cushing's Disease

Nicholas A. Tritos and Beverly M.K. Biller

Abstract Cyclic Cushing's disease (CD) is characterized by fluctuations in clinical or biochemical indices of hypercortisolism, and is often marked by periods of disease activity alternating with relative quiescence. Retrospectively collected data suggest that cyclic CD accounts for approximately 15–19% of all CD cases. The pathogenesis of this condition remains obscure.

Other than the presence of spontaneous fluctuations in its course, there are no distinguishing clinical or laboratory features of cyclic CD. However, the presence of varying degrees of hypercortisolism during its natural history frequently leads to major diagnostic difficulties, confounding the interpretation of diagnostic testing. Furthermore, assessment of the outcome of therapeutic interventions can be hampered by the intermittent nature of hypercortisolism inherent in cyclic CD.

Prospective studies may be helpful in further elucidating the natural history of cyclic CD and molecular studies will be needed to understand the pathophysiology of this enigmatic and challenging condition.

Keywords Hypercortisolism • Glucocorticoid hormonogenesis • Pituitary adenoma • Ectopic ACTH syndrome

Introduction

Over the past 5 decades, there have been many case reports and some series of patients with Cushing's syndrome (CS) or Cushing's disease (CD) who have experienced significant fluctuations in biochemical indices of disease activity in a

N.A. Tritos (✉)
Neuroendocrine Unit, Massachusetts General Hospital,
Zero Emerson Place, Suite #112, Boston, MA 02114, USA
e-mail: Ntritos@partners.org

periodic or irregular temporal pattern, a condition most commonly referred to as "cyclic CS (or CD)" [1–4].

Significant temporal variations in glucocorticoid hormonogenesis have been reported among patients with CS of diverse etiologies, including pituitary adenomas, the ectopic ACTH syndrome, or various adrenal pathologies [1, 5–8].

In this chapter, published data on the prevalence and clinical features of cyclic CD will be summarized. In addition, hypotheses regarding the pathophysiologic mechanisms leading to cyclic CD will be presented. The unique diagnostic and therapeutic challenges frequently posed by patients with cyclic CD will be discussed and suggestions for future study will be offered.

Definition and Prevalence

A variety of terms have been applied to denote patients with CD who have experienced substantial fluctuations in biochemical indices of disease activity with or without concurrent changes in clinical features, including "intermittent hypercortisolism," "fluctuating steroid excretion," "unpredictable hypersecretion of cortisol," "periodic hormonogenesis," and "cyclic or cyclical CD (or CS)" [9–15].

It should be noted that there is no universally agreed upon case definition for cyclic CD. It has previously been suggested that three peaks and two troughs of hypercortisolism are required at a minimum to define a patient as having cyclic CD [3]. In one recent study, however, it was suggested that the presence of only one cycle, defined as two peaks with an interim trough (or remission) of hypercortisolism, should suffice as a case definition [1]. In addition, in the same study, patients were considered to experience variability in hypercortisolism if spontaneous doubling or halving of mean serum cortisol, obtained from a five point cortisol day curve, was identified.

In this chapter, the term "cyclic CD" is consistently used to describe patients with spontaneous fluctuations in biochemical hypercortisolism (with or without concurrent changes in clinical findings), including at least two peaks and one trough in indices of disease activity. It should be recognized, however, that consensus regarding a more precise case definition will be very helpful to guide future research and practice.

There are no prospective studies of patients with cyclic CD. Case reports of patients with CD who had experienced marked spontaneous fluctuations in hypercortisolism were first published over 5 decades ago [10, 16]. In retrospect, Harvey Cushing's index patient, "Minnie G," may have had cyclic CD, as she was noted to experience a spontaneous clinical remission followed by symptomatic recurrence [17, 18]. At that time, however, there were no laboratory tests available to document variations in cortisolemia or cortisoluria. Subsequent reports presented data obtained through rather inaccurate tests of hypercortisolism, such as urine 17 hydroxysteroids, to define disease activity.

Although case reports originally suggested that cyclic CD is likely rare, more recently retrospective studies and case series have indicated that the prevalence of cyclic CD is approximately 15–19% among all CD patients [1, 19, 20]. In addition, in one study of CS patients, a higher prevalence of 36% was noted [21]. It is likely that these estimates are conservative, as they were all derived from retrospective reviews of case records.

Presentation of a Case

A 22-year-old woman presented with a history of recent-onset weight gain (130 lb in 2 years), facial rounding, and plethora. She had also experienced decrease in stamina, easy bruising, and emotional lability. Hydrochlorothiazide had been prescribed because of recently diagnosed hypertension. She had no history of major depression, anorexia, or alcohol abuse. On examination, her face appeared more round and plethoric when compared with photographs taken 2 years previously. Central obesity with supraclavicular fullness, violaceous striae (7-mm wide) and symmetric proximal muscle weakness were present.

Three late-night salivary cortisol tests, seven 24-h urine free cortisol tests, and two dexamethasone-suppressed corticotropin releasing hormone (CRH)-stimulation tests had all been normal, and her plasma adrenocorticotropin (ACTH) was not suppressed. Because of strong clinical suspicion for CS, she had been prescribed ketoconazole, which led to some improvement in her symptoms. However, the medication had to be discontinued because of an increase in liver enzymes.

She was referred to our institution for further evaluation, which included nightly (11 pm) saliva collections for cortisol assay over two 1-month periods. The results of these tests established the presence of intermittent (cyclic) hypercortisolism [Fig. 6.1a]. Magnetic resonance imaging (MRI) examination of her pituitary did not show a sellar mass. She subsequently underwent bilateral inferior petrosal sinus sampling (BIPSS) at a time when her disease was active, based on late-night salivary cortisol testing. During BIPSS, blood samples were obtained for ACTH assay before as well as after CRH administration, establishing the presence of a significant gradient between central and peripheral serum ACTH levels (peak left inferior petrosal ACTH level: 551 pg/ml, peak right inferior petrosal ACTH level: 19 pg/ml, and concurrent peripheral ACTH level: 17 pg/ml, yielding a maximal central to peripheral serum ACTH level ratio: 32:1, measured at 10 min after CRH administration).

On transsphenoidal exploration of her pituitary, a minute pituitary adenoma was resected, which demonstrated immunoreactivity for ACTH. Postoperatively, the patient's early morning serum cortisol levels as well as her 24 h urine free cortisol were repeatedly undetectable while she received low-dose dexamethasone (0.5 mg by mouth twice daily).

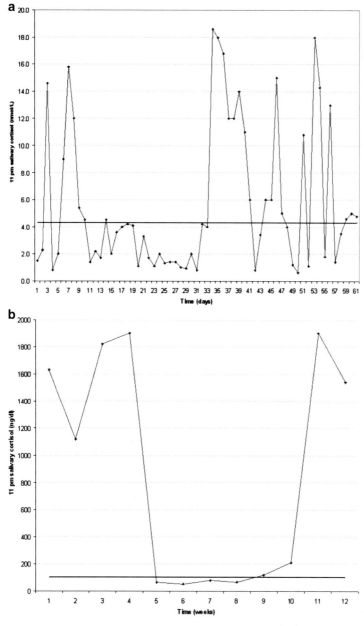

Fig. 6.1 Late-night (11 pm) salivary cortisol profile of two patients with Cushing's disease. The *horizontal black lines* depict the upper end of normal range. In (**a**), a 22-year woman presented with a history of recent-onset weight gain, facial rounding, plethora, easy bruising, muscle weakness, hypertension, and emotional lability (case presented in the text). Her symptoms did not show significant variation, despite the presence of substantial fluctuations in late-night salivary cortisol. In (**b**), an 81-year woman presented with recurrent episodes of profound fatigue and weakness, facial rounding, hypertension, edema, and hypokalemia lasting for approximately 5–6 weeks. Her symptoms correlated with episodes of hypercortisolism, demonstrated by late-night salivary cortisol testing

Clinical Features and Laboratory Findings

As exemplified by the case presentations, patients with cyclic CD do not have unique clinical features. A slightly older mean age at presentation as well as female gender predilection have been suggested [1]. However, the condition has been described across the lifespan in both genders (Table 6.1) [3].

Many patients with cyclic CD have significant variations in clinical activity of their disease, including periods of symptomatic exacerbation interspersed with relative remission of hypercortisolism [1, 3, 4]. Spontaneous periodic or irregularly occurring fluctuations in common manifestations of CD, including overweight and central adiposity, edema, hypertension, muscle weakness, leukocytosis, hypokalemia, or hyperglycemia, during the course of the illness have been noted. In addition, symptomatic hypercortisolism alternating with spontaneous hypoadrenalism has also been described [22].

A detailed discussion of the diagnostic performance of laboratory tests employed in the diagnosis and differential diagnosis of CD has been presented in a different chapter and will not be detailed herein. However, several points pertaining to cyclic CD should be made.

Patients with cyclic CD exhibit substantial fluctuations in cortisol levels over time, with or without concurrent variations in clinical symptoms. In earlier reports, disease activity was assessed using 24-h urine collections submitted for 17 hydroxysteroid or free cortisol assay measured by radioimmunoassay (RIA) [9, 10, 12, 16]. More recently, urine cortisol has been measured using more accurate methods, including liquid chromatography followed by tandem mass spectrometry (LC/MS/MS) or high pressure liquid chromatography (HPLC).

As 24-h urine collections are rather cumbersome to perform, it has been suggested that the urine cortisol to creatinine ratio, measured in early morning urine samples is a reliable index of disease activity, and is easier for the patient to collect on

Table 6.1 Clinical features among patients with cyclic Cushing's disease in published case series or reviews of five or more patients (duplicate reports were not included)

First author, year	Number of patients	Gender (F/M)	Approximate intercycle length (range)	Surgical management (%)	Prognosis
Atkinson et al. (1985) [21]	5	4/1	3–60 days	TSS (100%), bilateral adrenalectomy (40%)	NR
Atkinson et al. (2005) [14]	6	NR	NR	TSS (100%), bilateral adrenalectomy (65%)	NR
Meinardi et al. (2007) [3]	35	25/10	1–1,642 days	TSS (60%)	Recurrence in 11/21 (52%)
Alexandraki et al. (2009) [1]	30	26/4	0.2–26 years	TSS (63%), bilateral adrenalectomy (27%)	Cure in 6/19 (31.6%), recurrence in 4/19 (21%)

NR not reported, *TSS* transsphenoidal pituitary surgery

multiple days [23]. In addition, the mean of a five-point cortisol day curve established by measuring serum cortisol at specific time points through the day has been used to follow hypercortisolism over time [1]. The more recent introduction of sensitive and accurate salivary cortisol assays provides a reliable and convenient monitoring test of disease activity [11, 24]. In our department, measuring salivary cortisol between 11 pm and midnight in regular intervals has been used to establish and follow hypercortisolism in patients with suspected or established cyclic CD (Fig. 6.1).

Earlier case reports and case series suggested that hypercortisolism occurs with regular periodicity in each patient with cyclic CD [4]. Substantial variations in intercycle length between patients were noted, with a cycle length between 12 h and 85 days, or 12 h and 510 days indicated in different studies [3, 4]. More recent findings have indicated that many patients with cyclic CD exhibit irregular fluctuations in disease activity [1]. In addition, a mean period (intercycle length) of 3.8 years was recently reported in a group of cyclic CD patients [1]. However, as all these data have been collected retrospectively, the presence of ascertainment bias cannot be excluded.

There have been several reports of paradoxical responses of serum cortisol on dexamethasone suppression testing in patients with cyclic CD, with increases in serum cortisol noted after dexamethasone administration [25, 26]. Although the exact mechanisms underlying these observations have not been definitively established, it has been proposed that these findings may simply represent spontaneous fluctuations in cortisolemia.

As a corollary to these findings, the results of dexamethasone suppression testing should be viewed with extreme caution in patients with suspected cyclic CD. In addition, as with all dynamic tests used to investigate the presence or etiology of hypercortisolism, dexamethasone suppression testing should only be performed during periods of confirmed disease activity (based on the results of late-night salivary cortisol or urine free cortisol tests).

Similarly, BIPSS, used to establish the pituitary as the source of ACTH excess, should only be performed during a period of predicted hypercortisolism. Late-night salivary cortisol or 24-h urine free cortisol testing should be performed just before BIPSS to confirm the presence of disease activity. These steps are critical to the interpretation of BIPSS findings, since establishing a central source of ACTH excess rests upon the presence of adequate suppression of normal pituitary corticotrophs by hypercortisolemia during BIPSS. Data obtained through BIPSS performed in normal volunteers indicate that high central ACTH levels and high central to peripheral ACTH ratios may be present in this population, and may show considerable overlap with those of patients with Cushing's disease [27].

Pathophysiology

The mechanisms underlying the generation of rhythmic or irregular variations in disease activity in cyclic CD have not been established. In healthy individuals, cortisol secretion follows circadian, ultradian, and infradian rhythms [28]. Whether some patients with cyclic CD simply exhibit exaggerated variations of normal infradian or ultradian rhythms in cortisol secretion remains unclear.

Several pertinent hypotheses have been proposed to explain cyclic behavior in this condition, based on limited data from clinical case reports. Episodic growth or death of pituitary adenoma cells has been suggested by some investigators [29–31]. Others have proposed the presence of fluctuations in negative feedback control mechanisms of ACTH secretion by tumor cells as a potential explanation of cyclicity [32].

In addition, variations in hypothalamic control mechanisms of ACTH-producing pituitary adenomas have been postulated in other reports, including fluctuations in CRH secretion as a result of oscillations in central dopaminergic, serotoninergic, or γ-aminobutyric acid (GABA)-releasing pathways [33–35]. It is likely that diverse underlying mechanisms may be present in different patients. It is clear that more studies are needed to characterize the pathophysiology of cyclic CD.

Diagnostic Approach

The possibility of cyclic CD should be considered in patients with clinical findings suggestive of hypercortisolism, who appear to go through periods of spontaneous remission and recurrence. Consideration of cyclic CD is also important in patients with a clinical picture consistent with hypercortisolism, whose laboratory investigations, including late-night salivary cortisol or 24-h urine free cortisol, are normal on initial testing, such as in the case presented. In addition, patients with erratic or inconsistent results on these studies as well as patients with seemingly paradoxical responses on dexamethasone suppression testing should be suspected of having cyclic CD (Table 6.2).

A suggested approach to patients with possible cyclic hypercortisolism is shown in Fig. 6.2. In the presence of adequate clinical suspicion, it is important that serial laboratory testing be pursued even if initial investigations do not confirm hypercortisolism. Monitoring late-night (between 11 pm and midnight) salivary cortisol daily for several weeks, up to 1 month, is recommended as the initial approach in patients with suspected cyclic CD. In settings where salivary cortisol testing is not available, consecutive measurements of daily cortisol to creatinine ratios in early morning urine samples have been used to monitor cyclic cortisol excess.

If these results are unremarkable and clinical suspicion remains high, laboratory testing should be repeated every few months in an effort to detect the presence of hypercortisolism. Measurement of 24-h urine free cortisol is often used for confirmation once a temporal pattern of disease activity has been established, based on the results of multiple late-night salivary cortisol assays.

The possibility of a pseudo-Cushing's state should also be considered early during the course of investigation for suspected cyclic CD, and the presence of conditions known to be associated with hypercortisolemia, including major depression, anorexia, strenuous exercise, and alcohol excess among others, should be sought [36]. Use of the dexamethasone-suppressed CRH-stimulation test or the

Table 6.2 Clinical settings raising suspicion for cyclic hypercortisolism

Clinical findings suggestive of intermittent cortisol excess, with periods of spontaneous clinical remission and recurrence

Clinical picture consistent with hypercortisolism, with normal laboratory investigations

Suggestive clinical presentation and inconsistent or erratic results of tests aimed at demonstrating cortisol excess

Clinically suspected hypercortisolism and seemingly paradoxical responses on dexamethasone suppression testing

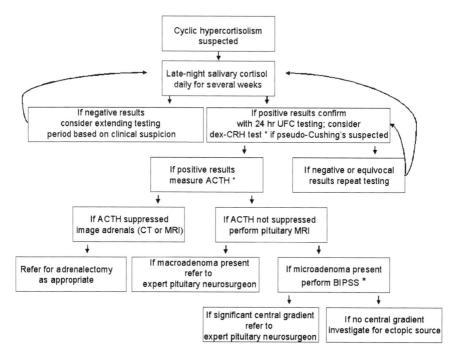

Fig. 6.2 A proposed algorithm for the approach to the patient with suspected cyclic hypercortisolism. Testing to be conducted during periods of biochemical hypercortisolism (*asterisks*). *ACTH* adrenocorticotropin, *CT* computed tomography, *Dex-CRH test* dexamethasone-suppressed corticotropin-releasing hormone stimulated test, *BIPSS* bilateral inferior petrosal sinus sampling, *MRI* magnetic resonance imaging, *UFC* urine free cortisol

measurement or midnight serum cortisol has been suggested to be accurate in distinguishing between endogenous hypercortisolism secondary to CS from that associated with pseudo-Cushing's states in several studies [37–39]. However, the diagnostic performance of these tests has not been unequivocally established and has not been specifically investigated in patients with known or suspected cyclic CD [40, 41]. Therefore, caution should be taken that a search for cortisol excess should not be abandoned in the face of negative results on either of these two tests, if clinical suspicion for cyclic CD remains high.

The possibility of exogenous glucocorticoid administration should be kept in mind during the evaluation of patients with suspected hypercortisolism. Intermittent use of prescription or over the counter medications containing glucocorticoids may mimic cyclic endogenous hypercortisolism. Therefore, obtaining a careful, thorough history on the use of all medications and supplements is very important.

Factitious hypercortisolism should also be considered in patients with suspected cyclic CD, particularly if cortisol has been measured by RIA [42, 43]. As urine or salivary cortisol tests are increasingly being performed by employing LC/MS/MS, which can distinguish between cortisol and synthetic glucocorticoids, this issue should cause less difficulty in the future, except for patients taking hydrocortisone surreptitiously or those who spike their collected specimens with hydrocortisone [3].

Once the presence of endogenous CS has been established, subsequent investigations should aim at establishing whether hypercortisolism is ACTH-dependent, and if so, whether it is of central (pituitary) origin (cyclic CD). Such a search is very relevant to the care of the patient with cyclic CS, as the presence of cyclicity has been found in patients with CS of diverse etiologies, including pituitary adenomas, the ectopic ACTH syndrome, as well as ACTH-independent adrenal adenoma or hyperplasia [3, 4].

As there are no specific imaging findings in patients with cyclic CD, appropriate imaging studies should be performed, as guided by the results of biochemical investigations, including MRI examination of the pituitary in patients with cyclic CS and nonsuppressed plasma ACTH levels.

While the general approach employed to establish the cause of hypercortisolism is not different from that used in all other patients with CS, it should again be emphasized that all such biochemical testing, including BIPSS, in patients with suspected cyclic CD should be conducted during a period of confirmed hypercortisolism.

Management

As with any patient who has CD, those with a confirmed cyclic pattern should be referred to a neurosurgeon with expertise in pituitary microsurgery [44, 45]. Retrospectively collected data have suggested that patients with cyclic CD may be less likely to experience a remission after selective pituitary adenomectomy and that an adenoma may be less likely to be found at surgery [1]. However, these findings have not been prospectively verified.

Postoperatively, our practice has been to place these patients on low-dose dexamethasone, while careful follow-up is maintained, including monitoring early morning serum cortisol, late-night salivary cortisol, and 24-h urine free cortisol at regular intervals, in order to establish whether remission has occurred. This can be difficult to ascertain in patients with cyclic CD because of the intrinsic fluctuations in hypercortisolism in this condition, which may falsely suggest that remission is present during a period of spontaneous quiescence.

Patients with active disease clearly persisting after transsphenoidal surgery are typically considered for a second surgical procedure by an experienced neurosurgeon [46]. Patients with persistent CD after second pituitary surgery are frequently considered for pituitary radiotherapy or, rarely, bilateral adrenalectomy [46]. The management of these patients parallels that of all other patients with CD, and the reader is referred to the pertinent chapters in this book for details.

The role of medical therapy in cyclic CD has not been examined in prospective studies. Earlier case reports have suggested a beneficial effect of bromocriptine, sodium valproate, or cyproheptadine on hypercortisolism in cyclic CD, by influencing dopaminergic, GABAergic, or serotoninergic pathways, respectively, which are thought to modulate ACTH secretion from tumorous corticotrophs [33–35]. These treatment options have not been confirmed to be effective in large groups of patients.

Recent preliminary studies have suggested a beneficial effect of two newer pituitary-directed therapies on hypercortisolism in CD, including the dopamine agonist cabergoline and the somatostatin receptor ligand pasireotide (SOM-230) [47, 48]. However, there are no published trials of these agents in cyclic CD patients. In addition, several agents inhibiting adrenal steroidogenesis, including ketoconazole, metyrapone, aminoglutethimide, or mitotane, have been shown to be of benefit in ameliorating hypercortisolism and have been used in CD patients failing pituitary surgery [46]. However, no case series of patients with cyclic CD treated with any of these agents have been published.

It should be noted that no medical therapy is currently FDA-approved specifically for use in patients with cyclic CD. However, based on available data in patients with CD in general, a trial of cabergoline or one of the adrenally acting agents (most commonly ketoconazole or metyrapone) is frequently considered in patients with cyclic CD failing pituitary surgery while awaiting the effects of radiotherapy, or occasionally as an alternative to radiotherapy. Patients with cyclic CD on medical therapy require close monitoring to detect the development of hypocortisolism, which might occur as a result of the additive effects of the agent used and spontaneous fluctuations in disease activity.

Summary and Future Directions

Several retrospective studies have suggested that cyclic CD, characterized by regular or irregular fluctuations in clinical or biochemical disease activity, may be more common than originally thought. The pathogenesis of this entity remains poorly understood.

Cyclic CD poses significant clinical challenges in diagnosis and management, requiring a systematic approach in order to optimize clinical outcomes. Prospective studies of patients with cyclic CD, using a uniform case definition and diagnostic approach, will likely be helpful in fully establishing the natural history of this condition and the effectiveness of currently available as well as novel therapies. In addition, molecular studies will likely be needed to elucidate the pathogenesis of this enigmatic condition.

References

1. Alexandraki KI, Kaltsas GA, Isidori AM, et al. The prevalence and characteristic features of cyclicity and variability in Cushing's disease. Eur J Endocrinol. 2009;160(6):1011–8.
2. Atkinson AB, McCance DR, Kennedy L, Sheridan B. Cyclical Cushing's syndrome first diagnosed after pituitary surgery: a trap for the unwary. Clin Endocrinol (Oxf). 1992;36(3):297–9.
3. Meinardi JR, Wolffenbuttel BH, Dullaart RP. Cyclic Cushing's syndrome: a clinical challenge. Eur J Endocrinol. 2007;157(3):245–54.
4. Shapiro MS, Shenkman L. Variable hormonogenesis in Cushing's syndrome. Q J Med. 1991;79(288):351–63.
5. Peri A, Bemporad D, Parenti G, Luciani P, Serio M, Mannelli M. Cushing's syndrome due to intermittent ectopic ACTH production showing a temporary remission during a pulmonary infection. Eur J Endocrinol. 2001;145(5):605–11.
6. Terzolo M, Ali A, Pia A, et al. Cyclic Cushing's syndrome due to ectopic ACTH secretion by an adrenal pheochromocytoma. J Endocrinol Invest. 1994;17(11):869–74.
7. Gunther DF, Bourdeau I, Matyakhina L, et al. Cyclical Cushing syndrome presenting in infancy: an early form of primary pigmented nodular adrenocortical disease, or a new entity? J Clin Endocrinol Metab. 2004;89(7):3173–82.
8. Green JR, van't Hoff W. Cushing's syndrome with fluctuation due to adrenal adenoma. J Clin Endocrinol Metab. 1975;41(2):235–40.
9. Bochner F, Burke CJ, Lloyd HM, Nurnberg BI. Intermittent Cushing's disease. Am J Med. 1979;67(3):507–10.
10. Bassoe HH, Emberland R, Stoa KF. Fluctuating steroid excretion in Cushing's syndrome. Acta Endocrinol (Copenh). 1958;28(2):163–8.
11. Hermus AR, Pieters GF, Borm GF, et al. Unpredictable hypersecretion of cortisol in Cushing's disease: detection by daily salivary cortisol measurements. Acta Endocrinol (Copenh). 1993;128(5):428–32.
12. Bailey RE. Periodic hormonogenesis – a new phenomenon. Periodicity in function of a hormone-producing tumor in man. J Clin Endocrinol Metab. 1971;32(3):317–27.
13. Oates TW, McCourt JP, Friedman WA, Agee OF, Rhoton AL, Thomas Jr WC. Cushing's disease with cyclic hormonogenesis and diabetes insipidus. Neurosurgery. 1979;5(5):598–603.
14. Atkinson AB, Kennedy A, Wiggam MI, McCance DR, Sheridan B. Long-term remission rates after pituitary surgery for Cushing's disease: the need for long-term surveillance. Clin Endocrinol (Oxf). 2005;63(5):549–59.
15. Sakiyama R, Ashcraft MW, Van Herle AJ. Cyclic Cushing's syndrome. Am J Med. 1984;77(5):944–6.
16. Birke G, Diczfalusy E. Fluctuation in the excretion of adrenocortical steroids in a case of Cushing's syndrome. J Clin Endocrinol Metab. 1956;16(2):286–90.
17. Lanzino G, Maartens NF, Laws Jr ER. Cushing's case XLV: Minnie G. J Neurosurg. 2002;97(1):231–4.
18. Cushing H. The basophil adenomas of the pituitary body. Ann R Coll Surg Engl. 1969;44(4):180–1.
19. Streeten DH, Anderson Jr GH, Dalakos T, Joachimpillai AD. Intermittent hypercortisolism: a disorder strikingly prevalent after hypophysial surgical procedures. Endocr Pract. 1997;3(3):123–9.
20. McCance DR, Gordon DS, Fannin TF, et al. Assessment of endocrine function after transsphenoidal surgery for Cushing's disease. Clin Endocrinol (Oxf). 1993;38(1):79–86.
21. Atkinson AB, Kennedy AL, Carson DJ, Hadden DR, Weaver JA, Sheridan B. Five cases of cyclical Cushing's syndrome. Br Med J (Clin Res Ed). 1985;291(6507):1453–7.
22. Liebowitz G, White A, Hadani M, Gross DJ. Fluctuating hyper-hypocortisolaemia: a variant of Cushing's syndrome. Clin Endocrinol (Oxf). 1997;46(6):759–63.
23. Mullan KR, Atkinson AB, Sheridan B. Cyclical Cushing's syndrome: an update. Curr Opin Endocrinol Diabetes Obes. 2007;14(4):317–22.

24. Mosnier-Pudar H, Thomopoulos P, Bertagna X, Fournier C, Guiban D, Luton JP. Long-distance and long-term follow-up of a patient with intermittent Cushing's disease by salivary cortisol measurements. Eur J Endocrinol. 1995;133(3):313–6.
25. Brown RD, Van Loon GR, Orth DN, Liddle GW. Cushing's disease with periodic hormonogenesis: one explanation for paradoxical response to dexamethasone. J Clin Endocrinol Metab. 1973;36(3):445–51.
26. Liberman B, Wajchenberg BL, Tambascia MA, Mesquita CH. Periodic remission in Cushing's disease with paradoxical dexamethasone response: an expression of periodic hormonogenesis. J Clin Endocrinol Metab. 1976;43(4):913–8.
27. Yanovski JA, Cutler Jr GB, Doppman JL, et al. The limited ability of inferior petrosal sinus sampling with corticotropin-releasing hormone to distinguish Cushing's disease from pseudo-Cushing states or normal physiology. J Clin Endocrinol Metab. 1993;77(2):503–9.
28. Curtis GC. Psychosomatics and chronobiology: possible implications of neuroendocrine rhythms. A review. Psychosom Med. 1972;34(3):235–56.
29. Alarifi A, Alzahrani AS, Salam SA, Ahmed M, Kanaan I. Repeated remissions of Cushing's disease due to recurrent infarctions of an ACTH-producing pituitary macroadenoma. Pituitary. 2005;8(2):81–7.
30. Mantero F, Scaroni CM, Albiger NM. Cyclic Cushing's syndrome: an overview. Pituitary. 2004;7(4):203–7.
31. Schweikert HU, Fehm HL, Fahlbusch R, et al. Cyclic Cushing's syndrome combined with cortisol suppressible, dexamethasone non-suppressible ACTH secretion: a new variant of Cushing's syndrome. Acta Endocrinol (Copenh). 1985;110(3):289–95.
32. Estopinan V, Varela C, Riobo P, Dominguez JR, Sancho J. Ectopic Cushing's syndrome with periodic hormonogenesis – a case suggesting a pathogenetic mechanism. Postgrad Med J. 1987;63(744):887–9.
33. Watanobe H, Aoki R, Takebe K, Nakazono M, Kudo M. In vivo and in vitro studies in a patient with cyclical Cushing's disease showing some responsiveness to bromocriptine. Horm Res. 1991;36(5–6):227–34.
34. Beckers A, Stevenaert A, Pirens G, Flandroy P, Sulon J, Hennen G. Cyclical Cushing's disease and its successful control under sodium valproate. J Endocrinol Invest. 1990;13(11):923–9.
35. Hsu TH, Gann DS, Tsan KW, Russell RP. Cyproheptadine in the control of Cushing's disease. Johns Hopkins Med J. 1981;149(2):77–83.
36. Nieman LK, Biller BM, Findling JW, et al. The diagnosis of Cushing's syndrome: an Endocrine Society Clinical Practice Guideline. J Clin Endocrinol Metab. 2008;93(5):1526–40.
37. Valassi E, Swearingen B, Lee H, et al. Concomitant medication use can confound interpretation of the combined dexamethasone-corticotropin releasing hormone test in Cushing's syndrome. J Clin Endocrinol Metab. 2009;94(12):4851–9.
38. Yanovski JA, Cutler Jr GB, Chrousos GP, Nieman LK. The dexamethasone-suppressed corticotropin-releasing hormone stimulation test differentiates mild Cushing's disease from normal physiology. J Clin Endocrinol Metab. 1998;83(2):348–52.
39. Yanovski JA, Cutler Jr GB, Chrousos GP, Nieman LK. Corticotropin-releasing hormone stimulation following low-dose dexamethasone administration. A new test to distinguish Cushing's syndrome from pseudo-Cushing's states. JAMA. 1993;269(17):2232–8.
40. Erickson D, Natt N, Nippoldt T, et al. Dexamethasone-suppressed corticotropin-releasing hormone stimulation test for diagnosis of mild hypercortisolism. J Clin Endocrinol Metab. 2007;92(8):2972–6.
41. Reimondo G, Bovio S, Allasino B, et al. The combined low-dose dexamethasone suppression corticotropin-releasing hormone test as a tool to rule out Cushing's syndrome. Eur J Endocrinol. 2008;159(5):569–76.
42. Cizza G, Nieman LK, Doppman JL, et al. Factitious Cushing syndrome. J Clin Endocrinol Metab. 1996;81(10):3573–7.
43. Cook DM, Meikle AW. Factitious Cushing's syndrome. J Clin Endocrinol Metab. 1985;61(2):385–7.

44. Barker 2nd FG, Klibanski A, Swearingen B. Transsphenoidal surgery for pituitary tumors in the United States, 1996–2000: mortality, morbidity, and the effects of hospital and surgeon volume. J Clin Endocrinol Metab. 2003;88(10):4709–19.
45. Gittoes NJ, Sheppard MC, Johnson AP, Stewart PM. Outcome of surgery for acromegaly – the experience of a dedicated pituitary surgeon. QJM. 1999;92(12):741–5.
46. Biller BM, Grossman AB, Stewart PM, et al. Treatment of adrenocorticotropin-dependent Cushing's syndrome: a consensus statement. J Clin Endocrinol Metab. 2008;93(7):2454–62.
47. Pivonello R, De Martino MC, Cappabianca P, et al. The medical treatment of Cushing's disease: effectiveness of chronic treatment with the dopamine agonist cabergoline in patients unsuccessfully treated by surgery. J Clin Endocrinol Metab. 2009;94(1):223–30.
48. Boscaro M, Ludlam WH, Atkinson B, et al. Treatment of pituitary-dependent Cushing's disease with the multireceptor ligand somatostatin analog pasireotide (SOM230): a multicenter, phase II trial. J Clin Endocrinol Metab. 2009;94(1):115–22.

Chapter 7
Differential Diagnosis of Cushing's Syndrome

Bradley R. Javorsky, Ty B. Carroll, and James W. Findling

Abstract Determining the cause of spontaneous Cushing's syndrome is essential so that appropriate therapy can be recommended. Most patients (80%) have an ACTH-secreting neoplasm (pituitary or ectopic), while the rest have an adrenal-dependent (ACTH-independent) etiology. After hypercortisolism has been convincingly established, plasma adrenocorticotropic hormone (ACTH) levels are obtained to subdivide Cushing's syndrome into ACTH-dependent (>20 pg/ml) or ACTH-independent (<5 pg/ml) categories. Corticotropin-releasing hormone (CRH) stimulation testing can help to define these categories when ACTH levels are equivocal (5–20 pg/ml). Since clinical features are unreliable in distinguishing between subtypes of ACTH-dependent and ACTH-independent Cushing's syndrome, additional biochemical, radiologic, and angiographic tests are needed. Diagnostic accuracy of high-dose dexamethasone suppression testing and CRH stimulation testing are poor when trying to refine the diagnosis of ACTH-dependent Cushing's syndrome. Bilateral inferior petrosal sinus ACTH sampling with CRH stimulation has become the gold standard in this setting and should be used when magnetic resonance images of the pituitary do not reveal an unequivocal pituitary abnormality in a patient with clinical and biochemical findings consistent with ACTH-dependent Cushing's syndrome. In patients with ACTH-independent Cushing's syndrome, computed tomography of the adrenal glands is performed and will demonstrate either a single nodule (benign or malignant) or bilateral nodular hyperplasia caused by several unique pathophysiological mechanisms.

Keywords Adrenocorticotropic hormone • Hypercortisolism • Dexamethasone suppression testing • Corticotrophin-releasing hormone • Adrenal glands

J.W. Findling (✉)
Department of Medicine, Endocrinology Center and Clinics,
Medical College of Wisconsin, Milwaukee, WI 53051, USA
e-mail: jfindling@mcw.edu

Introduction

During the past 30 years, the introduction of reliable plasma adrenocorticotropic hormone (ACTH) measurements, sensitive pituitary and adrenal imaging studies, and bilateral inferior petrosal sinus ACTH sampling with corticotropin-releasing hormone (CRH) stimulation (IPSS) have provided the diagnostic tools necessary to differentiate between the many causes of Cushing's syndrome [1]. The differential diagnostic testing for Cushing's syndrome should only be considered after the diagnosis of pathologic endogenous hypercortisolism has been well established. None of the differential diagnostic tests have any reasonable level of sensitivity or specificity for establishing the actual diagnosis of Cushing's syndrome [2]. For example, pituitary and adrenal imaging abnormalities are quite common in patients with no evidence of an endocrine disorder and plasma ACTH levels may even be elevated in some normal subjects due to the stress of venipuncture [3, 4]. Moreover, IPSS results in patients with Cushing's disease may overlap with those in normal subjects [5].

Etiologic Considerations (Table 7.1)

The majority (80%) of patients with spontaneous Cushing's syndrome have an ACTH-secreting neoplasm (ACTH-dependent Cushing's syndrome) either from a pituitary tumor (Cushing's disease) or a nonpituitary neoplasm (ectopic ACTH syndrome). Some patients with ectopic ACTH syndrome (e.g., bronchial carcinoids) may present with hypercortisolism several years before there is radiographic evidence of neoplasm (occult ectopic ACTH syndrome). These subtypes of ACTH-dependent Cushing's syndrome may be clinically and biochemically indistinguishable, and careful assessment of diagnostic studies and clinical expertise are required to differentiate them [6].

The most common cause of ACTH-independent Cushing's syndrome is prolonged exogenous glucocorticoid therapy. A very careful history is needed to be certain that patients with ACTH-independent Cushing's syndrome are not receiving

Table 7.1 Causes of Cushing's syndrome

ACTH-Dependent
ACTH-secreting pituitary tumor (Cushing's disease)
Ectopic ACTH secreting neoplasm
Ectopic CRH-secreting neoplasm (rare)
ACTH-Independent
Exogenous glucocorticoid therapy
Adrenal neoplasm (adenoma or carcinoma)
Bilateral nodular adrenal hyperplasia
Carney complex (protein kinase A mutation)
Aberrant adrenal receptors (e.g., GIP, vasopressin)
McCune–Albright syndrome (mutations of Gsα)

any type of exogenous corticosteroid treatment [7]. The majority of patients with adrenal-dependent (ACTH-independent) endogenous Cushing's syndrome have a solitary benign adrenocortical neoplasm, while a minority has adrenocortical carcinoma. In addition, there are many diverse causes of bilateral nodular hyperplasia associated with endogenous ACTH-independent hypercortisolism.

Differentiating ACTH-Dependent from ACTH-Independent Cushing's Syndrome

Plasma ACTH

The initial step in the differential diagnosis of spontaneous Cushing's syndrome is the measurement of plasma ACTH. The introduction of a sensitive and specific two-site immunometric assay for plasma ACTH has now provided clinicians with a reliable initial step in distinguishing patients with ACTH-independent Cushing's syndrome (subnormal ACTH) from those with ACTH-dependent Cushing's (normal or elevated plasma ACTH) [8]. If the morning plasma ACTH level is suppressed below the reference range (<5 pg/ml), patients should then undergo adrenal imaging by computed tomography (CT) scanning. By contrast, patients with plasma ACTH >20 pg/ml have an ACTH-secreting neoplasm. However, the recognition of mild (and often subclinical) Cushing's syndrome associated with incidentally discovered adrenal adenomas has complicated the differentiation between ACTH-dependent and ACTH-independent endogenous hypercortisolism. Many of these patients have intermittent and only modest increases in cortisol secretion and may not have full suppression of plasma ACTH. Some of these patients may have basal plasma ACTH levels between 5 and 20 pg/ml [9]. In these patients, a CRH stimulation test may be required for an accurate differential diagnosis.

CRH Stimulation Test

Reincke has reported the plasma ACTH response to human CRH (hCRH) in normal subjects compared to patients with subclinical Cushing's and those with overt adrenal Cushing's syndrome (Fig. 7.1). Patients with unequivocal ACTH-independent Cushing's syndrome will have basal plasma ACTH <5 pg/ml with minimal increase in plasma ACTH or cortisol after hCRH administration; however, subjects with subclinical Cushing's syndrome may have basal ACTH levels between 5 and 20 pg/ml and have a modest – albeit attenuated – plasma ACTH and cortisol increase following hCRH infusion. Unfortunately, there is limited data available on the normative ACTH response to CRH. Values will depend on the type of ACTH assay employed and the type of CRH (ovine or human) administered. In general,

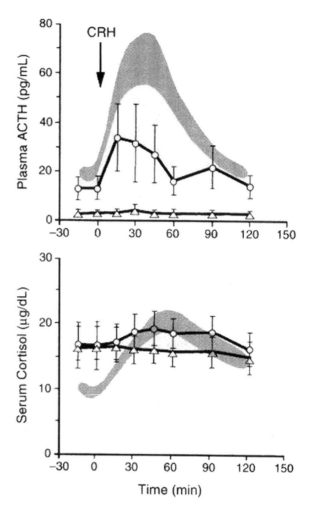

Fig. 7.1 Plasma ACTH and serum cortisol response to stimulation with human CRH (100 μg IV) in normal control subjects (mean ± SEM; shaded area), in six patients with subclinical Cushing's syndrome and in six patients with overt adrenal Cushing's syndrome. *Circles* preclinical Cushing's syndrome; *diamonds* adrenal Cushing's syndrome; *shaded areas* normal subjects (reprinted from Endocrinol Metab Clin North Am. Reincke, M, 2000:29:43–56 with permission from Elsevier)

patients with ACTH-independent Cushing's syndrome from mild hypercortisolism associated with nodular adrenal disease have peak plasma ACTH responses that are <30–40 pg/ml. By contrast, patients with ACTH-dependent Cushing's syndrome (usually due to Cushing's disease) have an exaggerated peripheral ACTH response to CRH as well as a significant increase in cortisol secretion.

It is not surprising that dexamethasone suppression testing (even high dose) does not reliably distinguish ACTH-dependent from ACTH-independent Cushing's syndrome [10]. This can be attributed to the fact that patients with predominantly adrenal-dependent Cushing's syndrome may have some degree of ACTH-dependency and suppression with high doses of dexamethasone may result in decreases but not complete suppression of cortisol secretion. However, as a rule, after either low-dose or high-dose dexamethasone suppression testing, plasma ACTH levels are usually undetectable in patients with adrenal-dependent Cushing's syndrome. And, as would be expected, the serum cortisol levels are not fully suppressed.

Imaging Studies

Imaging findings should not be used to distinguish ACTH-independent from ACTH-dependent Cushing's syndrome. Many patients with Cushing's disease will have CT evidence of nodular adrenal disease, presumably related to longstanding ACTH hypersecretion [11]. This nodular adrenal disease may be bilateral, but it is often unilateral. Patients with clinically significant Cushing's syndrome due to a cortisol-secreting adenoma (plasma ACTH <5 pg/ml) will usually have a small contralateral adrenal gland. However, the contralateral adrenal gland is usually normal in those subjects with subclinical adrenal-dependent Cushing's syndrome. Since small pituitary lesions are seen in as many as 10% of normal subjects, pituitary magnetic resonance imaging (MRI) alone should not be used to distinguish ACTH-dependent from ACTH-independent hypercortisolism. The differentiation of the subtype of Cushing's syndrome must be established biochemically.

ACTH-Dependent Cushing's Syndrome

Pituitary adenomas secreting ACTH (Cushing's disease) are responsible for at least 90% of cases of ACTH-dependent Cushing's syndrome. With the introduction of pituitary microsurgery in the 1970s as the treatment of choice for patients with Cushing's disease, it has become crucial to establish an accurate differential diagnosis in patients with ACTH-dependent Cushing's syndrome.

Cushing's disease and ectopic ACTH syndrome may be clinically indistinguishable. Since the pretest probability of Cushing's disease is so high, any diagnostic test must have very good accuracy. Radiological studies and dynamic tests of steroid secretion are also often inconclusive or misleading in separating these disease entities [1–5]. Because of its high sensitivity and specificity, IPSS has become the test of choice in the differential evaluation of ACTH-dependent Cushing's syndrome.

Clinical Features

The clinical signs and symptoms of hypercortisolism may be similar in patients with Cushing's disease or ectopic ACTH syndrome. Early reports describing patients with the ectopic ACTH syndrome made note of features not typically seen in patients with Cushing's disease such as the absence of classic physical signs of Cushing's syndrome, weight loss, and hyperpigmentation [12, 13]. A more recent analysis of clinical features notes patients with ectopic ACTH syndrome as being significantly older, more likely to be male, having a shorter duration of clinical findings, more likely to have hypokalemia, and having higher 24-h urinary free cortisol and plasma ACTH levels [1, 14]. A logistic regression model using only these clinical and simple biochemical variables has an overall

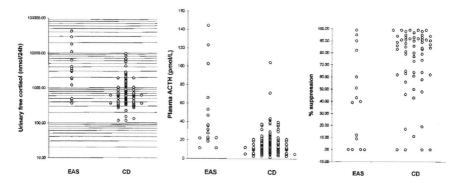

Fig. 7.2 Biochemical characteristics of patients with CD and EAS. *Left panel*, 24-h urinary free cortisol ($n=99$ CD; $n=15$ EAS); *middle panel*, plasma ACTH ($n=102$ CD; $n=17$ EAS); *right panel*, percent suppression with high-dose dexamethasone ($n=61$ CD; $n=15$ EAS). Used with permission from J Clin Endocrinol Metab. Aron et al. 1997:82:1780–5, Copyright 1997, The Endocrine Society

diagnostic accuracy of 91.2%; however, 26.7% of ectopic ACTH syndrome cases would be misdiagnosed using this model and a considerable amount of overlap is observed for cortisol and ACTH levels (Fig. 7.2) [15]. These findings underscore the need for additional diagnostic testing.

Biochemical Testing

Historically, clinicians have relied on provocative biochemical testing, in particular the high-dose dexamethasone suppression test (HDD) and CRH stimulation test, to distinguish Cushing's disease from ectopic ACTH production. These tests, however, have been associated with limited diagnostic accuracy [15–19].

Several variations of HDD have been developed in an attempt to differentiate Cushing's disease from ectopic ACTH syndrome. The idea behind the HDD is the concept that corticotroph cells, in contrast to ectopic ACTH-secreting tumors, retain a degree of sensitivity to glucocorticoid feedback. The original test designed by Liddle over 50 years ago, even before the ectopic ACTH syndrome had been described, used a protocol of 2 mg dexamethasone every 6 h for 48 h [20]. Urinary 17-hydroxysteroid was collected before and after dexamethasone administration. Suppression by 50% was felt to be consistent with Cushing's disease. This test has been modified in many ways since its introduction to improve accuracy and convenience. Urinary free cortisol levels have replaced measurement of 17-hydroxysteroid levels by most laboratories. Many investigators now use plasma cortisol levels (after 48 h of dexamethasone 2 mg every 6 h or after a single 8 mg evening dose of dexamethasone) rather than urinary measurements. Finally, protocols using 5–7 h continuous infusions of dexamethasone have been described [21, 22].

HDD test performance is suboptimal with a sensitivity of 79–85% and a specificity of 67–100% depending on the percent suppression of urinary or plasma cortisol levels used [23, 24] (Fig. 7.2). Variables that may account for low test performance include the importance of sample timing, incomplete urine collections, poor test adherence, and variable dexamethasone metabolism and absorption. Since the diagnostic accuracy of HDD is less than the pretest probability of Cushing's disease, HDD is no longer recommended for the differential diagnosis of ACTH-dependent Cushing's syndrome.

Almost since the isolation of CRH by Vale and colleagues in 1981, stimulation testing with this neuropeptide has been used in the differential diagnosis of ACTH-dependent Cushing's syndrome [22]. Orth et al. demonstrated that administration of CRH potently stimulates release of ACTH in normal subjects and patients with Cushing's disease [25]. In contrast to pituitary adenomas, nonpituitary ACTH-producing tumors respond poorly to CRH administration, presumably because of lower CRH receptor expression.

To distinguish between causes of ACTH-dependent Cushing syndrome, percent change between basal and peak ACTH or cortisol values are used after intravenous injection of CRH (1 µg/kg or 100 µg). Sensitivity and specificity of the CRH test depends on which criteria are chosen; ranges of 35–105% for the rise of ACTH above basal levels have been used resulting in sensitivities of 70–93% at high specificity. For cortisol, ranges of 14–50% have been used resulting in a sensitivity of only 50–91% [16, 26–28]. Furthermore, a combined analysis of all published series in a 1998 review by Newell-Price et al. indicated that 7–14% of all patients with Cushing's disease fail to respond to CRH if the best discriminating criteria are applied [28].

Imaging Studies

Imaging of the pituitary to identify patients with corticotroph adenomas is limited by the frequency of incidental pituitary lesions in the normal population. Depending on the series, anywhere from 1.5% to 26.7% (the majority falling between 8% and 14%) of subjects at autopsy are found to have incidental pituitary adenomas [29]. Similarly, MRI detects focal areas of decreased signal intensity in the pituitary in 10–38% of normal volunteers [4, 30]. Conversely, despite dramatic improvements in the quality of pituitary imaging, from sellar polytomography to CT to MRI, approximately 20–50% of patients with pathologically confirmed Cushing's disease do not have tumors seen on even the most sensitive studies [31].

ACTH-secreting pituitary adenomas are typically hypodense on noncontrasted MRI. The administration of contrast (gadolinium-diethylenetriaminepentaacetic acid) may identify an additional population of tumors [32]. Other techniques have been introduced to improve the sensitivity of MRI such as dynamic contrast enhancement (where images are obtained within seconds of contrast injection to take advantage of different dynamics of contrast enhancement between normal pituitary tissue and pituitary adenomas) and utilization of 1 mm spoiled gradient recalled acquisition in the steady-state sequences [31, 33]. These approaches have improved the sensitivity of detecting corticotroph adenomas, but at the expense of lower specificity.

In a study comparing MRI and IPSS, Kaskarelis et al. showed that the accuracy for detecting a pituitary source of ACTH was 50% for MRI and 88% for successful IPSS [34]. Of the 54 patients with confirmed final diagnoses, MRI resulted in 25 false negatives and 2 false positives, while IPSS had 2 false negatives and 3 false positives.

Inferior Petrosal Sinus ACTH Sampling

In light of the high pretest probability of Cushing's disease in patients with ACTH-dependent Cushing's syndrome, and the poor performance of biochemical testing and radiologic imaging, IPSS has emerged as the differential diagnostic test of choice. As previously noted, ACTH-dependent pathologic hypercortisolism must first be established before performing IPSS, as considerable overlap exists between patients with confirmed Cushing's disease and normal individuals or patients with "pseudo-Cushing" states [5].

Anterior pituitary hormones such as ACTH reach the systemic circulation via small hypophyseal and lateral adenohypophyseal veins that converge into the confluent pituitary veins, join the cavernous sinus on the same side, and empty into the inferior petrosal sinus. IPSS takes advantage of this anatomy to determine if there is a central to peripheral ACTH gradient. During the procedure, a skilled invasive radiologist catheterizes each inferior petrosal sinus and blood samples for ACTH are withdrawn in the basal state and then at 3, 5, and 10 min after intravenous administration of 1 μg/kg (or 100 μg) CRH from each inferior petrosal sinus and a peripheral vein (Fig. 7.3). Petrosal sinus to peripheral (IPS:P) ACTH ratios ≥2.0 at baseline or a peak ≥3.0 after CRH administration (at any of the time points) are diagnostic of Cushing's disease. Technical success rates are high (85–99%), and complications are uncommon, in institutions that perform IPSS regularly [35–38]. Minor groin hematomas occur 3–4% of the time, while more serious complications such as thromboembolism, venous subarachnoid hemorrhage, or brainstem injury have been rarely reported [35, 37, 39–41].

Anomalous venous drainage is well documented and may be responsible for false-negative IPSS results [42, 43]. In situations where the IPSS results suggest ectopic ACTH syndrome, measurement of prolactin in the inferior petrosal sinuses will help to validate the integrity of pituitary venous effluent. Normalization of the IPS:P ACTH ratio to the IPS:P prolactin ratio can increase the diagnostic accuracy of this test [44]. Normalized ratios greater than 0.8 are indicative of Cushing's disease, while ratios less than 0.6 are seen in patients with ectopic ACTH syndrome (Fig. 7.4). Therefore, we routinely store plasma samples during IPSS for possible measurement of prolactin in patients without a

7 Differential Diagnosis of Cushing's Syndrome

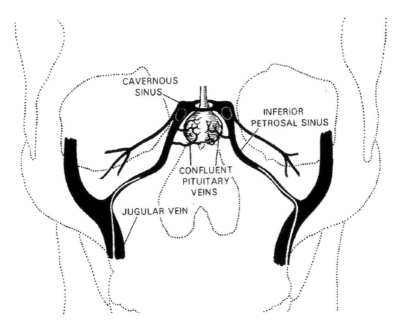

Fig. 7.3 Catheter placement for bilateral simultaneous blood sampling of the inferior petrosal sinuses. Confluent pituitary veins empty laterally into the cavernous sinuses, which drain into the inferior petrosal sinuses. Used with permission from N Engl J Med. Oldfield, et al. 1985;312:100–3. Copyright 1985, Massachusetts Medical Society, all rights reserved

pituitary ACTH gradient. False positive tests may be due to rare cases of CRH-secreting tumors or testing during a period of normocortisolemia in patients with intermittent ACTH secretion. To rule out the latter situation when interpreting IPSS results, we measure late night salivary cortisol levels prior to the procedure to confirm hypercortisolism.

Early series reported sensitivities and specificities of 100% [17, 36]. Subsequent studies have largely replicated these findings, reporting sensitivities ranging from 85% to 100% with specificities of 90–100% [17, 18, 23, 26, 42, 45–50]. A review of 21 studies found an overall sensitivity and specificity of 96 and 100%, respectively [51]. Lindsay and Nieman combined reports of 726 patients who had Cushing's disease and 112 who had ectopic ACTH syndrome, finding a diagnostic sensitivity and specificity for IPSS of 94% [2].

Use of desmopressin (a synthetic analog of vasopressin) during IPSS has also been investigated. Vasopressin receptors are present on corticotroph adenoma cells and only rarely on ectopic tumors producing ACTH. Furthermore, CRH is not available in all centers. In several studies using desmopressin, sensitivities were 92–95% with specificities of 100% [52]. When CRH and desmopressin were combined, sensitivity was 97–100% compared to 87% for CRH alone [53, 54]. Larger studies are needed to confirm these results.

When compared to other tests, IPSS is consistently found to be more accurate for separating pituitary-dependent ACTH excess from the ectopic ACTH syndrome.

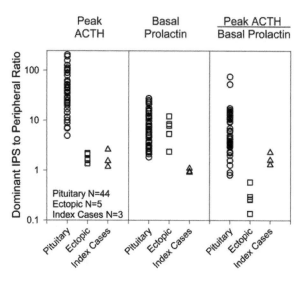

Fig. 7.4 IPS:P ratios for patients with proven Cushing's disease (pituitary; *circles*), ectopic ACTH syndrome (ectopic; *squares*), and the three index cases (*triangles*). The *left panel* is the post-CRH IPS to peripheral ACTH ratio. The *middle panel* is the basal (pre-CRH) IPS to peripheral prolactin ratio from the same sites as the ACTH ratios. The *right panel* is the *left panel* divided by the *middle panel* giving IPS:P ratios normalized to the ipsilateral prolactin ratio. Notice the overlap of the IPS-peripheral ACTH ratio for the ectopic ACTH and index cases, and also notice that the index cases had IPS-peripheral prolactin ratios that were lower than in pituitary and ectopic ACTH, and that normalizing the peak ACTH IPS:P ratio to the ipsilateral prolactin ratio led to results in index cases (with subsequently proven Cushing's disease) similar to prospectively proven pituitary Cushing's disease. Used with permission from J Clin Endocrinol Metab., Findling, et al. 2004;89:6005–9, Copyright 2004, The Endocrine Society

In a NIH series of patients with ectopic ACTH syndrome, 98% were found to have the expected findings with IPSS, while biochemical testing (2 day and overnight high-dose dexamethasone tests, and peripheral CRH administration) was at best 92% accurate [18]. Even more impressive differences between IPSS and high-dose dexamethasone or peripheral CRH testing were observed in a study by Wiggam et al. which compared IPSS (without CRH administration) to CRH testing and HDD in 44 patients with confirmed Cushing's disease and 1 patient with confirmed ectopic ACTH syndrome [19]. They showed that in patients with proven pituitary disease, only 48% met the criteria for HDD and 70% met the criteria for CRH testing (only 35% had a correct response to both tests). By contrast, IPSS successfully indicated Cushing's disease in 82% of cases. Presumably, if CRH had been administered during IPSS, the sensitivity would have been even higher.

Sampling at sites other than the inferior petrosal sinuses has been investigated in an effort to further improve diagnostic accuracy, increase availability, or further reduce the risk of complications. Compared to IPSS, jugular vein sampling has demonstrated a lower diagnostic sensitivity, suggesting the risks and costs of this procedure are not justified [17, 42, 55, 56]. Cavernous sinus sampling after CRH stimulation has sensitivities and specificities similar to IPSS; however, it is technically more challenging and transient cranial nerve palsies have been reported with this procedure [37, 57].

In addition to distinguishing between Cushing's disease and ectopic ACTH-secreting neoplasms, IPSS has been examined for its utility in lateralizing corticotroph adenomas within the pituitary. This would provide neurosurgeons with additional information when attempting to localize tumors too small to be seen on even the most sensitive imaging studies. Although theoretically possible in most individuals, lateralization data is confounded in persons with centrally located tumors, anomalous venous drainage patterns, or multifocal lesions [58]. Studies have reported variable rates of success, ranging from 50% to 100% [36, 59–61]. Lateralization data should, therefore, not replace a thorough surgical exploration of the entire pituitary gland.

Ectopic ACTH Syndrome

Approximately 10% of cases of endogenous ACTH-dependent Cushing's syndrome are secondary to the ectopic ACTH syndrome [13, 18, 62]. A wide variety of tumors have been reported to cause ectopic ACTH secretion. The most common of these tumors are neuroendocrine tumors of the lung; bronchial carcinoid tumors represent 25% of cases while small cell and adenocarcinomas of the lung together account for 20% [62]. The remaining half of ectopic ACTH syndrome is caused by tumors of the thymus, gastrointestinal tract, islet cell, pheochromocytoma, and medullary thyroid carcinomas (Fig. 7.5).

Localization of Ectopic ACTH-Secreting Neoplasms

As described above, only after a biochemical evaluation has confirmed ACTH-dependent hypercortisolism, and further differential diagnostic testing (i.e., IPSS) has suggested an ectopic source, should localization studies be undertaken. In 33–44% of cases, efforts to localize the source of ectopic ACTH-secretion are unsuccessful [63–65]. Initial imaging should begin with CT scan of the abdomen and chest. Additional imaging with MRI of the chest may provide localizing information in those patients without lesions seen on CT [66]. If no causative lesion is found using CT or MRI, somatostatin receptor scintigraphy may be useful; however, the relatively small size of the tumors is often at the limit of resolution for somatostatin receptor scintigraphy [51, 67]. Standard 18-fluorodeoxyglucose positron emission tomography scanning has not been found to be of additional benefit [65, 68]. Tumor markers including calcitonin, gastrin, glucagon, or somatostatin may be elevated in patients with ectopic ACTH syndrome but are rarely helpful in localization [67].

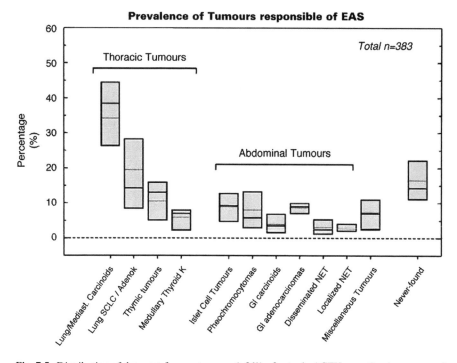

Fig. 7.5 Distribution of the most frequent source (>2%) of ectopic ACTH secretion in a group of 383 patients with EAS (used with permission from Isidori, AM and Lenzi, A. Arq Bras Endocrinol Metab 2007;51:1217–25)

ACTH-Independent Cushing's Syndrome

ACTH-independent hypercortisolism is caused by either exogenous steroid use or by autonomous adrenal production of cortisol. Distinguishing between these two etiologies is essential.

Exogenous Cushing's Syndrome

The exact prevalence of exogenous Cushing's syndrome is unknown. This is largely due to the lack of a uniformly accepted definition making estimates of prevalence difficult. Regardless, exogenous Cushing's syndrome is clearly much more common than all forms of endogenous hypercortisolism.

Exclusion of exogenous Cushing's syndrome should be the initial step in the investigation of all patients with suspected hypercortisolism [7]. Excluding exogenous glucocorticoid use is often straightforward; however, determining a source of exogenous steroid use can be challenging as even the use of nonoral glucocorticoids can lead to Cushing's syndrome. Intra-articular, inhaled, nasal, topical, and even topical ocular preparations have all been reported to cause exogenous Cushing's syndrome [69–71]. Another group of patients in whom the diagnosis of exogenous Cushing's syndrome is more difficult to secure are those unknowingly exposed to glucocorticoids through drugs of abuse or herbal remedies [72, 73]. As such, a thorough review of any and all over-the-counter, herbal, and traditional medicines, as well as drugs of abuse, should be obtained.

Biochemical evaluation of these patients will show variable cortisol levels depending on the cross reactivity of the cortisol assay with the glucocorticoid to which the patient is exposed. Patients exposed to hydrocortisone will have high plasma cortisol levels, but other synthetic steroids (i.e., prednisone and dexamethasone) have much lower cross reactivity and can lead to low plasma cortisol levels. As a result, traditional testing for cortisol excess is not helpful in patients with exogenous Cushing's syndrome. The diagnosis is secured in a patient with clinical features of steroid excess and a history of exposure to supraphysiological doses of glucocorticoids. Complementary biochemical testing can reveal suppressed ACTH levels and often low dehydroepiandrosterone sulfate (DHEA-S) levels.

Adrenal-Dependent Cushing's Syndrome

Adrenal-dependent (ACTH-independent) Cushing's syndrome accounts for 20% of endogenous hypercortisolism. Solitary cortisol-secreting adrenal adenomas account for 90% of these cases [51]. Adrenal carcinoma, ACTH-independent macronodular adrenal hyperplasia (AIMAH), primary pigmented nodular adrenal disease, and McCune–Albright syndrome constitute the remaining 10% of cases [74–77] (Table 7.1).

Differentiating between the causes of adrenal-dependent Cushing's syndrome is based mainly on clinical grounds and imaging characteristics as very few biochemical differences exist between these etiologies.

Solitary Adrenal Adenoma

Incidental adrenal adenomas occur in 4% of patients undergoing abdominal imaging and 5–20% of these individuals have biochemical hypercortisolism [78–86]. Once endogenous ACTH-independent hypercortisolism has been confirmed, CT imaging of the adrenal glands should be obtained as it is a sensitive tool to detect cortisol-secreting neoplasms. These lesions are generally unilateral, rounded, well circumscribed and measure >1 cm in diameter. Importantly, these lesions are generally lipid rich and have a low density (<10 Hounsfield Units) on CT scanning. The contralateral adrenal gland is often small, but may be normal in size.

Adrenocortical Carcinoma

Adrenocortical carcinoma is a rare malignancy with only two new cases per million population per year. It occurs with a bimodal age distribution peaking before age 5 and from ages 50–60 [87]. Adrenocortical carcinoma is often hormonally active with hyperaldosteronism, virilization, and Cushing's syndrome occurring most commonly. The timing of onset for stigmata of Cushing's syndrome is a diagnostic clue as patients with adrenocortical carcinoma can develop symptoms rapidly. Refractory hypertension, hypokalemia, muscle wasting, and weight loss are other features that should raise the suspicion for adrenocortical carcinoma. The survival in patients with adrenocortical carcinoma is generally very poor, as most patients are diagnosed with stage III and IV disease with 5-year survival rates of 30% and 15% respectively [88].

The identification of a unilateral, irregular adrenal mass in a patient with ACTH-independent Cushing's syndrome is essentially diagnostic of adrenocortical carcinoma [89]. These tumors are generally large by the time of diagnosis, and CT scanning can often identify additional metastatic disease, assisting in staging and therapeutic decision making.

ACTH-Independent Macronodular Adrenal Hyperplasia

AIMAH is a rare form of bilateral nodular adrenal disease that results from aberrant hormone receptor signaling. The receptors identified to cause this condition are a diverse group of hormone receptors including receptors for gastric inhibitory polypeptide, β-adrenergic, vasopressin, serotonin, angiotensin II, luteinizing hormone/human chorionic gonadotropin, and leptin [90]. This process is thought to begin with binding of the normal ligand to its inappropriately expressed receptor resulting in stimulation of the adrenal glands via downstream signaling. This leads to growth of large monoclonal and polyclonal nodules in both adrenal glands with resultant overproduction and secretion of cortisol [91, 92].

AIMAH presents, on average, at a more advanced age than Cushing's syndrome caused by unilateral adrenal disease. Patients present at a mean age of 51 years of age with equal male: female distribution [93]. A diagnostic clue in patients with AIMAH is a greater than normal cortisol response to ACTH administration.

Abdominal imaging in these patients often reveals bilateral massively enlarged adrenal glands. There may be numerous nodules up to 4 cm in size, or the adrenal gland can appear diffusely enlarged [94]. On pathological examination, the adrenal cortex shows diffuse internodular hyperplasia which is in contrast to conditions such as McCune–Albright syndrome where the internodular cortex is atrophic [95, 96].

Primary Pigmented Nodular Adrenocortical Disease

PPNAD is another rare adrenal disease that results in hypercortisolism. In this condition, multiple small, often coalescent, adrenal nodules form and develop autonomous function. The pathophysiology responsible for the nodule formation is not completely understood but appears to be due to mutations in the tumor suppressor protein kinase R1a subunit (PRKAR1A) [97]. Patients with Carney's complex, an autosomal dominant, inherited multiple neoplasia syndrome (that may present with acromegaly, calcifying Sertoli cells tumors, thyroid nodules, cutaneous and atrial myxomas, breast ductal adenomas, and psammomatous melanotic schwannomas, as well as PPNAD), account for 50% of patients with PPNAD with the remaining 50% being sporadic cases [97, 98].

PPNAD has a bimodal age distribution at presentation with most cases being diagnosed in the second and third decades of life [97]. Patients with PPNAD may not present with the typical stigmata of Cushing's syndrome. They are often lean and without central obesity. Common age-dependent features include short stature, osteoporosis, and severe muscle wasting [99]. A clinical feature that can help in diagnosis is that many patients with PPNAD have a paradoxical 50% or greater increase in cortisol production in 2-day-low and high-dose dexamethasone suppression testing [100].

Imaging reveals diverse findings. Some patients can have frankly enlarged adrenals bilaterally, while other can have essentially normal appearing glands on CT. Another well-known finding is a "string of beads" appearance of the adrenals. When examined pathologically there are darkly pigmented nodules ranging in size from microscopic to 1 cm. The intervening adrenal cortex is generally atrophic, which is in contrast to AIMAH [101].

McCune–Albright Syndrome

McCune–Albright syndrome, the result of a mutation in the α subunit of the stimulatory guanine nucleotide-binding protein (Gsα), is a familial form of adrenal-dependent Cushing's syndrome. This mutation leads to constitutive activation of the cyclic AMP pathway resulting in excessive cortisol secretion.

Patients with McCune–Albright syndrome generally present at a very young age with other manifestations such as polyostotic fibrous dysplasia, café au lait spots, and other autonomous endocrine hyperfunctions (i.e., premature puberty in girls and growth hormone excess).

The mutation in Gsα leads to a genetic mosaic with adrenal nodules containing the mutation. The adrenal cortex between nodules is atrophic and does not contain the Gsα mutation.

Subclinical Cushing's Syndrome

An important caveat to the differential diagnosis of adrenal-dependent Cushing's syndrome is patients with mild or subclinical Cushing's syndrome. Although there is no consensus upon diagnostic criteria for mild cortisol excess, most agree that inappropriate and autonomous cortisol secretion in a patient with an incidentally discovered adrenal nodule, is consistent with subclinical Cushing's syndrome. These individuals often lack the classic stigmata of Cushing's syndrome, and as such any patient with an incidentally discovered adrenal nodule should be evaluated for autonomous cortisol secretion. Urine free cortisol is a poorly sensitive tool for this evaluation and is positive in only 32% of patients with subclinical Cushing's syndrome [80]. There are conflicting data regarding the diagnostic performance of late-night salivary for subclinical Cushing's syndrome [102, 103]. The 1-mg overnight dexamethasone suppression test and suppression of morning ACTH appear to perform best in the diagnosis of mild cortisol excess [80].

The complete clinical implications of subclinical Cushing's syndrome have not been fully elucidated. However, patients with mild cortisol excess have been found to have lower bone density and a greater risk of fracture [104]. These patients also have higher rates of obesity, glucose intolerance and metabolic syndrome. Additionally, small studies have shown a benefit in these metabolic findings after adrenalectomy [105].

Algorithm for Cushing's Syndrome Differential Diagnosis (Fig. 7.6)

After hypercortisolism has been convincingly demonstrated, plasma ACTH levels should be obtained to distinguish between ACTH-dependent and ACTH-independent Cushing's syndrome. A plasma ACTH level ≥20 pg/ml indicates an ACTH-dependent source. In this circumstance, a dedicated MRI of the sella should be obtained to look for a pituitary adenoma. Generally speaking, patients with clinical and biochemical findings consistent with Cushing's disease, and an unequivocal mass in the pituitary, can be directly referred to an experienced neurosurgeon for consideration of transsphenoidal tumor resection. However, if there is an equivocal or absent pituitary lesion on imaging, or the patient has atypical clinical features, it is recommended that patients be referred to a specialized center for IPSS. Patients found to have a pituitary source of excess ACTH should then be referred to a neurosurgeon. If there is no central to peripheral gradient on IPSS, a search for an ectopic source of ACTH should be pursued.

An ACTH level ≤5 pg/ml on initial testing is indicative of ACTH-independent hypercortisolism. The next step is to obtain an adrenal CT for differential diagnosis of adrenal-dependent Cushing's syndrome.

The most challenging diagnostic scenario occurs when ACTH levels are between 5 and 20 pg/ml. Patients with ACTH levels in this range should be evaluated by an experienced clinician familiar with the differential diagnosis of Cushing's syndrome. CRH stimulation is generally the next step in the diagnostic algorithm.

7 Differential Diagnosis of Cushing's Syndrome

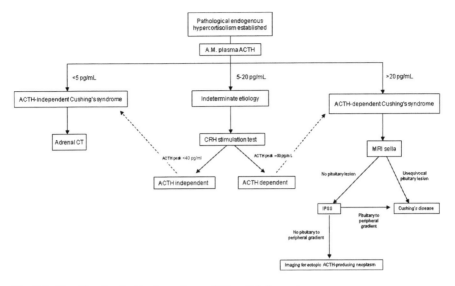

Fig. 7.6 Algorithm for Cushing's syndrome differential diagnosis

References

1. Findling JW, Raff H. Diagnosis and differential diagnosis of Cushing's syndrome. Endocrinol Metab Clin North Am. 2001;30:729–47.
2. Lindsay JR, Nieman LK. Differential diagnosis and imaging in Cushing's syndrome. Endocrinol Metab Clin North Am. 2005;34:403–21. x.
3. Thompson GB, Young Jr WF. Adrenal incidentaloma. Curr Opin Oncol. 2003;15:84–90.
4. Hall WA, Luciano MG, Doppman JL, et al. Pituitary magnetic resonance imaging in normal human volunteers: occult adenomas in the general population. Ann Intern Med. 1994; 120:817–20.
5. Yanovski JA, Cutler Jr GB, Doppman JL, et al. The limited ability of inferior petrosal sinus sampling with corticotropin-releasing hormone to distinguish Cushing's disease from pseudo-Cushing states or normal physiology. J Clin Endocrinol Metab. 1993;77:503–9.
6. Raff H, Findling JW. A physiologic approach to diagnosis of the Cushing syndrome. Ann Intern Med. 2003;138:980–91.
7. Nieman LK, Biller BM, Findling JW, et al. The diagnosis of Cushing's syndrome: an Endocrine Society Clinical Practice Guideline. J Clin Endocrinol Metab. 2008;93: 1526–40.
8. Raff H, Findling JW. A new immunoradiometric assay for corticotropin evaluated in normal subjects and patients with Cushing's syndrome. Clin Chem. 1989;35:596–600.
9. Reincke M, Nieke J, Krestin GP, et al. Preclinical Cushing's syndrome in adrenal "incidentalomas": comparison with adrenal Cushing's syndrome. J Clin Endocrinol Metab. 1992;75:826–32.
10. Flack MR, Oldfield EH, Cutler Jr GB, et al. Urine free cortisol in the high-dose dexamethasone suppression test for the differential diagnosis of the Cushing syndrome. Ann Intern Med. 1992;116:211–7.
11. Findling JW, Doppman JL. Biochemical and radiologic diagnosis of Cushing's syndrome. Endocrinol Metab Clin North Am. 1994;23:511–37.

12. Meador CK, Liddle GW, Island DP, et al. Cause of Cushing's syndrome in patients with tumors arising from "nonendocrine" tissue. J Clin Endocrinol Metab. 1962;22:693–703.
13. Wajchenberg BL, Mendonca BB, Liberman B, et al. Ectopic adrenocorticotropic hormone syndrome. Endocr Rev. 1994;15:752–87.
14. Howlett TA, Grossman A, Rees LH, Besser GM. Differential diagnosis of Cushing's syndrome. Lancet. 1986;2:871.
15. Aron DC, Raff H, Findling JW. Effectiveness versus efficacy: the limited value in clinical practice of high dose dexamethasone suppression testing in the differential diagnosis of adrenocorticotropin-dependent Cushing's syndrome. J Clin Endocrinol Metab. 1997;82:1780–5.
16. Kaye TB, Crapo L. The Cushing syndrome: an update on diagnostic tests. Ann Intern Med. 1990;112:434–44.
17. Findling JW, Kehoe ME, Shaker JL, Raff H. Routine inferior petrosal sinus sampling in the differential diagnosis of adrenocorticotropin (ACTH)-dependent Cushing's syndrome: early recognition of the occult ectopic ACTH syndrome. J Clin Endocrinol Metab. 1991;73:408–13.
18. Ilias I, Torpy DJ, Pacak K, et al. Cushing's syndrome due to ectopic corticotropin secretion: twenty years' experience at the National Institutes of Health. J Clin Endocrinol Metab. 2005;90:4955–62.
19. Wiggam MI, Heaney AP, McIlrath EM, et al. Bilateral inferior petrosal sinus sampling in the differential diagnosis of adrenocorticotropin-dependent Cushing's syndrome: a comparison with other diagnostic tests. J Clin Endocrinol Metab. 2000;85:1525–32.
20. Liddle GW. Tests of pituitary-adrenal suppressibility in the diagnosis of Cushing's syndrome. J Clin Endocrinol Metab. 1960;20:1539–60.
21. Biemond P, de Jong FH, Lamberts SW. Continuous dexamethasone infusion for seven hours in patients with the Cushing syndrome. A superior differential diagnostic test. Ann Intern Med. 1990;112:738–42.
22. Croughs RJ, Docter R, de Jong FH. Comparison of oral and intravenous dexamethasone suppression tests in the differential diagnosis of Cushing's syndrome. Acta Endocrinol (Copenh). 1973;72:54–62.
23. Tabarin A, Greselle JF, San-Galli F, et al. Usefulness of the corticotropin-releasing hormone test during bilateral inferior petrosal sinus sampling for the diagnosis of Cushing's disease. J Clin Endocrinol Metab. 1991;73:53–9.
24. Dichek HL, Nieman LK, Oldfield EH, et al. A comparison of the standard high dose dexamethasone suppression test and the overnight 8-mg dexamethasone suppression test for the differential diagnosis of adrenocorticotropin-dependent Cushing's syndrome. J Clin Endocrinol Metab. 1994;78:418–22.
25. Orth DN, DeBold CR, DeCherney GS, et al. Pituitary microadenomas causing Cushing's disease respond to corticotropin-releasing factor. J Clin Endocrinol Metab. 1982;55:1017–9.
26. Invitti C, Pecori Giraldi F, de Martin M, Cavagnini F. Diagnosis and management of Cushing's syndrome: results of an Italian multicentre study. Study Group of the Italian Society of Endocrinology on the Pathophysiology of the Hypothalamic-Pituitary-Adrenal Axis. J Clin Endocrinol Metab. 1999;84:440–8.
27. Pecori Giraldi F, Invitti C, Cavagnini F. Study Group of the Italian Society of Endocrinology on the Pathophysiology of the Hypothalamic-pituitary-adrenal axis. The corticotropin-releasing hormone test in the diagnosis of ACTH-dependent Cushing's syndrome: a reappraisal. Clin Endocrinol (Oxf). 2001;54:601–7.
28. Newell-Price J, Morris DG, Drake WM, et al. Optimal response criteria for the human CRH test in the differential diagnosis of ACTH-dependent Cushing's syndrome. J Clin Endocrinol Metab. 2002;87:1640–5.
29. Molitch ME, Russell EJ. The pituitary "incidentaloma". Ann Intern Med. 1990;112:925–31.
30. Chong BW, Kucharczyk W, Singer W, George S. Pituitary gland MR: a comparative study of healthy volunteers and patients with microadenomas. AJNR Am J Neuroradiol. 1994;15:675–9.

31. Patronas N, Bulakbasi N, Stratakis CA, et al. Spoiled gradient recalled acquisition in the steady state technique is superior to conventional postcontrast spin echo technique for magnetic resonance imaging detection of adrenocorticotropin-secreting pituitary tumors. J Clin Endocrinol Metab. 2003;88:1565–9.
32. Doppman JL, Frank JA, Dwyer AJ, et al. Gadolinium DTPA enhanced MR imaging of ACTH-secreting microadenomas of the pituitary gland. J Comput Assist Tomogr. 1988;12:728–35.
33. Tabarin A, Laurent F, Catargi B, et al. Comparative evaluation of conventional and dynamic magnetic resonance imaging of the pituitary gland for the diagnosis of Cushing's disease. Clin Endocrinol (Oxf). 1998;49:293–300.
34. Kaskarelis IS, Tsatalou EG, Benakis SV, et al. Bilateral inferior petrosal sinuses sampling in the routine investigation of Cushing's syndrome: a comparison with MRI. AJR Am J Roentgenol. 2006;187:562–70.
35. Miller DL, Doppman JL. Petrosal sinus sampling: technique and rationale. Radiology. 1991;178:37–47.
36. Oldfield EH, Doppman JL, Nieman LK, et al. Petrosal sinus sampling with and without corticotropin-releasing hormone for the differential diagnosis of Cushing's syndrome. N Engl J Med. 1991;325:897–905.
37. Lefournier V, Gatta B, Martinie M, et al. One transient neurological complication (sixth nerve palsy) in 166 consecutive inferior petrosal sinus samplings for the etiological diagnosis of Cushing's syndrome. J Clin Endocrinol Metab. 1999;84:3401–2.
38. Jehle S, Walsh JE, Freda PU, Post KD. Selective use of bilateral inferior petrosal sinus sampling in patients with adrenocorticotropin-dependent Cushing's syndrome prior to transsphenoidal surgery. J Clin Endocrinol Metab. 2008;93:4624–32.
39. Miller DL, Doppman JL, Peterman SB, et al. Neurologic complications of petrosal sinus sampling. Radiology. 1992;185:143–7.
40. Blevins Jr LS, Christy JH, Khajavi M, Tindall GT. Outcomes of therapy for Cushing's disease due to adrenocorticotropin-secreting pituitary macroadenomas. J Clin Endocrinol Metab. 1998;83:63–7.
41. Obuobie K, Davies JS, Ogunko A, Scanlon MF. Venous thrombo-embolism following inferior petrosal sinus sampling in Cushing's disease. J Endocrinol Invest. 2000;23:542–4.
42. Doppman JL, Oldfield EH, Nieman LK. Bilateral sampling of the internal jugular vein to distinguish between mechanisms of adrenocorticotropic hormone-dependent Cushing syndrome. Ann Intern Med. 1998;128:33–6.
43. Mamelak AN, Dowd CF, Tyrrell JB, et al. Venous angiography is needed to interpret inferior petrosal sinus and cavernous sinus sampling data for lateralizing adrenocorticotropin-secreting adenomas. J Clin Endocrinol Metab. 1996;81:475–81.
44. Findling JW, Kehoe ME, Raff H. Identification of patients with Cushing's disease with negative pituitary adrenocorticotropin gradients during inferior petrosal sinus sampling: prolactin as an index of pituitary venous effluent. J Clin Endocrinol Metab. 2004;89:6005–9.
45. Kaltsas GA, Giannulis MG, Newell-Price JD, et al. A critical analysis of the value of simultaneous inferior petrosal sinus sampling in Cushing's disease and the occult ectopic adrenocorticotropin syndrome. J Clin Endocrinol Metab. 1999;84:487–92.
46. Bessac L, Bachelot I, Vasdev A, et al. Catheterization of the inferior petrosal sinus. Its role in the diagnosis of Cushing's syndrome. Experience with 23 explorations. Ann Endocrinol (Paris). 1992;53:16–27.
47. Bonelli FS, Huston 3rd J, Carpenter PC, et al. Adrenocorticotropic hormone-dependent Cushing's syndrome: sensitivity and specificity of inferior petrosal sinus sampling. AJNR Am J Neuroradiol. 2000;21:690–6.
48. Colao A, Faggiano A, Pivonello R, et al. Inferior petrosal sinus sampling in the differential diagnosis of Cushing's syndrome: results of an Italian multicenter study. Eur J Endocrinol. 2001;144:499–507.
49. Colao A, Merola B, Tripodi FS, et al. Simultaneous and bilateral inferior petrosal sinus sampling for the diagnosis of Cushing's syndrome: comparison of multihormonal assay,

baseline multiple sampling and ACTH-releasing hormone test. Horm Res. 1993;40: 209–16.
50. Lopez J, Barcelo B, Lucas T, et al. Petrosal sinus sampling for diagnosis of Cushing's disease: evidence of false negative results. Clin Endocrinol (Oxf). 1996;45:147–56.
51. Newell-Price J, Trainer P, Besser M, Grossman A. The diagnosis and differential diagnosis of Cushing's syndrome and pseudo-Cushing's states. Endocr Rev. 1998;19:647–72.
52. Castinetti F, Nagai M, Dufour H, et al. Gamma knife radiosurgery is a successful adjunctive treatment in Cushing's disease. Eur J Endocrinol. 2007;156:91–8.
53. Tsagarakis S, Vassiliadi D, Kaskarelis IS, et al. The application of the combined corticotropin-releasing hormone plus desmopressin stimulation during petrosal sinus sampling is both sensitive and specific in differentiating patients with Cushing's disease from patients with the occult ectopic adrenocorticotropin syndrome. J Clin Endocrinol Metab. 2007;92:2080–6.
54. Tsagarakis S, Kaskarelis IS, Kokkoris P, et al. The application of a combined stimulation with CRH and desmopressin during bilateral inferior petrosal sinus sampling in patients with Cushing's syndrome. Clin Endocrinol (Oxf). 2000;52:355–61.
55. Ilias I, Chang R, Pacak K, et al. Jugular venous sampling: an alternative to petrosal sinus sampling for the diagnostic evaluation of adrenocorticotropic hormone-dependent Cushing's syndrome. J Clin Endocrinol Metab. 2004;89:3795–800.
56. Erickson D, Huston 3rd J, Young Jr WF, et al. Internal jugular vein sampling in adrenocorticotropic hormone-dependent Cushing's syndrome: a comparison with inferior petrosal sinus sampling. Clin Endocrinol (Oxf). 2004;60:413–9.
57. Oliverio PJ, Monsein LH, Wand GS, Debrun GM. Bilateral simultaneous cavernous sinus sampling using corticotropin-releasing hormone in the evaluation of Cushing disease. AJNR Am J Neuroradiol. 1996;17:1669–74.
58. Laws Jr ER. Multiple pituitary adenomas. J Neurosurg. 2000;93:909–11.
59. Miller DL, Doppman JL, Nieman LK, et al. Petrosal sinus sampling: discordant lateralization of ACTH-secreting pituitary microadenomas before and after stimulation with corticotropin-releasing hormone. Radiology. 1990;176:429–31.
60. McCance DR, McIlrath E, McNeill A, et al. Bilateral inferior petrosal sinus sampling as a routine procedure in ACTH-dependent Cushing's syndrome. Clin Endocrinol (Oxf). 1989;30:157–66.
61. Lefournier V, Martinie M, Vasdev A, et al. Accuracy of bilateral inferior petrosal or cavernous sinuses sampling in predicting the lateralization of Cushing's disease pituitary microadenoma: influence of catheter position and anatomy of venous drainage. J Clin Endocrinol Metab. 2003;88:196–203.
62. Isidori AM, Lenzi A. Ectopic ACTH syndrome. Arq Bras Endocrinol Metabol. 2007;51:1217–25.
63. Doppman JL, Nieman L, Miller DL, et al. Ectopic adrenocorticotropic hormone syndrome: localization studies in 28 patients. Radiology. 1989;172:115–24.
64. Findling JW, Tyrrell JB. Occult ectopic secretion of corticotropin. Arch Intern Med. 1986;146:929–33.
65. Torpy DJ, Chen CC, Mullen N, et al. Lack of utility of (111)In-pentetreotide scintigraphy in localizing ectopic ACTH producing tumors: follow-up of 18 patients. J Clin Endocrinol Metab. 1999;84:1186–92.
66. Doppman JL, Pass HI, Nieman LK, et al. Detection of ACTH-producing bronchial carcinoid tumors: MR imaging vs CT. AJR Am J Roentgenol. 1991;156:39–43.
67. Isidori AM, Kaltsas GA, Pozza C, et al. The ectopic adrenocorticotropin syndrome: clinical features, diagnosis, management, and long-term follow-up. J Clin Endocrinol Metab. 2006;91:371–7.
68. Pacak K, Ilias I, Chen CC, et al. The role of [(18)F]fluorodeoxyglucose positron emission tomography and [(111)In]-diethylenetriaminepentaacetate-D-Phe-pentetreotide scintigraphy in the localization of ectopic adrenocorticotropin-secreting tumors causing Cushing's syndrome. J Clin Endocrinol Metab. 2004;89:2214–21.
69. Abraham G. Exogenous Cushing's syndrome induced by surreptitious topical glucocorticosteroid overdose in infants with diaper dermatitis. J Pediatr Endocrinol Metab. 2007;20:1169–71.

70. Chiang MY, Sarkar M, Koppens JM, et al. Exogenous Cushing's syndrome and topical ocular steroids. Eye. 2006;20:725–7.
71. Hopkins RL, Leinung MC. Exogenous Cushing's syndrome and glucocorticoid withdrawal. Endocrinol Metab Clin North Am. 2005;34:371–84. ix.
72. Azizi F, Jahed A, Hedayati M, et al. Outbreak of exogenous Cushing's syndrome due to unlicensed medications. Clin Endocrinol (Oxf). 2008;69:921–5.
73. Razenberg AJ, Elte JW, Rietveld AP, et al. A "smart" type of Cushing's syndrome. Eur J Endocrinol. 2007;157:779–81.
74. Newell-Price J, Bertagna X, Grossman AB, Nieman LK. Cushing's syndrome. Lancet. 2006;367:1605–17.
75. Ambrosi B, Bochicchio D, Ferrario R, et al. Screening tests for Cushing's syndrome. Clin Endocrinol (Oxf). 1990;33:809–11.
76. Lindholm J, Juul S, Jorgensen JO, et al. Incidence and late prognosis of Cushing's syndrome: a population-based study. J Clin Endocrinol Metab. 2001;86:117–23.
77. Etxabe J, Vazquez JA. Morbidity and mortality in Cushing's disease: an epidemiological approach. Clin Endocrinol (Oxf). 1994;40:479–84.
78. Ambrosi B, Peverelli S, Passini E, et al. Abnormalities of endocrine function in patients with clinically "silent" adrenal masses. Eur J Endocrinol. 1995;132:422–8.
79. Terzolo M, Pia A, Ali A, et al. Adrenal incidentaloma: a new cause of the metabolic syndrome? J Clin Endocrinol Metab. 2002;87:998–1003.
80. Terzolo M, Bovio S, Reimondo G, et al. Subclinical Cushing's syndrome in adrenal incidentalomas. Endocrinol Metab Clin North Am. 2005;34:423–39. x.
81. Grumbach MM, Biller BM, Braunstein GD, et al. Management of the clinically inapparent adrenal mass ("incidentaloma"). Ann Intern Med. 2003;138:424–9.
82. Osella G, Terzolo M, Borretta G, et al. Endocrine evaluation of incidentally discovered adrenal masses (incidentalomas). J Clin Endocrinol Metab. 1994;79:1532–9.
83. Kloos RT, Gross MD, Francis IR, et al. Incidentally discovered adrenal masses. Endocr Rev. 1995;16:460–84.
84. Barzon L, Sonino N, Fallo F, et al. Prevalence and natural history of adrenal incidentalomas. Eur J Endocrinol. 2003;149:273–85.
85. Caplan RH, Strutt PJ, Wickus GG. Subclinical hormone secretion by incidentally discovered adrenal masses. Arch Surg. 1994;129:291–6.
86. Terzolo M, Osella G, Ali A, et al. Subclinical Cushing's syndrome in adrenal incidentaloma. Clin Endocrinol (Oxf). 1998;48:89–97.
87. Flack MR, Chrousos GP. Neoplasms of the adrenal cortex. In: Holland R, editor. Cancer medicine. 4th ed. New York: Lea and Fibinger; 1996. p. 1563–70.
88. Latronico AC, Chrousos GP. Extensive personal experience: adrenocortical tumors. J Clin Endocrinol Metab. 1997;82:1317–24.
89. Barzilay JI, Pazianos AG. Adrenocortical carcinoma. Urol Clin North Am. 1989;16:457–68.
90. Costa MH, Lacroix A. Cushing's syndrome secondary to ACTH-independent macronodular adrenal hyperplasia. Arq Bras Endocrinol Metabol. 2007;51:1226–37.
91. Gicquel C, Bertagna X, Le Bouc Y. Recent advances in the pathogenesis of adrenocortical tumours. Eur J Endocrinol. 1995;133:133–44.
92. Beuschlein F, Reincke M, Karl M, et al. Clonal composition of human adrenocortical neoplasms. Cancer Res. 1994;54:4927–32.
93. Zeiger MA, Nieman LK, Cutler GB, et al. Primary bilateral adrenocortical causes of Cushing's syndrome. Surgery. 1991;110:1106–15.
94. Lacroix A, Bourdeau I. Bilateral adrenal Cushing's syndrome: macronodular adrenal hyperplasia and primary pigmented nodular adrenocortical disease. Endocrinol Metab Clin North Am. 2005;34:441–58. x.
95. Weinstein LS, Shenker A, Gejman PV, et al. Activating mutations of the stimulatory G protein in the McCune-Albright syndrome. N Engl J Med. 1991;325:1688–95.
96. Boston BA, Mandel S, LaFranchi S, Bliziotes M. Activating mutation in the stimulatory guanine nucleotide-binding protein in an infant with Cushing's syndrome and nodular adrenal hyperplasia. J Clin Endocrinol Metab. 1994;79:890–3.

97. Stratakis CA, Kirschner LS, Carney JA. Clinical and molecular features of the Carney complex: diagnostic criteria and recommendations for patient evaluation. J Clin Endocrinol Metab. 2001;86:4041–6.
98. Kirschner LS, Taymans SE, Stratakis CA. Characterization of the adrenal gland pathology of Carney complex, and molecular genetics of the disease. Endocr Res. 1998;24:863–4.
99. Horvath A, Stratakis C. Primary pigmented nodular adrenocortical disease and Cushing's syndrome. Arq Bras Endocrinol Metabol. 2007;51:1238–44.
100. Stratakis CA, Sarlis N, Kirschner LS, et al. Paradoxical response to dexamethasone in the diagnosis of primary pigmented nodular adrenocortical disease. Ann Intern Med. 1999;131:585–91.
101. Carney JA, Gordon H, Carpenter PC, et al. The complex of myxomas, spotty pigmentation, and endocrine overactivity. Medicine (Baltimore). 1985;64:270–83.
102. Nunes ML, Vattaut S, Corcuff JB, et al. Late-night salivary cortisol for diagnosis of overt and subclinical Cushing's syndrome in hospitalized and ambulatory patients. J Clin Endocrinol Metab. 2009;94:456–62.
103. Masserini B, Morelli V, Bergamaschi S, et al. The limited role of midnight salivary cortisol levels in the diagnosis of subclinical hypercortisolism in patients with adrenal incidentaloma. Eur J Endocrinol. 2009;160:87–92.
104. Chiodini I, Viti R, Coletti F, et al. Eugonadal male patients with adrenal incidentalomas and subclinical hypercortisolism have increased rate of vertebral fractures. Clin Endocrinol (Oxf). 2009;70:208–13.
105. Mitchell IC, Auchus RJ, Juneja K, et al. "Subclinical Cushing's syndrome" is not subclinical: improvement after adrenalectomy in 9 patients. Surgery. 2007;142:900–5.

Chapter 8
Radiologic Imaging Techniques in Cushing's Disease

Otto Rapalino and Pamela Schaefer

Abstract Neuroimaging studies play a central role in the clinical diagnosis and management of patients with Cushing's disease. Modalities such as magnetic resonance imaging (MRI), computed tomography (CT), and positron emission tomography (PET) are available to identify the presence of a pituitary lesion, which in turn allows for surgical treatment of this condition. All of these techniques have different strengths and weaknesses and can serve complementary roles in the evaluation of pituitary pathology in patients with Cushing's disease. However, despite advances in diagnostic imaging, there are still some patients in whom a structural abnormality cannot be identified. This chapter aims to give the reader a practical but thorough overview of the imaging techniques available for the diagnosis of Cushing's disease, including their advantages and limitations.

Keywords Pituitary pathology • Neuroimaging • Diagnostic imaging • Magnetic resonance imaging • Computed tomography • Positron emission tomography • Adrenocorticotropic hormone

Introduction

Current imaging techniques used in the evaluation of patients with Cushing's disease include computed tomography (CT), magnetic resonance imaging (MRI), and positron emission tomography (PET) techniques. Plain radiographs at best can demonstrate enlargement of the sella and are rarely performed nowadays.

O. Rapalino
Neuroradiology Division, Department of Radiology, Massachusetts General Hospital,
55 Fruit Street, Gray Building 273A, Boston, MA 02067, USA
e-mail: orapalino@partners.org

Intraoperative ultrasound (IOUS) can sometimes be used in an attempt to identify pituitary adenomas in patients with Cushing's disease during surgical resection [1, 2].

Pituitary Imaging

Computed Tomography

Non-contrast-enhanced sellar CT imaging with thin high-resolution images can be helpful for preoperative planning prior to resection. The addition of intravenous contrast material improves the visualization of vascular structures and sellar contents (Table 8.1). Contrast-enhanced CT imaging of the sella turcica is typically performed as an alternative study for evaluation of sellar pathology in patients with contraindications for MR imaging. The precontrast CT protocol typically consists of thin collimated axial, coronal, and sagittal images (Fig. 8.1). Postcontrast CT imaging can be performed as a single postcontrast scan (e.g., routine or CTA protocols) or as a dynamic CT study with multiple consecutive acquisitions (Table 8.2). CT imaging allows the evaluation of the extent of pneumatization of the sphenoid sinus, presence of a sellar bulge, sphenoid sinus dominance, relationship of intrasinus septations with carotid and optic canals, presence of osseous dehiscence of these canals, vascular anomalies (particular when a CT angiogram is performed), intercarotid distance, and the presence of paranasal sinus mucosal inflammatory changes (Fig. 8.1) [1–4]. Additional findings important for the surgical approach such as location of the optic chiasm, size of tuberculum sella and position of the supraclinoid internal carotid arteries can also be evaluated with CT [1–4].

Computed Tomography can also be used for detection of pituitary microadenomas, with sensitivity values ranging from 42% [5, 6] up to 69% [7, 8]. Teasdale et al. [8] reported that high-resolution CT has a sensitivity of approximately 69% (20/29

Table 8.1 CT imaging of the sellar region: Pearls and pitfalls

Pearls
- Non-contrast-enhanced CT imaging is the best imaging modality for presurgical evaluation of osseous anatomy and pathological changes in the sellar and parasellar compartments
- Contrast-enhanced CT imaging, particularly using a dynamic protocol, is useful for the assessment of sellar contents as an alternative modality in patients with contraindications for MRI

Pitfalls
- CT imaging, despite current technical improvements, remains less accurate than MRI for detection of microadenomas, particularly ACTH-producing microadenomas
- Beam hardening and scatter-related artifacts limit the evaluation of the sellar contents, resulting in artifactual foci of apparent decreased enhancement within the gland

8 Radiologic Imaging Techniques in Cushing's Disease

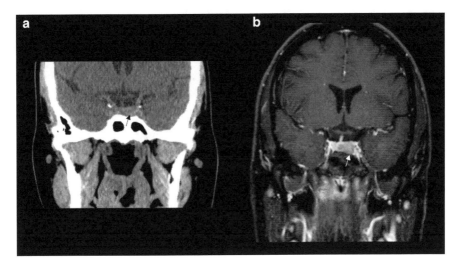

Fig. 8.1 Sellar CT and pituitary MRI of a patient with Cushing's disease. (**a**) Unenhanced coronal CT image at the level of the pituitary gland. There is poor visualization of a 14×10 mm macroadenoma clearly seen on the Gadolinium-enhanced T1-weighted coronal MR image (**b**)

Table 8.2 CT protocols

Protocol	Contrast administration	Scanning protocol	Indication
Sellar CT without contrast	No	Thin axial, reformatted 1-mm coronal and sagittal images	Presurgical evaluation of sella turcica and paranasal sinuses
Nondynamic postcontrast sellar CT	Yes	Similar images acquired 20–480 s after injection depending on desired effect (arterial versus parenchymal enhancement)	Routine postcontrast protocol for patients with contraindications for MR imaging
Dynamic sellar CT	Yes	Baseline precontrast scan. Then, every 2 s after injection during the first 4 scans and then at progressively longer intervals every 8–30 s [11]	High-resolution CT imaging in patients with contraindications for MR imaging

microadenomas identified at surgery) and a false-positive rate of approximately 28% (8/28 with normal histology) [8]. These authors also described a better correlation between the CT abnormalities and the pathological findings with microadenomas larger than 6 mm [8].

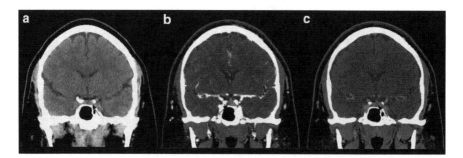

Fig. 8.2 Coronal precontrast (**a**) arterial phase (**b**), and venous phase (**c**) images through the pituitary gland of a patient with Cushing's disease: A small focus of decreased attenuation and decreased enhancement is noted in the left paramedian region of the pituitary gland on precontrast and venous phase images, respectively (*arrows*) that correlated with petrosal venous sampling and pathological findings consistent with a microadenoma. Arterial phase images demonstrate artifactual decreased enhancement on the right

Microadenomas can appear as foci of relatively decreased/delayed enhancement in comparison with the remaining gland [9, 10] or may show variable early enhancement [11] (Fig. 8.2). For contrast-enhanced studies, the best contrast ratio between the normal gland and the microadenoma is typically seen approximately 50 s after injection [9]. CT is also useful for evaluation of osseous scalloping or osseous destruction produced by macroadenomas or pituitary carcinomas [12]. Unfortunately, CT evaluation of the sellar contents is limited by the frequent presence of streak and beam hardening artifacts, confusing the interpretation of hypodensities in the pituitary gland (Table 8.1).

The use of Multidetector CT (MDCT) technology has improved the spatial and temporal resolution of the evaluation of pituitary pathology compared to conventional CT [9, 13]. Miki et al. reported that MDCT provides better visualization of the lateral margin of sellar tumors (important for the identification of cavernous sinus invasion) and associated osseous changes (e.g., erosion of the sellar floor) [13].

MDCT has also allowed the use of dynamic CT imaging which appears to be more sensitive for detection of microadenomas, with sensitivity values as high as 82–88% [14]. The dynamic CT protocol consists of the acquisition of 1.5-mm thick coronal CT images immediately before and after the administration of intravenous contrast (e.g., one pre- and eight postcontrast images at progressively longer intervals ranging from 2 to 30 s) at the same level through the pituitary gland [11].

Magnetic Resonance Imaging

MRI is the best imaging modality for detection of intrasellar and suprasellar pathology [7, 15–18] as well as involvement of the cavernous sinus [19] and hypothalamus. MR imaging also offers exquisite anatomic detail of the sellar and parasellar

8 Radiologic Imaging Techniques in Cushing's Disease

Table 8.3 MR protocol for pituitary imaging

Sequence	Slice thickness	Duration	Comments
Sagittal precontrast T1-weighted SE	3–5 mm	3 min	
Coronal precontrast T1-weighted SE	3-mm	3–4 min	
Coronal precontrast T2-weighted TSE/FSE	3-mm	3–4 min	Useful for evaluation of cystic lesions
Gadolinium administration – 0.1 mmol/kg			
Coronal dynamic pre- and postcontrast T1-weighted TSE/FSE	2-mm	20–30 s per acquisition	Increases the sensitivity for detection of microadenomas
Coronal FS postcontrast T1-weighted SE	3-mm	4 min	
Sagittal FS postcontrast T1-weighted SE	3-mm	4 min	

SE spin echo, *TSE* turbo spin echo, *FSE* fast spin echo, *FS* fat suppressed

structures that is very helpful for preoperative planning. The typical MRI protocol for pituitary imaging is shown in Table 8.3 [68].

The most common pathologic conditions responsible for Cushing's disease that can identified on MRI are micro-or macroadenomas (<10 and ≥10 mm, respectively). In the appropriate clinical situation, the MRI can be used to demonstrate pituitary hyperplasia [20] and pituitary carcinomas [21, 22].

Microadenomas represent the most common pathological substrate of Cushing's disease [accounting for approximately 80–90% of adrenocorticotropic hormone (ACTH)-producing adenomas] [23]. In general, microadenomas are typically identified as foci of relatively delayed/decreased enhancement within the pituitary gland (with the normal gland showing early homogeneous enhancement) [24] (Fig. 8.3). Unfortunately, MRI shows marked intraobserver and interobserver variability for the initial diagnosis and imaging follow-up of pituitary microadenomas [25].

Conventional contrast-enhanced pituitary MR imaging has a lower accuracy for detection of corticotropin-secreting microadenomas in comparison with non-ACTH-producing microadenomas [26]. Peck et al. [27] reported that conventional Gadolinium-enhanced MRI has sensitivity and specificity values of approximately 71% and 87% [27], respectively, for detection of ACTH-producing microadenomas. Colombo et al. reported an accuracy of 65–75% for their detection with MRI [28]. Newton et al. reported that MRI identified the correct location of microadenomas in 4/6 cases of Cushing's disease (66.7% of cases) [26]. The two undetected cases by MRI in this series included a false-positive (MR abnormality did not correspond to microadenoma detected during surgery) and a false-negative (suspected by venous sampling and contrast-enhanced CT) case [26]. The decreased sensitivity of contrast-enhanced MRI for detection of microadenomas is partially related to the similar signal intensity of ACTH-producing microadenomas with the rest of the pituitary gland on pre- and postcontrast images [29] (Fig. 8.4). Up to 47 and 14% of ACTH-producing microadenomas can be isointense to the rest of the pituitary gland on pre and postcontrast images, respectively [6, 29].

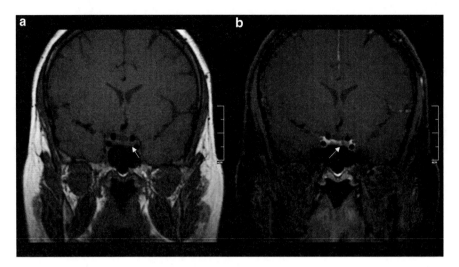

Fig. 8.3 Pituitary MRI of a young patient with Cushing's disease (3 T study). (**a**) Precontrast coronal T1-weighted image showing a subtle area of slightly decreased signal within the left side of the pituitary gland. (**b**) Gadolinium-enhanced coronal T1-weighted image at the same level demonstrates a 3-mm area of relatively delayed enhancement within the left side of the gland, consistent with a microadenoma

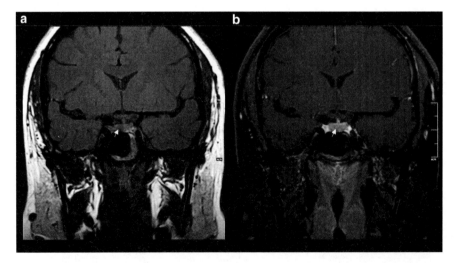

Fig. 8.4 False-positive 3 T pituitary MRI from the same patient in Fig. 9.2. (**a**) Unenhanced coronal T1-weighted image demonstrates an apparent area of decreased signal within the right side of the gland. (**b**) Gadolinium-enhanced T1-weighted image at the same level shows a subtle area of delayed enhancement colocalized with the previous abnormality. Inferior Petrosal Sinus Sampling (IPSS) showed a slight asymmetry towards the left. Tissue compatible with a microadenoma was found in surgery in the left side of the gland

Table 8.4 MR imaging of Cushing's disease: Pearls and pitfalls

Pearls
- Most accurate imaging modality for pre- and postoperative assessment of intrasellar contents
- Combination of dynamic gadolinium-enhanced and high-field MR techniques improve the accuracy for detection of ACTH-producing microadenomas

Pitfalls
- About 30% of ACTH-producing microadenomas are not detected with conventional MRI techniques
- Postoperative imaging is limited by the development of granulation tissue and fibrosis similar in appearance to residual adenoma

Dynamic contrast-enhanced MR imaging of the pituitary gland slightly increases the sensitivity for detection of microadenomas [30] (Table 8.4). Dynamic MRI of the pituitary gland involves the acquisition of high-resolution T1-weighted MR images of the pituitary gland before and repeatedly after contrast administration (every 30 s). This technique increases the sensitivity for detection of pituitary microadenomas up to 95%, with a false-positive rate of 16% [31, 32].

A clinical research study by Kanou et al. using 1.5 T MRI demonstrated that 14.3% of microadenomas can only be identified using dynamic MR techniques [33]. The earlier images (between 1 and 4 min after injection) of these dynamic series are the best for identification of microadenomas due to marked difference in enhancement between the lesion (relatively little enhancement) and the surrounding normal pituitary gland (avid enhancement) [34]. ACTH-producing microadenomas have been described as demonstrating a "simultaneous" pattern of enhancement with progressive increase of enhancement during the first minute and a plateau of enhancement during the next 2 min [33].

Contrast-enhanced MR imaging at 3 T is even more sensitive than 1.5 T MRI for detection of pituitary microadenomas, and recent studies support contrast-enhanced 3 T MR imaging as the study of choice for patients with Cushing's disease with negative or equivocal 1.5 T MR studies [35–37]. Erickson et al. [35] described sensitivities twice as high on 3 T (67–70%) in comparison with 1.5 T (30%). Subtracted and dynamic postcontrast images did not show a higher sensitivity (22–50% and 63–67%, respectively) than conventional postcontrast nondynamic images (44–70%) at 3 T in this study [35]. Wolfsberger et al. reported that 3 T MRI has also a higher sensitivity and specificity for detection of cavernous sinus invasion (83 and 84%, respectively) compared to 1.5 T studies (67 and 58%) [38]. 3 T MR imaging is also helpful as an intraoperative tool to maximize resection of pituitary neoplasms [39] and for the detection of rare cases of ectopic ACTH-producing pituitary adenomas (e.g., located in the sphenoid or cavernous sinuses) [40–43].

One of the difficulties arising from the increased sensitivity of advanced imaging techniques is the potential confounder of "incidentalomas." Incidental microadenomas can be found in up to 31% of autopsy specimens [44], approximately 39.5%

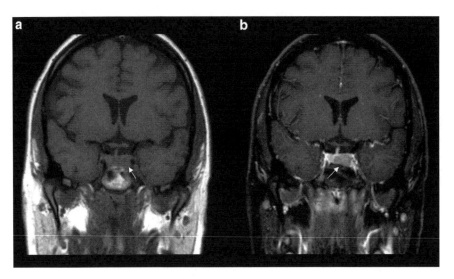

Fig. 8.5 Pituitary MRI of a middle-age man with Cushing's disease (1.5 T study). Unenhanced (**a**) and Gadolinium-enhanced (**b**) T1-weighted MR images through the pituitary gland demonstrate a 14×10-mm hypo-enhancing lesion within the left side of the pituitary gland consistent with a macro-adenoma

and 13.8% of these stain for Prolactin and ACTH, respectively [44, 45]. Similarly, using Gadolinium-enhanced MRI, hypoenhancing foci compatible with microadenomas are found in up to 34% of normal volunteers [44, 46]. Considering the relatively high prevalence of incidental microadenomas, many individuals will demonstrate small sellar abnormalities in MRI scans without associated clinical consequences [44]. Rates of approximately 10–12% of false-positive MR scans (with focal MR abnormalities that were pathologically proven not to be ACTH-producing microadenomas or were artifactual in nature) have been reported in the literature in patients with Cushing's disease [28, 31, 47]. Thus, a sensitive scan may identify a lesion that is an "incidentaloma" rather than the source of Cushing's disease. Adrenal insufficiency following transsphenoidal adenomectomy [48] or pathological confirmation of an ACTH-staining adenoma are the only methods for confirming that a lesion seen on MRI was truly the source of the Cushing's disease.

Macroadenomas are adenomas measuring at least 10 mm in maximal dimension and are responsible for 10–20% of cases of Cushing's disease [49] (Fig. 8.5). ACTH-producing macroadenomas rarely present as giant adenomas (>5 cm of maximal dimension) and constitute approximately 3% of giant adenomas [50]. Macroadenomas can extend into the cavernous sinus, sphenoid sinus, clivus and suprasellar cistern with compression of the optic chiasm [51]. Encasement of the cavernous segments of the internal carotid arteries rarely results in significant narrowing [51]. Macroadenomas typically exhibit signal characteristics similar to microadenomas but with more variable [34] and earlier [52] enhancement. Macroadenomas may show intratumoral hemorrhage (10–15%) [51] or intratumoral cystic changes [34].

8 Radiologic Imaging Techniques in Cushing's Disease

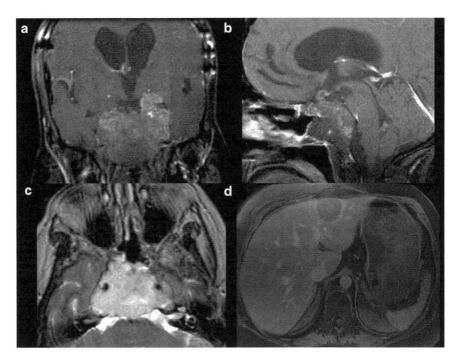

Fig. 8.6 Pituitary and liver MR studies of a 35-year-old patient with an ACTH-producing pituitary carcinoma with liver metastases. Gadolinium-enhanced coronal (**a**) and sagittal (**b**) T1-weighted as well as unenhanced axial T2-weighted images (**c**) demonstrate a large mass replacing the sella turcica with extensive invasion of the central skull base and cavernous sinuses bilaterally. Gadolinium-enhanced axial T1-weighted image through the liver (**d**) shows a peripherally enhancing metastatic lesion in the left lobe of the liver (pathology proven)

Pituitary hyperplasia is a rare cause of Cushing's disease [53–55]. In general, there are two types of pituitary hyperplasia: Diffuse and Nodular [55]. ACTH-producing hyperplasia is typically of the nodular type [55]. There have also been reports of coexistence of ACTH-producing microadenomas and corticotroph hyperplasia [55]. Pituitary hyperplasia typically presents in MRI as a uniform enlargement of the gland (simulating hypophysitis) or as an intrasellar mass lesion poorly differentiated from the rest of the pituitary gland [56–59].

Malignant ACTH-producing pituitary tumors are rare and typically produce invasion of the parasellar compartments as well as distant metastases [60] (Fig. 8.6). Twenty-two percent of pituitary carcinomas secrete ACTH (Fig. 9.5) while 50% are considered nonfunctional [60].

Ultrasound

Intraoperative ultrasound (IOUS) has been used in the past for the detection and localization of microadenomas during surgery with a reported sensitivity of up to

Table 8.5 Pet imaging of Cushing's disease: Pearls and pitfalls

Pearls
- PET imaging complements MRI, improves the overall accuracy of the imaging evaluation and reduces the number of false-positive lesions
- The combination of [^{11}C] methionine – PET with 3 T MRI has so far shown the highest reported accuracy for detection of ACTH-producing microadenomas

Pitfalls
- False-positive cases in PET imaging have been reported [66], highlighting the need to correlate with other imaging modalities (e.g. MRI) to achieve an accurate diagnosis

82% [61, 62]. Watson et al. reported that IOUS has a sensitivity of 73% and a positive predictive value of 84% for detection of microadenomas previously undetected by MRI [62].

Positron Emission Tomography

Different radiotracers have been developed and incorporated in the diagnostic imaging of pituitary tumors, particularly ACTH-producing adenomas. The most commonly used radiotracers include ^{18}fluoro-deoxy-glucose (^{18}FDG) (glucose analog) and [^{11}C] Methionine [63]. FDG-PET has been described as a complementary imaging tool to CT and MRI in the evaluation of pituitary adenomas in patients with Cushing's disease, with sensitivity values of approximately 60% [64] for detection of ACTH-secreting microadenomas (Table 8.5). Alzahrani et al. reported the detection of an occult microadenoma using FDG-PET/CT among four cases with negative MRI (approximately 25% of negative MRI cases) [64]. Pituitary micro- or macroadenomas usually show increased FDG uptake [65]. FDG-PET is also helpful to improve the specificity of the imaging evaluation by reducing the number of false-positive cases [66].

In a recent study, Ikeda et al. [67] demonstrated that the combination of Methionine (MET)-PET and 3 T MRI is very accurate for detection of ACTH-producing pituitary adenomas, with accuracy rates up to 100% [67]. In the same study, accuracy rates for FDG-PET/3 T MRI and conventional MR imaging were 73% and 40%, respectively [67].

Summary

Several types of imaging modalities are currently available for the noninvasive diagnostic evaluation of patients with Cushing's disease. These imaging modalities each have their particular strengths and weaknesses, complementing each other to provide a noninvasive window to the sellar region. MR imaging (particularly using dynamic techniques and 3 T systems) is the best imaging tool for visualization of sellar and parasellar contents. Ultrasound is sometimes used for intraoperative imaging. CT imaging is very helpful for preoperative evaluation of the osseous anatomy and pathological changes. PET imaging, especially with [^{11}C] Methionine and in combination with 3 T MRI, is highly accurate for detection of ACTH-producing microadenomas. Despite the availability of these noninvasive imaging modalities, a pituitary adenoma cannot be identified in a small proportion of patients with Cushing's disease, and additional more invasive methods (e.g., petrosal venous sampling) are required to guide the surgical treatment of these occult ACTH-producing microadenomas.

References

1. Hamid O, El Fiky L, Hassan O, Kotb A, El Fiky S. Anatomic variations of the sphenoid sinus and their impact on trans-sphenoid pituitary surgery. Skull Base. 2008;18:9–15.
2. Unal B, Bademci G, Bilgili YK, Batay F, Avci E. Risky anatomic variations of sphenoid sinus for surgery. Surg Radiol Anat. 2006;28:195–201.
3. Kazkayasi M, Karadeniz Y, Arikan OK. Anatomic variations of the sphenoid sinus on computed tomography. Rhinology. 2005;43:109–14.
4. Meloni F, Mini R, Rovasio S, Stomeo F, Teatini GP. Anatomic variations of surgical importance in ethmoid labyrinth and sphenoid sinus. A study of radiological anatomy. Surg Radiol Anat. 1992;14:65–70.
5. Kulkarni MV, Lee KF, McArdle CB, Yeakley JW, Haar FL. 1.5-T MR imaging of pituitary microadenomas: technical considerations and CT correlation. AJNR Am J Neuroradiol. 1988;9:5–11.
6. Buchfelder M, Nistor R, Fahlbusch R, Huk WJ. The accuracy of CT and MR evaluation of the sella turcica for detection of adrenocorticotropic hormone-secreting adenomas in Cushing disease. AJNR Am J Neuroradiol. 1993;14:1183–90.
7. Katz SB, Laperie RC, Moncet D, et al. Diagnostic imaging in Cushing's disease and its correlation with postsurgical clinical course. Medicina (B Aires). 1998;58:477–82.
8. Teasdale E, Teasdale G, Mohsen F, Macpherson P. High-resolution computed tomography in pituitary microadenoma: is seeing believing? Clin Radiol. 1986;37:227–32.
9. Abe T, Izumiyama H, Fujisawa I. Evaluation of pituitary adenomas by multidirectional multislice dynamic CT. Acta Radiol. 2002;43:556–9.
10. Thuomas KA. Pituitary microadenoma. MR appearance and correlation with CT. Acta Radiol. 1999;40:663.
11. Bonneville JF, Cattin F, Gorczyca W, Hardy J. Pituitary microadenomas: early enhancement with dynamic CT–implications of arterial blood supply and potential importance. Radiology. 1993;187:857–61.
12. Davis PC, Hoffman Jr JC, Spencer T, Tindall GT, Braun IF. MR imaging of pituitary adenoma: CT, clinical, and surgical correlation. AJR Am J Roentgenol. 1987;148:797–802.
13. Miki Y, Kanagaki M, Takahashi JA, et al. Evaluation of pituitary macroadenomas with multi-detector-row CT (MDCT): comparison with MR imaging. Neuroradiology. 2007;49:327–33.
14. Stadnik T, Spruyt D, van Binst A, Luypaert R, d'Haens J, Osteaux M. Pituitary microadenomas: diagnosis with dynamic serial CT, conventional CT and T1-weighted MR imaging before and after injection of gadolinium. Eur J Radiol. 1994;18:191–8.
15. Tripathi S, Ammini AC, Bhatia R, et al. Cushing's disease: pituitary imaging. Australas Radiol. 1994;38:183–6.

16. Jagannathan J, Sheehan JP, Jane Jr JA. Evaluation and management of Cushing syndrome in cases of negative sellar magnetic resonance imaging. Neurosurg Focus. 2007;23:E3.
17. Bonneville JF, Cattin F, Bonneville F, Schillo F, Jacquet G. Pituitary gland imaging in Cushing's disease. Neurochirurgie. 2002;48:173–85.
18. Escourolle H, Abecassis JP, Bertagna X, et al. Comparison of computerized tomography and magnetic resonance imaging for the examination of the pituitary gland in patients with Cushing's disease. Clin Endocrinol (Oxf). 1993;39:307–13.
19. Knappe UJ, Jaursch-Hancke C, Schonmayr R, Lorcher U. Assessment of normal perisellar anatomy in 1.5 T T2-weighted MRI and comparison with the anatomic criteria defining cavernous sinus invasion of pituitary adenomas. Cen Eur Neurosurg. 2009;70:130–6.
20. Kovacs K. The pathology of Cushing's disease. J Steroid Biochem Mol Biol. 1993;45:179–82.
21. Tonner D, Belding P, Moore SA, Schlechte JA. Intracranial dissemination of an ACTH secreting pituitary neoplasm – a case report and review of the literature. J Endocrinol Invest. 1992;15:387–91.
22. Caduff F, Staub JJ, Nordmann A, Radu EW, Landolt H. [The diagnosis of Cushing's syndrome. Results of diagnostic assessment of 20 patients with Cushing's syndrome of variable etiology (1979–1989)]. Schweiz Med Wochenschr. 1991;121:10–20.
23. Choi WHaMCB. Pituitary Tumors. In: Lu JJ, Brady LW, eds. *Radiation oncology : an evidence-based approach*. Berlin: Springer; 2008;xx, 675 p.
24. Dwyer AJ, Frank JA, Doppman JL, et al. Pituitary adenomas in patients with Cushing disease: initial experience with Gd-DTPA-enhanced MR imaging. Radiology. 1987;163:421–6.
25. Bahurel-Barrera H, Assie G, Silvera S, Bertagna X, Coste J, Legmann P. Inter- and intraobserver variability in detection and progression assessment with MRI of microadenoma in Cushing's disease patients followed up after bilateral adrenalectomy. Pituitary. 2008;11:263–9.
26. Newton DR, Dillon WP, Norman D, Newton TH, Wilson CB. Gd-DTPA-enhanced MR imaging of pituitary adenomas. AJNR Am J Neuroradiol. 1989;10:949–54.
27. Peck WW, Dillon WP, Norman D, Newton TH, Wilson CB. Imaging of pituitary microadenomas at 1.5 T: experience with Cushing disease. AJR Am J Roentgenol. 1989;152:145–51.
28. Colombo N, Loli P, Vignati F, Scialfa G. MR of corticotropin-secreting pituitary microadenomas. AJNR Am J Neuroradiol. 1994;15:1591–5.
29. Vest-Courtalon C, Ravel A, Perez N, et al. Pituitary gland MRI and Cushing disease: report of 14 operated patients. J Radiol. 2000;81:781–6.
30. Davis WL, Lee JN, King BD, Harnsberger HR. Dynamic contrast-enhanced MR imaging of the pituitary gland with fast spin-echo technique. J Magn Reson Imaging. 1994;4:509–11.
31. Friedman TC, Zuckerbraun E, Lee ML, Kabil MS, Shahinian H. Dynamic pituitary MRI has high sensitivity and specificity for the diagnosis of mild Cushing's syndrome and should be part of the initial workup. Horm Metab Res. 2007;39:451–6.
32. Xing B, Deng K, Ren ZY, et al. Magnetic resonance imaging characteristics and surgical results of adrenocorticotropin-secreting pituitary adenomas. Chin Med Sci J. 2008;23:44–8.
33. Kanou Y, Arita K, Kurisu K, Tomohide A, Iida K. Clinical implications of dynamic MRI for pituitary adenomas: clinical and histologic analysis. J Clin Neurosci. 2002;9:659–63.
34. FitzPatrick M, Tartaglino LM, Hollander MD, Zimmerman RA, Flanders AE. Imaging of sellar and parasellar pathology. Radiol Clin North Am. 1999;37:101–21. x.
35. Erickson D, Erickson B, Watson R, et al. 3 Tesla magnetic resonance imaging with and without corticotropin releasing hormone stimulation for the detection of microadenomas in Cushing's syndrome. Clin Endocrinol (Oxf). 2010;72(6):793–9.
36. Kim LJ, Lekovic GP, White WL, Karis J. Preliminary experience with 3-tesla MRI and Cushing's disease. Skull Base. 2007;17:273–7.
37. Yoneoka Y, Watanabe N, Matsuzawa H, et al. Preoperative depiction of cavernous sinus invasion by pituitary macroadenoma using three-dimensional anisotropy contrast periodically rotated overlapping parallel lines with enhanced reconstruction imaging on a 3-tesla system. J Neurosurg. 2008;108:37–41.

38. Wolfsberger S, Ba-Ssalamah A, Pinker K, et al. Application of three-tesla magnetic resonance imaging for diagnosis and surgery of sellar lesions. J Neurosurg. 2004;100:278–86.
39. Pamir MN, Peker S, Ozek MM, Dincer A. Intraoperative MR imaging: preliminary results with 3 tesla MR system. Acta Neurochir Suppl. 2006;98:97–100.
40. Slonim SM, Haykal HA, Cushing GW, Freidberg SR, Lee AK. MRI appearances of an ectopic pituitary adenoma: case report and review of the literature. Neuroradiology. 1993;35:546–8.
41. Koizumi M, Usui T, Yamada S, et al. Successful treatment of Cushing's disease caused by ectopic intracavernous microadenoma. Pituitary. 2008
42. Kim LJ, Klopfenstein JD, Cheng M, et al. Ectopic intracavernous sinus adrenocorticotropic hormone-secreting microadenoma: could this be a common cause of failed transsphenoidal surgery in Cushing disease? Case report. J Neurosurg. 2003;98:1312–7.
43. Ohnishi T, Arita N, Yoshimine T, Mori S. Intracavernous sinus ectopic adrenocorticotropin-secreting tumours causing therapeutic failure in transsphenoidal surgery for Cushing's disease. Acta Neurochir (Wien). 2000;142:855–64.
44. Molitch ME. Pituitary tumours: pituitary incidentalomas. Best Pract Res Clin Endocrinol Metab. 2009;23:667–75.
45. Buurman H, Saeger W. Subclinical adenomas in postmortem pituitaries: classification and correlations to clinical data. Eur J Endocrinol. 2006;154:753–8.
46. Hall WA, Luciano MG, Doppman JL, Patronas NJ, Oldfield EH. Pituitary magnetic resonance imaging in normal human volunteers: occult adenomas in the general population. Ann Intern Med. 1994;120:817–20.
47. Salenave S, Gatta B, Pecheur S, et al. Pituitary magnetic resonance imaging findings do not influence surgical outcome in adrenocorticotropin-secreting microadenomas. J Clin Endocrinol Metab. 2004;89:3371–6.
48. Hermus AR, Pieters GF, Pesman GJ, et al. Coexistence of hypothalamic and pituitary failure after successful pituitary surgery in Cushing's disease? J Endocrinol Invest. 1987;10:365–9.
49. De Martin M, Pecori Giraldi F, Cavagnini F. Cushing's disease. Pituitary. 2006;9:279–87.
50. Chacko G, Chacko AG, Lombardero M, et al. Clinicopathologic correlates of giant pituitary adenomas. J Clin Neurosci. 2009;16:660–5.
51. Rennert J, Doerfler A. Imaging of sellar and parasellar lesions. Clin Neurol Neurosurg. 2007;109:111–24.
52. Swallow CE, Osborn AG. Imaging of sella and parasellar disease. Semin Ultrasound CT MR. 1998;19:257–71.
53. Haap M, Gallwitz B, Meyermann R, Mittelbronn M. Cushing's disease associated with both pituitary microadenoma and corticotroph hyperplasia. Exp Clin Endocrinol Diabetes. 2009;117:289–93.
54. Kovacs K, Horvath E, Coire C, et al. Pituitary corticotroph hyperplasia preceding adenoma in a patient with Nelson's syndrome. Clin Neuropathol. 2006;25:74–80.
55. Horvath E, Kovacs K, Scheithauer BW. Pituitary hyperplasia. Pituitary. 1999;1:169–79.
56. Papakonstantinou O, Bitsori M, Mamoulakis D, Bakantaki A, Papadaki E, Gourtsoyiannis N. MR imaging of pituitary hyperplasia in a child with growth arrest and primary hypothyroidism. Eur Radiol. 2000;10:516–8.
57. Young M, Kattner K, Gupta K. Pituitary hyperplasia resulting from primary hypothyroidism mimicking macroadenomas. Br J Neurosurg. 1999;13:138–42.
58. Wolansky LJ, Leavitt GD, Elias BJ, Lee HJ, Dasmahapatra A, Byrne W. MRI of pituitary hyperplasia in hypothyroidism. Neuroradiology. 1996;38:50–2.
59. Dadachanji MC, Bharucha NE, Jhankaria BG. Pituitary hyperplasia mimicking pituitary tumor. Surg Neurol. 1994;42:397–9.
60. McCutcheon IE. Pituitary tumors in oncology. In: DeMonte F, editor. Tumors of the brain and spine. New York: Springer; 2007. p. xii. 364.
61. Ram Z, Shawker TH, Bradford MH, Doppman JL, Oldfield EH. Intraoperative ultrasound-directed resection of pituitary tumors. J Neurosurg. 1995;83:225–30.

62. Watson JC, Shawker TH, Nieman LK, DeVroom HL, Doppman JL, Oldfield EH. Localization of pituitary adenomas by using intraoperative ultrasound in patients with Cushing's disease and no demonstrable pituitary tumor on magnetic resonance imaging. J Neurosurg. 1998;89:927–32.
63. Pacak K, Eisenhofer G, Goldstein DS. Functional imaging of endocrine tumors: role of positron emission tomography. Endocr Rev. 2004;25:568–80.
64. Alzahrani AS, Farhat R, Al-Arifi A, Al-Kahtani N, Kanaan I, Abouzied M. The diagnostic value of fused positron emission tomography/computed tomography in the localization of adrenocorticotropin-secreting pituitary adenoma in Cushing's disease. Pituitary. 2009;12: 309–14.
65. Ryu SI, Tafti BA, Skirboll SL. Pituitary adenomas can appear as hypermetabolic lesions in F-FDG PET imaging. J Neuroimaging. 2010;20(4):393–6.
66. De Souza B, Brunetti A, Fulham MJ, et al. Pituitary microadenomas: a PET study. Radiology. 1990;177:39–44.
67. Ikeda H, Abe T, Watanabe K. Usefulness of composite methionine-positron emission tomography/3.0-tesla magnetic resonance imaging to detect the localization and extent of early-stage Cushing adenoma. J Neurosurg. 2010;112(4):750–5.
68. Hallam DK. Pituitary. In: Haacke EM, Lin W, editors. Current protocols in magnetic resonance imaging. New York: Wiley; 2001. Wiley InterScience (Online service).

Chapter 9
Surgical Treatment of Cushing's Disease

Travis S. Tierney and Brooke Swearingen

Abstract Modern transsphenoidal surgery for Cushing's disease is usually curative, achieving durable remission in 70–90% of cases. Comparison of remission and recurrence rates between series in the literature is difficult as many employ different remission criteria. Complication rates are low, but include hypopituitarism, diabetes insipidus, and CSF rhinorhhea. Improved remission rates can be obtained with early re-exploration after initial unsuccessful procedures, and reoperation remains an option after recurrence. This chapter reviews current surgical techniques, including microscopic and endoscopic approaches.

Keywords Adrenocorticotropic hormone • Hypercortisolemia • Hypophysectomy • Pituitary adenoma • Transsphenoidal surgery

Introduction

Modern transsphenoidal surgery for Cushing's disease is usually curative, achieving durable remission in 70–90% of cases. About 70% of patients with endogenous hypercortisolemia (Cushing's syndrome) harbor an adrenocorticotropic hormone-secreting pituitary tumor (Cushing's disease) [1]. Virtually, all of these tumors are benign (fewer than 1 in 500 metastasize [2, 3]) and most are smaller than 10 mm in diameter (fewer than 15% are macroadenomas [4, 5]). In USA about 400 cases of Cushing's disease come to medical attention each year [6, 7]. The great majority are women, with an incidence three- to tenfold that of men [8, 9].

B. Swearingen (✉)
Department of Neurosurgery, Massachusetts General Hospital
and Harvard Medical School, 15 Parkman Street, Boston, MA 02114, USA
e-mail: bswearingen@partners.org

Usually, Cushingoid signs (e.g., truncal obesity, proximal muscle wasting, violaceous striae, hypertension, hyperglycemia, hirsutism, and easily bruised, thinned skin) prompt a thorough endocrine evaluation that often begins with a 24-h urine or midnight salivary cortisol level screening to confirm the diagnosis of hypercortisolemia [10]. The diagnostic evaluation has been recently reviewed and is discussed at length in Chaps. 4 and 7 [11, 12]. Standard high-resolution gadolinium-contrasted spin-echo MRI with dedicated fine cuts through the sella will reveal a well-defined pituitary mass in about 50–70% of case with biochemically confirmed Cushing's disease, as discussed in Chap. 8 [13]. Newer dynamic gadolinium imaging techniques with spoiled gradient sequences may improve this sensitivity [14, 15]. With equivocal imaging, bilateral inferior petrosal sinus sampling with corticotropin-releasing hormone stimulation may be undertaken to centralize, and possibly lateralize, the ACTH source prior to surgery [16, 17].

Indications for Surgery

Transsphenoidal surgery for Cushing's disease has a superior remission rate with an acceptably low risk of complications, as compared to either medical or radiation therapy, and is the initial treatment of choice in most cases. Contraindications to transsphenoidal surgery may be either anatomic or medical. Anatomic abnormalities that may make the transsphenoidal approach more difficult or less effective include a vascular abnormality of the carotid artery that obstructs access to the sella, such as tortuous medial loop or intracavernous aneurysm of the carotid artery [18], or tumor located exclusively in the cavernous sinus [19]. Significant lateral or anterior intracranial extension of the less common Cushing's macroadenoma may necessitate a transcranial approach. Medical contraindications would include the presence of such severe comorbidities that the risk of anesthesia is unacceptable; in these cases pretreatment with pharmacologic therapy or primary radiotherapy may be alternatives.

Untreated Cushing's disease causes significant morbidity and mortality [20, 21]. The long-term effects of prolonged hypercortisolemia are well-known and include the development of malignant hypertension and cardiovascular disease that statistically contribute to increased mortality risk [1, 22, 23]. Even patients with so-called subclinical hypercortisolemia [24] seem to be at a significantly higher risk of developing hyperglycemia [25–27], heart disease [28], and osteoporosis [29]. Because successful treatment of Cushing's disease is believed to mitigate many of these risks [21, 30–33], surgical intervention is usually indicated as soon as the diagnosis is definitively established.

Medical treatment of Cushing's disease may be undertaken in selected patients as a bridge to definitive microsurgery to improve preoperative risk. However, medical pretreatment has not been systematically compared to immediate surgery, and the adverse long-term side effects of agents traditionally used to block excess corticosteroid production usually make their chronic use undesirable [34]. Historically, several oral agents were used as adjuvants to pituitary irradiation and together achieved remissions that approached modern rates of cure for microsurgery [35–37], but many patients developed permanent panhypopituitarism as a result of pituitary irradiation [38], and a few underwent malignant progression [39]. Recently, somatostatin analogues [40] and dopamine agonists [41] have shown a promising safety and efficacy profile in clinical trials for de novo and persistent Cushing's disease. These and other recent medical advances in the treatment Cushing's disease are discussed in Chap. 12.

Surgical Techniques

Since Jules Hardy first reported the excision of a pituitary microadenoma using the operative microscope in the mid-1960s, three basic approaches to the sella have evolved. These include the traditional sublabial transseptal route [42], the direct transnasal approach [43], and endonasal endoscopy [44]. The sublablial approach provides a wide field of view with microscopic visualization associated with some increased incisional morbidity and pain from the incision itself. It is still used by some experienced pituitary surgeons [45] for the excellent exposure it provides. The direct endonasal approach usually offers almost equivalent visualization without the morbidity associated with the sublabial incision [46]. Endoscopic approaches have recently gained favor; they offer wider visualization of the sella without the morbidity of the sublabial incision, but generally cannot provide binocular vision or depth of field; remission rates appear similar.

For both endoscopic and microscopic surgery, preoperative screening, anesthesia, and positioning are the similar. The patient is placed supine in a semiflexed position with the head just slightly above the right atrium. Some surgeons employ three-point skeletal fixation, especially if surgical navigation is used, but securing the head on a gel headrest usually provides adequate fixation as well as small degree of intraoperative neck flexibility that is occasionally useful in visualizing corners of the sella. Oxymetazoline hydrochloride is applied to the nasal mucosal and the nose and upper lip are prepped. A small area in the lower right abdominal quadrant is prepared for later fat graft harvest.

Direct Endonasal Approach

For the microscopic transnasal approach, a speculum is inserted through the vestibule of the naris in line with the middle turbinate along the posterior nasal septum, and lidocaine with epinephrine is infiltrated submucosally. An incision is made through the mucosa to bone. The posterior nasal septum is fractured and deviated laterally with its attached mucosa, avoiding a submucosal dissection and the need for postoperative nasal packing. A self-retaining speculum is centered directly over the anterior wall of the sphenoid and aimed approximately at the floor of the sella by lateral fluoroscopy. This allows for a direct midline orientation to be maintained, which is critical in Cushing's disease with a normal-sized sella. The sphenoid is opened with the drill and Kerrison punch and any underlying septae are drilled away. The pattern of septal anatomy on a coronal CT is often useful defining the sphenoidal anatomy, or imaged-guided frameless stereotaxy can also be used.

Once the sella is clearly visualized, a high-speed diamond drill is used to thin the anterior floor. A direct midline approach is essential to avoid vascular injury [47]. The floor of the sella is opened to the fullest extent laterally to the cavernous sinus on either side.

A durotomy is made centrally. The surface of the gland is exposed as widely as possible and is inspected for any sign of adenoma. The gland is hemisected and biopsies are taken from each quadrant, concentrating on the side predicted by the lateralization of the IPSS. It is sometimes useful to prepare an intraoperative cytological smear of any suspicious material, as this minimizes handling of the minute and friable tissue, and may allow a tissue diagnosis to be made even if no material is available for paraffin sectioning. The gland is systematically sampled for frozen section analysis when no clear evidence of tumor is found. If multiple biopsies are negative for tumor, the contralateral lobe is inspected. If still no tumor is found, many surgeons perform a hemihypophysectomy on the suspected side.

Hemostasis is obtained, and the tumor bed packed with a small piece of abdominal fat. The sellar floor can be reconstructed with bone or cartilage harvested from the septum, titanium mesh, or various artificial materials. It is not necessary to routinely pack the sphenoid sinus, but a thin layer of fibrin glue can be used to cover the anterior wall of the sella of the risk of postoperative CSF leak is thought to be high. The speculum is removed from the naris, the mucosal flap is inspected for bleeding, the middle turbinate is medialized, and the nasal septum is repositioned in the midline. No nasal packing is usually necessary.

Endoscopic Approach

Although the direct endonasal microscopic technique provides superb optics and binocular vision, endoscopic approaches, which offer a wider field of view, have been widely publicized and appear to have similar remission rates in experienced hands [48, 49]. Here, an endoscope is introduced along the nasal septum medial to the middle turbinate. Since no speculum is used, occasionally the middle turbinate may require removal for satisfactory access. A mucosal incision is then made down to bone. The septum is either fractured just medial to the point where it joins the prow of the sphenoid, or the ostia is enlarged medially. Either the nasal septum together with overlying mucosa of the contralateral naris is pushed off the midline, or the initial opening may be made unilaterally by enlarging the sphenoid ostia expanded medially to create an anterior sphenoidotomy. Underlying septae are drilled away to expose the face of the sella. Any mucosal bleeding can usually be controlled with bipolar cautery. At this point, the endoscope is either rigidly fixed in place with an endoscope holder, or manipulated intraoperatively by an assistant, again allowing two-handed intrasellar surgery to proceed in much the same way as previously described. Although initial techniques employed a monocular endoscope, which did not compare with the optics and binocular vision of the operating microscope, recent technologic advances have now incorporated hi-definition optics, and three-dimensional video microscopy is under development. Recently, several centers have reported their experience with pure endoscopic approaches for Cushing's disease [44, 50–57]. Initial remission rates and complications are comparable to standard transsphenoidal surgery, but long-term follow-up will be necessary to determine whether one technique is optimal.

Surgical Remission and Long-Term Outcome

We reviewed surgical outcomes for over 2,600 patients reported in 21 retrospective series published within the last 10 years that had at least 40 patients and a minimum 12 month mean follow-up time [5, 21, 58–70]. Outcomes of studies reporting data exclusively from children with Cushing's disease [71–73] are discussed in Chap. 14. Except the 15 series that have included data from patients under 18 years, we do not explicitly review surgical outcomes for pediatric Cushing's disease. This review is complicated by the fact that there is no single, generally accepted standard for remission of disease, and different studies employ differing criteria.

Overall, simple unweighted average rates of remission (i.e., the percentage of patients with normal to low cortisol levels after initial surgery) and recurrence (i.e., the percentage of patients once in remission with new hypercortisolemia) were 82 and 11%, respectively (see Table 9.1). The significant variability between studies likely reflects some combination of differing biochemical definitions of remission, follow-up, patient selection and surgical expertise. For example, the highest rate of initial remission (97%) following transsphenoidal surgery for Cushing's disease occurred in a series reporting outcomes exclusively from patients with well-defined intraoperative adenomas [70]. Conversely, series with rates of remission lower than 75% included large numbers of patients with macroadenomas and/or tumor invasion of the cavernous sinus [5, 58, 61, 64–66]. Several studies have shown that dural sinus invasion correlates with persistent disease after primary surgery [5, 79–81]. Most [5, 21, 62, 65, 67, 75, 76, 82] but not all studies [60, 63, 64, 68, 69] showed that patients with smaller tumors tended to achieve higher rates of remission. The lowest overall rates of remission occurred for patients who underwent repeat transsphenoidal surgery for either persistent (simple unweighted average 50%, range 0–100% of case) or recurrent (simple unweighted average 62%, range 37–100% of case) disease (Table 9.2). Some evidence from single institutions [61, 62] suggests a trend toward higher remission rates with increasing experience, but not all long-term series confirm this [5, 60], and no large-scale surveillance data on disease remission as a function of experience has been published, as the administrative

Table 9.1 Cushing's disease: outcomes after microsurgery in series with more than 40 patients published since 1999[a]

Study, year [ref.]	Cases (N)	Follow-up (years)	Remission rate (%)	Recurrence % (N) YTR
Jagannathan, 2009 [70]	261	7 Mean	97 Initial	2.4 (6) 4.7 mean
Fomekong, 2009 [69]	40	7.2 Mean	80 Overall	9.4 (3) 4.5 mean
			75 Initial micro	
			92 Initial macro	
Atkinson, 2008 [55]	42	2.5 Median	86 Initial	11.1 (4) 4.8 mean
Hofmann, 2008 [5]	426	5.6 Median	69 Initial	14.3 (42) 6.1 mean
Prevedello, 2008 [74]	167	3.3 Mean	80 Initial	12.8 (19) 4.2 mean
Acebes, 2007 [68]	44	4.1 Mean	89 Initial	7.7 (3) 4.6 mean
Rollin, 2007 [67]	108	6 Mean	85 Initial	6.8 (6) 3.7 mean
			29 Redo	
Esposito, 2006 [75]	40	2.8 Mean	93 Initial	3.1 (1) 1.7
			45 Redo	
Atkinson, 2005 [66]	63	9.6 Median	71 Initial	22.2 (10) 5.3 mean
Hammer, 2004 [76]	289	11.1 Median	82 Initial	9 (13) 4.9 median
Salenave, 2004 [77]	54	1.7 Median	85 Initial	19.6 (9) 1.4 mean
Chen, 2003 [65]	174	>5	74 Initial	6.3 (8) 3.5 median
Flitsch, 2003 [78]	147	5.1 Mean	93 Initial	6.5 (9) 3.7 mean
Pereira, 2003 [64]	78	7.2 Median	72 Initial	9.0 (5) 7.0 median
Shimon, 2002 [63]	82	4.2 Mean	78 Initial	5 (3) 2, 4 and 5
			62 Redo	
Rees, 2002 [62]	53	6 Median	77 Initial	4.8 (2) 1.1 and 3
Yap, 2002 [61]	97	3.1 Median	69 Initial	11.5 (7) 3.0 mean
Chee, 2001 [60]	61	7.3 Median	79 Initial	14.6 (7) 6.3 mean
Barbetta, 2001 [59]	68	4.8 Median	90 Initial	21 (13) 3.0 mean
Swearingen, 1999 [21]	161	8.0 Median	85 Overall	7 (10) 5.7 mean
			90 Initial micro	
			65 Initial macro	
Invitti, 1999 [58]	236	2.3	69 Initial	17 (22/129) 9.6 mean

[a]When more than one series have been published from the same institution or surgeon, the most recent paper is cited. All series had a least 1 year of follow-up

databases used to ascertain disease experience do not include remission data. Stricter remission criteria naturally contribute to apparently lower rates of initial remission [5, 61, 62], but no single biochemical definition of remission has been shown to ideally predict which patients may eventually recur and require further intervention. Utz et al. [92] extensively reviewed this contentious issue and ultimately recommended long-term serial testing for all patients as the only definitive way to diagnose recurrence. Perhaps the most pragmatic use of immediate postoperative testing is to identity those patients with persistent hypercortisolemia (i.e., surgical failures) for earlier intervention.

Several studies show that early reexploration can achieve remission in over 50% of cases after an initially unsuccessful operation [21, 63, 84–88]. Usually, a partial

Table 9.2 Cushing's disease: outcomes after repeat microsurgery for persistent or recurrent disease

Study, year [ref.]	Cases (N)	% Cured
Persistent disease		
Friedman, 1989 [83]	31	71 (22)
Trainer 1993 [84]	10	60 (6)
Ram, 1994 [85]	17	53 (9)
Knappe, 1996 [86]	16	56 (9)
Shimon, 2002 [63]	10	60 (6)
Pereira, 2003 [64]	10	40 (4)
Locatelli, 2005 [87]	12	67 (8)
Esposito, 2006 [75]	11	45 (5)
Rollin, 2007 [67]	5	0
Prevedello, 2008 [74]	4	25 (1)
Aghi, 2008 [88]	10	70 (7)
Hofmann, 2008 [5]	15	20 (3)
Fomekong, 2009 [69]	14	29 (4)
Jagannathan, 2009 [70]	9	100 (9)
Recurrent disease		
Knappe, 1996 [86]	24	71 (17)
Shimon, 2002 [63]	3	66 (2)
Pereira, 2003 [64]	4	75 (3)
Hofmann, 2006 [89]	13	46 (6)
Rollin, 2007 [67]	4	50 (2)
Aghi, 2008 [88]	13	77 (10)
Hofmann, 2008 [5]	35	37 (13)
Patil, 2008 [90]	36	61 (22)
Fomekong, 2009 [69]	3	66 (2)
Jagannathan, 2009 [70]	6	100 (6)
Persistent v Recurrent NS[a]		
Invitti, 1999 [58]	21	43 (9)
Chee, 2001 [60]	13	38 (5)
Benveniste, 2005 [91]	42	57 (24)

[a]*NS*: not stated

hypophysectomy or selective adenomectomy is undertaken based on initial IPSS lateralization [87] or guided by the use of intraoperative ultrasonography [93]. Early repeat surgery appears to carry greater risks of CSF leak [60, 85–87] and anterior pituitary dysfunction compared with primary surgery (range between 15 [88] and 50% [83]). These higher rates of hypopituitarism following immediate reoperation, however, are still lower than the long-term risk of hypopituitarism associated with contemporary radiation therapy [94–96]. Advocates of an early reoperation after failed surgery cite the ease of working within a fresh surgical field together with a chance of achieving the most rapid cortisol control as primary advantages of the technique [85, 87]. Conversely, data is now emerging on the phenomena of "delayed remission," where a small (about 6%) but significant number of patients initially thought to harbor persistent disease later spontaneously become normo- or hypocortisolemic [97, 98]. It is important to identify these patients before proceeding to additional and possibly unnecessary treatment.

Determination of Remission

There is no generally accepted "gold standard" for remission after successful transsphenoidal surgery. Multiple surgical series have employed various criteria to assess postoperative hypoadrenalism as an indicator of possible long-term remission. These issues have been reviewed in detail [92, 99]. A number of questions remain: (1) what is the optimal test for remission? (2) At what point should testing be done? (3) Is immediate postoperative glucocorticoid replacement necessary, and will this interfere with postoperative testing?

A summary of remission criteria and timing of testing from a number of major series is shown in Table 9.3. In general, most series combine a measurement of fasting serum cortisol with additional testing of the HPA axis, at variable intervals after surgery. We currently utilize remission criteria of a fasting serum cortisol level of <5 μg/day obtained within 1–2 days after the procedure, in association with a subnormal 24-h urine cortisol level, realizing that approximately 6% of patients will experience a delayed decline in cortisol levels [98]. A recent paper has suggested that midnight salivary cortisol levels may ultimately provide a more sensitive indicator of long-term remission [123]; their utility in the immediate postoperative period is not yet clear. Many of the early studies employed prophylactic postoperative steroid replacement to prevent a postoperative adrenal crisis. Some studies have since suggested that replacement can be withheld for a few days if the patient is monitored carefully while postoperative testing is under way (for a discussion of this approach see Chap. 10). Our current length of stay after transsphenoidal surgery is 1–2 days, and most postoperative testing is done on an outpatient basis. We, therefore, continue to use low dose dexamethasone replacement in the immediate postoperative period (0.5–1.0 mg daily), while early testing is performed; this dose of dexamethasone is unlikely to be suppressive of the HPA axis and will not interfere with cortisol assays. If the patient is in remission, we transition to prednisone at replacement doses after testing is completed. Alternatively, replacement with prednisone or hydrocortisone can be begun in the immediate postoperative period if it discontinued for at least 24 h prior to testing.

Assessment of HPA Axis and Withdrawal of Replacement

Normalization of the HPA after successful surgery can require an extended period (6–12 months.) A rapid return to eucortisolemia may represent an early recurrence. In some cases, normalization never occurs and lifelong replacement is required. Various studies have utilized a number of fasting cortisol threshold levels for the determination of the adequacy of adrenal reserve, in combination with ACTH stimulation or ITT. There is very little data specifically referring to postoperative Cushing's disease, and CD will confound the determination of postoperative adrenal insufficiency both through the stress of transsphenoidal surgery and the presence of

Table 9.3 Remission criteria after transsphenoidal surgery for CD (after Utz [92] and Czepielewski [99])

First author, year [ref.]	Timing of postoperative test	Biochemical tests	Remission threshold values
Hardy, 1962 [100]	ND	Cortisol	Normal
		Urinary 17-OHCS	Normal
		UFC	Normal
Boggan, 1983 [101]	6 Weeks	ACTH	Normal
		Cortisol	Normal
		LD-DST	Normal suppression
Fahlbusch, 1986 [102]	5–6 days	LD-DST (2 or 3 mg)	<2 μg/day
		Adrenal insufficiency	ND
Chandler, 1987 [103]	Within 1 week	Cortisol	<20.5 μg/day
		UFC	<130 μg/day
Nakane, 1987 [104]	ND	Cortisol	<20 μg/day
		ACTH	<100 μg/mL
Schrell, 1987 [105]	7–10 days	ACTH (am)	<50 pg/mL
		Cortisol (am)	<21 μg/day
		LD-DST (2 mg)	Normal suppression
Guilhaume, 1988 [106]	3–6 Months	UFC	<90 μg/day
		8 pm cortisol	<100 ng/mL
Mampalam, 1988 [107]	ND	Cortisol	Normal
		ACTH	Normal
		LD-DST	Normal suppression
Pieters, 1989 [108]	1 day	AM cortisol	<7 μg/day
Arnott, 1990 [109]	1–4 Week	UFC	<490 nmol/day
Burke, 1990 [110]	4 Weeks	UFC	<280 nmol/day
		12 am cortisol	<280 nmol/L
Tindall, 1990 [111]	1–24 Weeks	Cortisol	Normal
		UFC	Normal
Ludecke, 1991 [112]	16 h	Cortisol	Subnormal
		ACTH	Subnormal
Lindholm, 1992 [113]	ND	UFC or	<235 nmol/day
		ACTH stimulation	Low
McCance, 1993 [114]	1–4 days	AM cortisol	<550 nmol/L
		LD-DST (2 mg)	<60 nmol/L
		UFC	<50 nmol/L
Trainer, 1993 [84]	1 day	AM cortisol	<50 nmol/L
Ram, 1994 [85]	ND	AM cortisol	<5 μg/day
		UFC	<90 μg/day
Bochicchio, 1995 [115]	Within 6 months	LD-DST	Normal suppression
Bakiri, 1996 [116]	ND	Circadian rhythm	Normal
		LD-DST	Normal suppression
Knappe, 1996 [86]	ND	ND	ND
Sonino, 1996 [117]	5–15 days	UFC	<248 nmol/day
		LD-DST	Normal suppression

(continued)

Table 9.3 (continued)

First author, year [ref.]	Timing of postoperative test	Biochemical tests	Remission threshold values
Blevins, 1998 [118]	6 Months	Cortisol or	<5 µg/day
		UFC and	<15 µg/day
		LD-DST	Normal suppression
Invitti, 1999 [58]	ND	UFC	Low/normal
		AM cortisol	Low/normal
		AM ACTH	Low/normal
Swearingen, 1999 [21]	1–10 days	AM cortisol	<138 nmol/L
		UFC	<55 nmol/day
Barbetta, 2001 [59]	1 Month	Cortisol	Normal
		UFC	Normal
Chee, 2001 [60]	2 Weeks	AM cortisol	Normal
		12 am cortisol	<200 nmol/L
		LD-DST (2 mg)	cortisol <100 nmol/L and ACTH <5 ng/L
Estrada, 2001 [119]	8–12 days	Cortisol Q6h × 4	Normal
		UFC	<331 nmol/day
Rees, 2002 [62]	1–7 days	AM cortisol	<50 nmol/L
Shimon, 2002 [63]	4–6 Weeks	UFC	Normal
		LD-DST	<5 µg/day
Yap, 2002 [61]	3–4 days	AM cortisol	<50 nmol/L
Chen, 2003 [65]	2 days	LD-DST (1 mg)	<8 µg/day
Pereira, 2003 [64]	6 Months	LD-DST (1 mg)	<100 nmol/L
		UFC × 2	Normal
Hammer, 2004 [76]	1 Week	AM cortisol or	≤5 µg/day
	within 6 months	LD-DST (1 mg) or	≤5 µg/day
		UFC	Normal
Rollin, 2004 [120]	1–12 days	Cortisol	<5 µg/day
		LD-DST (1 mg)	<3 µg/day
Storr, 2005 [121]	1–8 days	Cortisol	<50 nmol/L
Atkinson, 2005 [66]	4–5 days	AM cortisol	<300 nmol/L
		UFC	Normal
		LD-DST (2 mg)	Normal suppression
Esposito, 2006 [75]	1–2 days	AM cortisol	<140 nmol/L
Acebes, 2007 [68]	24 h	ACTH	<7.55 pmol/L
		Cortisol	<585 nmol/L
Pouration, 2007 [122]	72 h	AM cortisol	≤2 µg/day
Patil, 2007 [7]	72 h	AM cortisol	≤2 µg/day
Hofmann, 2008 [5]	1 Week	ODST	≤2 µg/day
	3 Months	AM cortisol	≤18 ng/mL
	5 days	UFC	<90 µg/day
Carrasco, 2008 [123]	6–12 Months	Midnight salivary cortisol	<2 ng/mL

ND: not defined

preexisting long-term adrenal suppression. Current practice is generally extrapolated from (1) data correlating immediate postoperative basal cortisol levels in non-CD patients with delayed ACTH stimulation testing and/or ITT, and (2) the correlation of basal cortisol levels with ACTH stimulation and/or ITT separate from the stress of surgery in non-CD patients. After pituitary surgery, an early study reported that a fasting cortisol level of 9 μg/day several days postoperative predicted an adequate response to a later ITT [124]. More recent studies reported that basal cortisol levels of 14.5 μg/day [125] and 15 μg/day [126] were sufficient when obtained in the immediate postoperative period. Patients with CD were excluded from these studies. In the determination of non-postoperative adrenal insufficiency, 15% of patients with documented adrenal insufficiency had morning cortisol levels between 9 and 19 μg/day [127]. Others have suggested that fasting cortisol levels of 11 μg/day [128] or 15 μg/day [129] predict an adequate response to ITT. These issues have recently been reviewed and a meta-analysis performed, which concluded that a basal cortisol level of 13 μg/day was sufficient [130]. It was later reported, however, that using this threshold for basal cortisol in the immediate postoperative period would have led to an underdiagnosis of adrenal insufficiency by ITT at 1 month of 23%, and it was suggested that a higher level was appropriate [131]. In the preoperative non-CD group, there were no patients with a basal cortisol of ≥18 who failed ITT. We currently employ a threshold value for the fasting cortisol level of 18 μg/day to assess adequacy of adrenal reserve. Intermediate values require ACTH stimulation testing or ITT, after sufficient time has elapsed for adrenal atrophy to develop from central adrenal insufficiency.

Postoperative Complications

We reviewed the complication rates in surgical series published within the last 10 years that presented at least 40 patients and a minimum 12 month mean follow-up. Overall, morbidity and mortality were low (Table 9.4). In recent series, 30-day mortality ranged between 0 and 1.9%. In all reported cases, deaths occurred as a direct result of cardiac-related complications, further emphasizing the high comorbid medical risks known to be associated with Cushing's disease.

Hormone Insufficiency

The endocrine management of the postoperative patient as practiced at one major center is discussed in detail in Chap. 10. Surgery may result in insufficiency in both anterior and posterior hormone function. Long-term hypopituitarism, defined as hormone replacement of at least one pituitary axis, occurred in 1–25% of patients in most series. The variability between studies may in part be accounted for by differences in surgical technique and stringency and timing of postoperative testing.

Table 9.4 Cushing's disease: complications after microsurgery in large series since published since 1999[a]

Study, year [ref.]	Diabetes insipidus % (# cases) Transient	Diabetes insipidus % (# cases) Permanent	Hypopituitarism	CSF leak	Epistaxis	30-Day mortality
Jagannathan, 2009 [70]	6 (16)	0.4 (1)	NS	1.5 (4)	0.4 (1)	0
Fomekong, 2009 [69]	32.5 (13)	15 (5)	NS	10 (4)	2.5 (1)	0
Atkinson, 2008 [55]	14 (6)	0	NS	12 (5)	NS	0
Hofmann, 2008 [5]	0.9 (4)	NS	0.9 (4)	0.5 (2)	NS	0.7 (3)
Prevedello, 2008 [74]	6 (10)	5 (8)	13.2 (22)	1.8 (3)	NS	0
Acebes, 2007 [68]	NS	NS	NS	NS	NS	NS
Rollin, 2007 [67]	58 (60)	1 (1)	31 (32)	NS	NS	1.0 (1)
Esposito, 2006 [75]	10 (4)	2.5 (1)	0	2.5 (1)	NS	0
Atkinson, 2005 [66]	29 (18)	6.3 (4)	14.3 (9)	11.1 (7)	NS	1.6 (1)
Hammer, 2004 [76]	NS	3.1 (9)	9.3 (27)	3.9 (11)		1.0 (3)
Chen, 2003 [65]	NS	NS	5.7 (10)	0	NS	0
Salenave, 2004 [77]	5.5 (3)	NS	20.4 (11)	3.7 (2)	NS	0
Flitsch, 2001, 2003 [78]	NS	3.4 (5)	11.6 (17)	2.0 (3)	0.6 (1)	0
Pereira, 2003 [64]	NS	NS	NS	NS	NS	1.2 (1)
Shimon, 2002 [63]	NS	4.9 (4)	2.4 (2)	6.1 (5)	NS	NS
Rees, 2002 [62]	38 (20)	9 (5)	12	11 (6)	NS	1.9 (1)
Yap, 2002 [61]	42 (41)	8 (8)	22 (22)	8 (8)	6 (6)	1 (1)
Chee, 2001 [60]	21 (13)	NS	19.7 (12)	13.1 (8)	1.6 (1)	0
Swearingen, 1999 [21]	NS	3.6 (7)	24.4 (47)	2.6 (5)	0.5 (1)	0
Semple, 1999 [132]	8.5	0.95 (1)	NS	0.95 (1)	0.95 (1)	0.95 (1)

[a]When more than one series have been published from the same institution or surgeon, the most recent paper is cited
NS: not stated

These rates remain considerably lower than those following either modern fractionated radiotherapy or stereotactic radiosurgery for refractory Cushing's disease [94–96]. Even experienced centers differ in their management of postoperative adrenal replacement. Routine glucocorticoid replacement (which we employ) may make determination of remission more difficult, but minimizes the risk of hypoadrenalism in the outpatient setting. Hypotension that does not immediately respond to IV fluid should be aggressively treated with high-dose IV hydrocortisone to avoid an adrenal crisis. Transient postoperative diabetes insipidus is not uncommon, but permanent DI is unusual (Table 9.4), and can be managed with intermittent vasopressin. SIADH occurs in a significant fraction of patients and requires monitoring of serum sodium levels for 10–14 days after surgery. Mild cases can usually be managed with fluid restriction, although profound hyponatremia may require furosemide diuresis with 3% saline replacement, or the use of an ADH inhibitor.

Venous Thrombosis

Deep vein thrombosis following transsphenoidal surgery may occur at a somewhat higher rate than with other intracranial procedures (reported ranges between 0.6 [74] and 6% [62]), as Cushing's disease is associated with hypercoaguability. Unless contraindicated, elastic stockings and sequential compression devices are employed. Prophylactic subcutaneous low-molecular-weight heparin can also be used, while some have even recommended low-dose aspirin [132].

Neurologic Complications

Damage to visual pathways or injury to the carotid arteries is fortunately rare, occurring in less than 1% of cases in recent series that have reported it [7, 133].

Cerebrospinal Fluid Rhinorrhea

CSF rhinorrhea can be confirmed with laboratory testing for tau protein, which is present in spinal fluid but not nasal secretions. Management options include 2–3 days of CSF diversion through a lumbar drain with extended antibiotic coverage to avoid meningitis. A persistent CSF leak is an indication for reexploration and repacking of the tumor bed and sphenoid. This approach may be advisable, since it speeds healing, decreases hospital stay, and possibly reduces the risk of meningitis compared with CSF diversion.

Epistaxis

Some degree of epistaxis is expected, especially since routine nasal packing is no longer employed. Delayed epistaxis, occurring 2–3 weeks postoperative, is most commonly from a branch of the sphenopalatine artery and responds to packing or endoscopic cauterization. Severe bleeding, especially intraoperatively, should be evaluated with urgent carotid angiography or CT angiography to exclude a pseudoaneurysm in the cavernous carotid artery [47].

Infection

Chronic sphenoid sinusitis may occur in up to 10% cases following transsphenoidal surgery [133] and usually responds to antibiotics, although repeat cases may require eventual operative drainage [134]. Meningitis is rare, but is usually seen in association with an undetected CSF leak.

Recurrent Disease

The management of recurrent disease is discussed in detail in Chap. 13. Series with the longest follow-up clearly show that overall remission rates continuously fall over time [5, 21, 64, 66, 76, 135]. In the studies reviewed here, hypercortisolemia initially cured by transsphenoidal surgery reappeared in 2.4–22.2% of patients 3–10 years after their initial surgery (Table 9.1). In one study [64], a patient experienced recurrence after more than 20 years, strongly suggesting the need for lifelong cortisol monitoring of all patients with Cushing's disease. In many cases of recurrent disease, no well-defined tumor is seen on MRI imaging [89, 90]. Repeat IPSS in not useful for predicting laterality in repeat surgery [89].

Surgical options include total or partial hypophysectomy or selective adenomectomy if possible. For relapse, more aggressive resection has been shown to lead to higher rates of remission. For example in an early surgical series of recurrent Cushing's, Knappe and Lüdecke [86] reported a 71% remission rate following aggressive hypophysectomies, but at the cost of panhypopituitarism in 46% of their patients. In more recent series where patients underwent selective adenomectomy [5, 88–91], new hypopituitarism was rare, but rates of remission were also somewhat more modest (Table 9.2). Most centers favor selective adenomectomy over hypophysectomy when a discreet mass is found intraoperatively. Several series report recurrent tumor near the original operative site [80, 89, 104], and it is likely that most recurrent tumor arises from cells remaining from the initial operation. De novo disease occurrence could be postulated, but it seems reasonable in all cases of recurrent disease to review the previous operative note for localization clues, especially when no well-defined tumor is found on MRI or IPSS lateralization data is equivocal. When extension into the dura or wall of the cavernous sinus is identified intraoperatively, patients were traditionally considered to be surgically incurable [19]. However, recent publications have described techniques for directly entering the cavernous sinus with apparently successful removal of invasive tumor [136, 137]. In general, however, the presence intracavernous tumor is an indication for stereotactic radiation treatment.

Summary

Transsphenoidal microsurgery remains the most effective treatment for Cushing's disease. Initial remission rates between 85 and 90% can be expected when a discreet pituitary microadenoma is seen on preoperative imaging, in the hands of an experienced surgeon. Compared with other treatment modalities, surgery also offers the best chance of achieving rapid cortisol control and avoiding the long-term risk of hypopituitarism. At high-volume centers, both recurrence rates and complications are low. Options for patients who fail repeat surgery include pituitary irradiation together with ongoing medical therapy or bilateral adrenalectomy.

References

1. Newell-Price J, Bertagna X, Grossman AB, Nieman LK. Cushing's syndrome. Lancet. 2006;367:1605–17.
2. Ragel BT, Couldwell WT. Pituitary carcinoma: a review of the literature. Neurosurg Focus. 2004;16:E7.
3. van der Klaauw AA, Kienitz T, Strasburger CJ, Smit JW, Romijn JA. Malignant pituitary corticotroph adenomas: report of two cases and a comprehensive review of the literature. Pituitary. 2009;12:57–69.
4. Woo YS et al. Clinical and biochemical characteristics of adrenocorticotropin-secreting macroadenomas. J Clin Endocrinol Metab. 2005;90:4963–9.
5. Hofmann BM, Hlavac M, Martinez R, Buchfelder M, Muller OA, Fahlbusch R. Long-term results after microsurgery for Cushing disease: experience with 426 primary operations over 35 years. J Neurosurg. 2008;108:9–18.
6. Lindholm J et al. Incidence and late prognosis of Cushing's syndrome: a population-based study. J Clin Endocrinol Metab. 2001;86:117–23.
7. Patil CG, Lad SP, Harsh GR, Laws Jr ER, Boakye M. National trends, complications, and outcomes following transsphenoidal surgery for Cushing's disease from 1993 to 2002. Neurosurg Focus. 2007;23:E7.
8. Mindermann T, Wilson CB. Age-related and gender-related occurrence of pituitary adenomas. Clin Endocrinol (Oxf). 1994;41:359–64.
9. Pecori Giraldi F, Moro M, Cavagnini F. Gender-related differences in the presentation and course of Cushing's disease. J Clin Endocrinol Metab. 2003;88:1554–8.
10. Carroll T, Raff H, Findling JW. Late-night salivary cortisol for the diagnosis of Cushing syndrome: a meta-analysis. Endocr Pract. 2009;15:335–42.
11. Nieman LK et al. The diagnosis of Cushing's syndrome: an Endocrine Society Clinical Practice Guideline. J Clin Endocrinol Metab. 2008;93:1526–40.

12. Boscaro M, Arnaldi G. Approach to the patient with possible Cushing's syndrome. J Clin Endocrinol Metab. 2009;94:3121–31.
13. Kaskarelis IS et al. Bilateral inferior petrosal sinuses sampling in the routine investigation of Cushing's syndrome: a comparison with MRI. AJR Am J Roentgenol. 2006;187:562–70.
14. Tabarin A et al. Comparative evaluation of conventional and dynamic magnetic resonance imaging of the pituitary gland for the diagnosis of Cushing's disease. Clin Endocrinol (Oxf). 1998;49:293–300.
15. Patronas N et al. Spoiled gradient recalled acquisition in the steady state technique is superior to conventional postcontrast spin echo technique for magnetic resonance imaging detection of adrenocorticotropin-secreting pituitary tumors. J Clin Endocrinol Metab. 2003;88: 1565–9.
16. Oldfield EH et al. Petrosal sinus sampling with and without corticotropin-releasing hormone for the differential diagnosis of Cushing's syndrome. N Engl J Med. 1991;325:897–905.
17. Lad SP, Patil CG, Laws Jr ER, Katznelson L. The role of inferior petrosal sinus sampling in the diagnostic localization of Cushing's disease. Neurosurg Focus. 2007;23:E2.
18. Berker M, Aghayev K, Saatci I, Palaoglu S, Onerci M. Overview of vascular complications of pituitary surgery with special emphasis on unexpected abnormality. Pituitary. 2010;13: 160–7.
19. Wilson CB, Mindermann T, Tyrrell JB. Extrasellar, intracavernous sinus adrenocorticotropin-releasing adenoma causing Cushing's disease. J Clin Endocrinol Metab. 1995;80: 1774–7.
20. Etxabe J, Vazquez JA. Morbidity and mortality in Cushing's disease: an epidemiological approach. Clin Endocrinol (Oxf). 1994;40:479–84.
21. Swearingen B et al. Long-term mortality after transsphenoidal surgery for Cushing disease. Ann Intern Med. 1999;130:821–4.
22. Mancini T, Kola B, Mantero F, Boscaro M, Arnaldi G. High cardiovascular risk in patients with Cushing's syndrome according to 1999 WHO/ISH guidelines. Clin Endocrinol (Oxf). 2004;61:768–77.
23. Dekkers OM et al. Mortality in patients treated for Cushing's disease is increased, compared with patients treated for nonfunctioning pituitary macroadenoma. J Clin Endocrinol Metab. 2007;92:976–81.
24. Leibowitz G et al. Pre-clinical Cushing's syndrome: an unexpected frequent cause of poor glycaemic control in obese diabetic patients. Clin Endocrinol (Oxf). 1996;44:717–22.
25. Catargi B et al. Occult Cushing's syndrome in type-2 diabetes. J Clin Endocrinol Metab. 2003;88:5808–13.
26. Chiodini I et al. Association of subclinical hypercortisolism with type 2 diabetes mellitus: a case-control study in hospitalized patients. Eur J Endocrinol. 2005;153:837–44.
27. Taniguchi T, Hamasaki A, Okamoto M. Subclinical hypercortisolism in hospitalized patients with type 2 diabetes mellitus. Endocr J. 2008;55:429–32.
28. Tsuiki M, Tanabe A, Takagi S, Naruse M, Takano K. Cardiovascular risks and their long-term clinical outcome in patients with subclinical Cushing's syndrome. Endocr J. 2008;55:737–45.
29. Di Somma C et al. Severe impairment of bone mass and turnover in Cushing's disease: comparison between childhood-onset and adulthood-onset disease. Clin Endocrinol (Oxf). 2002; 56:153–8.
30. Bourdeau I et al. Loss of brain volume in endogenous Cushing's syndrome and its reversibility after correction of hypercortisolism. J Clin Endocrinol Metab. 2002;87:1949–54.
31. Faggiano A et al. Cardiovascular risk factors and common carotid artery caliber and stiffness in patients with Cushing's disease during active disease and 1 year after disease remission. J Clin Endocrinol Metab. 2003;88:2527–33.
32. Scommegna S et al. Bone mineral density at diagnosis and following successful treatment of pediatric Cushing's disease. J Endocrinol Invest. 2005;28:231–5.
33. Patil CG, Lad SP, Katznelson L, Laws Jr ER. Brain atrophy and cognitive deficits in Cushing's disease. Neurosurg Focus. 2007;23:E11.

34. Sonino N, Boscaro M, Paoletta A, Mantero F, Ziliotto D. Ketoconazole treatment in Cushing's syndrome: experience in 34 patients. Clin Endocrinol (Oxf). 1991;35:347–52.
35. Orth DN, Liddle GW. Results of treatment in 108 patients with Cushing's syndrome. N Engl J Med. 1971;285:243–7.
36. Luton JP et al. Treatment of Cushing's disease by O, p'DDD. Survey of 62 cases. N Engl J Med. 1979;300:459–64.
37. Ross WM, Evered DC, Hunter P, Benaim M, Cook D, Hall R. Treatment of Cushing's disease with adrenal blocking drugs and megavoltage therapy to the pituitary. Clin Radiol. 1979;30:149–53.
38. Castinetti F et al. Long-term results of stereotactic radiosurgery in secretory pituitary adenomas. J Clin Endocrinol Metab. 2009;94:3400–7.
39. Minniti G, Traish D, Ashley S, Gonsalves A, Brada M. Risk of second brain tumor after conservative surgery and radiotherapy for pituitary adenoma: update after an additional 10 years. J Clin Endocrinol Metab. 2005;90:800–4.
40. Boscaro M et al. Treatment of pituitary-dependent Cushing's disease with the multireceptor ligand somatostatin analog pasireotide (SOM230): a multicenter, phase II trial. J Clin Endocrinol Metab. 2009;94:115–22.
41. Pivonello R et al. The medical treatment of Cushing's disease: effectiveness of chronic treatment with the dopamine agonist cabergoline in patients unsuccessfully treated by surgery. J Clin Endocrinol Metab. 2009;94:223–30.
42. Hardy J. Transphenoidal microsurgery of the normal and pathological pituitary. Clin Neurosurg. 1969;16:185–217.
43. Griffith HB, Veerapen R. A direct transnasal approach to the sphenoid sinus. Technical note. J Neurosurg. 1987;66:140–2.
44. Jho HD. Endoscopic transsphenoidal surgery. J Neurooncol. 2001;54:187–95.
45. Kerr PB, Oldfield EH. Sublabial-endonasal approach to the sella turcica. J Neurosurg. 2008;109:153–5.
46. Dusick JR, Esposito F, Mattozo CA, Chaloner C, McArthur DL, Kelly DF. Endonasal transsphenoidal surgery: the patient's perspective-survey results from 259 patients. Surg Neurol. 2006;65:332–41. discussion 341–332.
47. Oskouian RJ, Kelly DF, Laws Jr ER. Vascular injury and transsphenoidal surgery. Front Horm Res. 2006;34:256–78.
48. Jho HD, Carrau RL. Endoscopy assisted transsphenoidal surgery for pituitary adenoma. Technical note. Acta Neurochir (Wien). 1996;138:1416–25.
49. Jho HD. Endoscopic pituitary surgery. Pituitary. 1999;2:139–54.
50. Kabil MS, Eby JB, Shahinian HK. Fully endoscopic endonasal vs. transseptal transsphenoidal pituitary surgery. Minim Invasive Neurosurg. 2005;48:348–54.
51. Netea-Maier RT et al. Transsphenoidal pituitary surgery via the endoscopic technique: results in 35 consecutive patients with Cushing's disease. Eur J Endocrinol. 2006;154:675–84.
52. Rudnik A, Kos-Kudla B, Larysz D, Zawadzki T, Bazowski P. Endoscopic transsphenoidal treatment of hormonally active pituitary adenomas. Neuro Endocrinol Lett. 2007;28:438–44.
53. Dehdashti AR, Gentili F. Current state of the art in the diagnosis and surgical treatment of Cushing disease: early experience with a purely endoscopic endonasal technique. Neurosurg Focus. 2007;23:E9.
54. Dehdashti AR, Ganna A, Karabatsou K, Gentili F. Pure endoscopic endonasal approach for pituitary adenomas: early surgical results in 200 patients and comparison with previous microsurgical series. Neurosurgery. 2008;62:1006–15. discussion 1015–1007.
55. Atkinson JL et al. Sublabial transseptal vs transnasal combined endoscopic microsurgery in patients with Cushing disease and MRI-depicted microadenomas. Mayo Clin Proc. 2008;83:550–3.
56. Gondim JA et al. Endoscopic endonasal transsphenoidal surgery: surgical results of 228 pituitary adenomas treated in a pituitary center. Pituitary. 2010;13:68–77.
57. Wagenmakers MA, Netea-Maier RT, van Lindert EJ, Timmers HJ, Grotenhuis JA, Hermus AR. Repeated transsphenoidal pituitary surgery (TS) via the endoscopic technique: a good

therapeutic option for recurrent or persistent Cushing's disease (CD). Clin Endocrinol (Oxf). 2009;70:274–80.
58. Invitti C, Pecori Giraldi F, de Martin M, Cavagnini F. Diagnosis and management of Cushing's syndrome: results of an Italian multicentre study. Study Group of the Italian Society of Endocrinology on the Pathophysiology of the Hypothalamic-Pituitary-Adrenal Axis. J Clin Endocrinol Metab. 1999;84:440–8.
59. Barbetta L, Dall'Asta C, Tomei G, Locatelli M, Giovanelli M, Ambrosi B. Assessment of cure and recurrence after pituitary surgery for Cushing's disease. Acta Neurochir (Wien). 2001;143:477–81. discussion 481–472.
60. Chee GH, Mathias DB, James RA, Kendall-Taylor P. Transsphenoidal pituitary surgery in Cushing's disease: can we predict outcome? Clin Endocrinol (Oxf). 2001;54:617–26.
61. Yap LB, Turner HE, Adams CB, Wass JA. Undetectable postoperative cortisol does not always predict long-term remission in Cushing's disease: a single centre audit. Clin Endocrinol (Oxf). 2002;56:25–31.
62. Rees DA, Hanna FW, Davies JS, Mills RG, Vafidis J, Scanlon MF. Long-term follow-up results of transsphenoidal surgery for Cushing's disease in a single centre using strict criteria for remission. Clin Endocrinol (Oxf). 2002;56:541–51.
63. Shimon I, Ram Z, Cohen ZR, Hadani M. Transsphenoidal surgery for Cushing's disease: endocrinological follow-up monitoring of 82 patients. Neurosurgery. 2002;51:57–61. discussion 61–52.
64. Pereira AM et al. Long-term predictive value of postsurgical cortisol concentrations for cure and risk of recurrence in Cushing's disease. J Clin Endocrinol Metab. 2003;88:5858–64.
65. Chen JC, Amar AP, Choi S, Singer P, Couldwell WT, Weiss MH. Transsphenoidal microsurgical treatment of Cushing disease: postoperative assessment of surgical efficacy by application of an overnight low-dose dexamethasone suppression test. J Neurosurg. 2003;98: 967–73.
66. Atkinson AB, Kennedy A, Wiggam MI, McCance DR, Sheridan B. Long-term remission rates after pituitary surgery for Cushing's disease: the need for long-term surveillance. Clin Endocrinol (Oxf). 2005;63:549–59.
67. Rollin G, Ferreira NP, Czepielewski MA. Prospective evaluation of transsphenoidal pituitary surgery in 108 patients with Cushing's disease. Arq Bras Endocrinol Metabol. 2007;51: 1355–61.
68. Acebes JJ, Martino J, Masuet C, Montanya E, Soler J. Early post-operative ACTH and cortisol as predictors of remission in Cushing's disease. Acta Neurochir (Wien). 2007;149:471–7. discussion 477–479.
69. Fomekong E, Maiter D, Grandin C, Raftopoulos C. Outcome of transsphenoidal surgery for Cushing's disease: a high remission rate in ACTH-secreting macroadenomas. Clin Neurol Neurosurg. 2009;111:442–9.
70. Jagannathan J et al. Outcome of using the histological pseudocapsule as a surgical capsule in Cushing disease. J Neurosurg. 2009;111:531–9.
71. Joshi SM et al. Cushing's disease in children and adolescents: 20 years of experience in a single neurosurgical center. Neurosurgery. 2005;57:281–5. discussion 281–285.
72. Kanter AS et al. Single-center experience with pediatric Cushing's disease. J Neurosurg. 2005;103:413–20.
73. Batista DL, Courcoutsakis N, Riar J, Keil MF, Stratakis CA. Severe obesity confounds the interpretation of low-dose dexamethasone test combined with the administration of ovine corticotrophin-releasing hormone in childhood Cushing syndrome. J Clin Endocrinol Metab. 2008;93:4323–30.
74. Prevedello DM, Pouratian N, Sherman J, et al. Management of Cushing's disease: outcome in patients with microadenoma detected on pituitary magnetic resonance imaging. J Neurosurg. 2008;109:751–9.
75. Esposito F et al. Clinical review: early morning cortisol levels as a predictor of remission after transsphenoidal surgery for Cushing's disease. J Clin Endocrinol Metab. 2006;91:7–13.

76. Hammer GD et al. Transsphenoidal microsurgery for Cushing's disease: initial outcome and long-term results. J Clin Endocrinol Metab. 2004;89:6348–57.
77. Salenave S et al. Pituitary magnetic resonance imaging findings do not influence surgical outcome in adrenocorticotropin-secreting microadenomas. J Clin Endocrinol Metab. 2004;89: 3371–6.
78. Flitsch J, Knappe UJ, Ludecke DK. The use of postoperative ACTH levels as a marker for successful transsphenoidal microsurgery in Cushing's disease. Zentralbl Neurochir. 2003;64: 6–11.
79. Meij BP, Lopes MB, Ellegala DB, Alden TD, Laws Jr ER. The long-term significance of microscopic dural invasion in 354 patients with pituitary adenomas treated with transsphenoidal surgery. J Neurosurg. 2002;96:195–208.
80. Dickerman RD, Oldfield EH. Basis of persistent and recurrent Cushing disease: an analysis of findings at repeated pituitary surgery. J Neurosurg. 2002;97:1343–9.
81. De Tommasi C, Vance ML, Okonkwo DO, Diallo A, Laws Jr ER. Surgical management of adrenocorticotropic hormone-secreting macroadenomas: outcome and challenges in patients with Cushing's disease or Nelson's syndrome. J Neurosurg. 2005;103:825–30.
82. Cannavo S et al. Long-term results of treatment in patients with ACTH-secreting pituitary macroadenomas. Eur J Endocrinol. 2003;149:195–200.
83. Friedman RB et al. Repeat transsphenoidal surgery for Cushing's disease. J Neurosurg. 1989;71:520–7.
84. Trainer PJ et al. Transsphenoidal resection in Cushing's disease: undetectable serum cortisol as the definition of successful treatment. Clin Endocrinol (Oxf). 1993;38:73–8.
85. Ram Z, Nieman LK, Cutler Jr GB, Chrousos GP, Doppman JL, Oldfield EH. Early repeat surgery for persistent Cushing's disease. J Neurosurg. 1994;80:37–45.
86. Knappe UJ, Ludecke DK. Persistent and recurrent hypercortisolism after transsphenoidal surgery for Cushing's disease. Acta Neurochir Suppl. 1996;65:31–4.
87. Locatelli M, Vance ML, Laws ER. Clinical review: the strategy of immediate reoperation for transsphenoidal surgery for Cushing's disease. J Clin Endocrinol Metab. 2005;90:5478–82.
88. Aghi MK et al. Management of recurrent and refractory Cushing's disease with reoperation and/or proton beam radiosurgery. Clin Neurosurg. 2008;55:141–4.
89. Hofmann BM, Hlavac M, Kreutzer J, Grabenbauer G, Fahlbusch R. Surgical treatment of recurrent Cushing's disease. Neurosurgery. 2006;58:1108–18. discussion 1108–1118.
90. Patil CG, Veeravagu A, Prevedello DM, Katznelson L, Vance ML, Laws Jr ER. Outcomes after repeat transsphenoidal surgery for recurrent Cushing's disease. Neurosurgery. 2008;63:266–70. discussion 270–261.
91. Benveniste RJ, King WA, Walsh J, Lee JS, Delman BN, Post KD. Repeated transsphenoidal surgery to treat recurrent or residual pituitary adenoma. J Neurosurg. 2005;102:1004–12.
92. Utz AL, Swearingen B, Biller BM. Pituitary surgery and postoperative management in Cushing's disease. Endocrinol Metab Clin North Am. 2005;34:459–78. xi.
93. Watson JC, Shawker TH, Nieman LK, DeVroom HL, Doppman JL, Oldfield EH. Localization of pituitary adenomas by using intraoperative ultrasound in patients with Cushing's disease and no demonstrable pituitary tumor on magnetic resonance imaging. J Neurosurg. 1998; 89:927–32.
94. Estrada J et al. The long-term outcome of pituitary irradiation after unsuccessful transsphenoidal surgery in Cushing's disease. N Engl J Med. 1997;336:172–7.
95. Petit JH et al. Proton stereotactic radiotherapy for persistent adrenocorticotropin-producing adenomas. J Clin Endocrinol Metab. 2008;93:393–9.
96. Vance ML. Cushing's disease: radiation therapy. Pituitary. 2009;12:11–4.
97. Marko NF, Weil RJ. Surgery: remission after transsphenoidal surgery for Cushing disease. Nat Rev Endocrinol. 2010;6:307–9.
98. Valassi E, Biller BM, Swearingen B, Pecori Giraldi F, Losa M, Mortini P, et al. Delayed remission after transsphenoidal surgery in patients with Cushing's disease. J Clin Endocrinol Metab. 2010;95:601–10.

99. Czepielewski MA, Rollin G, Casagrande A, Ferriera NP. Criteria of cure and remission in Cushing's disease: an update. Arq Bras Endocrinol Metab. 2007;51:1362–72.
100. Hardy J. L'exerese des adenomes hypophysiares par voie transsphenoidale. Union Med Can. 1962;91:933–45.
101. Boggan JE, Tyrrell B, Wilson CB. Transsphenoidal microsurgical management of Cushing's disease. J Neurosurg. 1983;59:195–200.
102. Fahlbusch R, Buchfelder M, Muller OA. Transsphenoidal surgery for Cushing's disease. J R Soc Med. 1986;79:262–9.
103. Chandler WF, Schteingart DE, Lloyd RV, McKeever PE, Ibarra-Perez G. Surgical treatment of Cushing's disease. J Neurosurg. 1987;66:204–12.
104. Nakane T, Kuwayama A, Watanabe M, Takahashi T, Kato T, Ichihara K, et al. Long-term results of transsphenoidal adenomectomy in patients with Cushing's disease. Neurosurgery. 1987;21:218–22.
105. Schrell U, Fahlbusch R, Buchfelder M, Riedl S, Stalla GK, Muller OA. Corticotropin-releasing hormone stimulation test before and after transsphenoidal microadenomectomy in 30 patients with Cushing's disease. J Clin Endocrinol Metab. 1987;64:1150–9.
106. Guilhaume B, Bertagna X, Thomsen M, Bricaire C, Vila-Porcile E, Olivier L, et al. Transsphenoidal pituitary surgery for the treatment of Cushing's disease: results in 64 patients and long-term followup studies. J Clin Endocrinol Metab. 1987;6:1056–64.
107. Mampalam TJ, Tyrrell B, Wilson CB. Transsphenoidal surgery for Cushing's disease. Ann Intern Med. 1988;109:487–93.
108. Pieters GFFM, Hermus ARMM, Meijer E, Smals AG, Kloppenborg PW. Predictive factors for initial cure and relapse rate after pituitary surgery for Cushing's disease. J Clin Endocrinol Metab. 1989;69:1122–6.
109. Arnott RD, Pestell RG, Mckelvie PA, Henderson JK, McNeill PM, Alford FP. A critical evaluation of transsphenoidal pituitary surgery in the treatment of Cushing's disease: prediction of outcome. Acta Endocrinol. 1990;123:423–30.
110. Burke CW, Adams CBT, Esiri MM, Morris C, Bevan JS. Transsphenoidal surgery for Cushing's disease: does what is removed determine the outcome? Clin Endocrinol. 1990;33:525–37.
111. Tindall GT, Herring CJ, Clark RV, Adams DA, Watts NB. Cushing's disease: results of transsphenoidal surgery with an emphasis on surgical failures. J Neurosurg. 1990;92:363–9.
112. Ludecke DK. Transnasal microsurgery of Cushing's disease. Pathol Res Pract. 1991;187:608–12.
113. Lindholm J. Endocrine function in patients with Cushing's disease before and after treatment. Clin Endocrinol. 1992;36:151–9.
114. McCance DR, Russell CF, Kennedy TL, Hadden DR, Kennedy L, Atkinson AB. Bilateral adrenalectomy: low mortality and morbidity in Cushing's disease. Clin Endocrinol. 1993;39:315–21.
115. Bochicchio D, Losa M, Buchfelder M. Factors influencing the immediate and late outcome of Cushing's disease by transsphenoidal surgery: a retrospective study by the European Cushing's Disease study Group. J Clin Endocrinol Metab. 1995;80:3114–20.
116. Bakiri F, Tatai S, Aouali R, Semrouni M, Derome P, Chitour F, et al. Treatment of Cushing's disease by transsphenoidal, pituitary microsurgery: prognosis factors and long-term follow-up. J Endocrinol Invest. 1996;19:572–80.
117. Sonino N, Zielezny M, Fava GA, Fallo F, Boscaro M. Risk factors and long-term outcome in pituitary-dependent Cushing's disease. J Clin Endocrinol Metab. 1996;81:2647–52.
118. Blevins Jr LS, Christy JH, Khajavi M, Tindall GT. Outcomes of therapy for Cushing's disease due to adrenocorticotropin-secreting pituitary macroadenoma. J Clin Endocrinol Metab. 1998;83:63–71.
119. Estrada J, Garcia-Uria JL, Lamas C, et al. The complete normalization of the adrenocortical function as the criteria of cure after transsphenoidal surgery for Cushing's disease. J Clin Endocrinol Metab. 2001;86:5695–9.

120. Rollin GAFS, Ferreira NP, Junges M, et al. Dynamics of serum cortisol levels after transsphenoidal surgery in a cohort of patients with Cushing's disease. J Clin Endocrinol Metab. 2004;89:1131–9.
121. Storr HL, Afshar F, Matson M, Sabin I, Davies KM, Evanson J, et al. Factors influencing cure by transsphenoidal selective adenomectomy in pediatric Cushing's disease. Eur J Endocrinol. 2005;152:825–33.
122. Pouratian N, Prevedello DM, Jagannathan J, Lopes MB, Vance ML, Laws Jr ER. Outcomes and management of patients with Cushing's disease without pathological confirmation of tumor resection after transsphenoidal surgery. J Clin Endocrinol Metab. 2007;92:3383–8.
123. Carrasco CA, Coste J, Guignat L, Groussin L, Dugue MA, Gaillard S, et al. Midnight salivary cortisol determination for assessing the outcome of transsphenoidal surgery in Cushing's disease. J Clin Endocrinol Metab. 2008;93:4228–34.
124. Watts NB, Tindall GT. Rapid assessment of corticotropin reserve after pituitary surgery. JAMA. 1988;259:708–11.
125. Jayasena CN, Gadhvi KA, Gobel B, et al. Day 5 morning cortisol predicts hypothalamic-pituitary-adrenal function after transsphenoidal surgery for pituitary tumors. Clinical Chem. 2009;55:972–7.
126. Marko NE, Gonugunta VA, Hamrahian AH, Usmani A, Mayberg M, Weil RJ. Use of morning serum cortisol level after transsphenoidal surgery to predict the need for long-term glucocorticoid supplementation. J Neurosurg. 2009;111:540–4.
127. Snow K, Jiang NS, Kao PC, Scheithauer BW. Biochemical evaluation of adrenal dysfunction: the laboratory perspective. Mayo Clin Proc. 1992;67:1055–65.
128. Haag E, Asplund K, Lithner E. Value of basal plasma cortisol assays in the assessment of pituitary-adrenal insufficiency. Clin Endocrinol. 1987;26:221–6.
129. Stewart PM, Corrie J, Seckl JR, et al. A rational approach for assessing the hypothalamic-pituitary-adrenal axis. Lancet. 1988;1:1208–10.
130. Kazlauskaite R, Evans AT, Villabona CV, et al. Corticotropin tests for hypothalamic-pituitary-adrenal insufficiency: a metaanalysis. J Clin Endocrinol Metab. 2008;93:4245–53.
131. Karaca Z, Tanriverdi F, Atmaca H, et al. Can basal cortisol measurements be an alternative to the insulin tolerance test in the assessment of the hypothalamic-pituitary-adrenal axis before and after pituitary surgery? Eur J Endocrinol. 2010;163:377–82.
132. Semple PL, Laws Jr ER. Complications in a contemporary series of patients who underwent transsphenoidal surgery for Cushing's disease. J Neurosurg. 1999;91:175–9.
133. Ciric I, Ragin A, Baumgartner C, Pierce D. Complications of transsphenoidal surgery: results of a national survey, review of the literature, and personal experience. Neurosurgery. 1997;40:225–36. discussion 236–227.
134. Batra PS, Citardi MJ, Lanza DC. Isolated sphenoid sinusitis after transsphenoidal hypophysectomy. Am J Rhinol. 2005;19:185–9.
135. Patil CG et al. Late recurrences of Cushing's disease after initial successful transsphenoidal surgery. J Clin Endocrinol Metab. 2008;93:358–62.
136. Kitano M, Taneda M, Shimono T, Nakao Y. Extended transsphenoidal approach for surgical management of pituitary adenomas invading the cavernous sinus. J Neurosurg. 2008;108:26–36.
137. Koizumi M, et al. Successful treatment of Cushing's disease caused by ectopic intracavernous microadenoma. Pituitary. 2010;13:95–104.

Chapter 10
Postoperative Management and Assessment of Cure

Mary Lee Vance

Abstract Cushing's disease is best treated with surgical removal of the ACTH-producing adenoma. The optimal outcome is a decline in serum cortisol to subnormal, ideally to <1 μg/dl, immediately after surgery. Different remission criteria have been proposed, with alternatives in testing and use of postoperative glucocorticoid replacement; this chapter outlines our post-operative management algorithm as currently practiced. Classical management and an "ideal" situation are discussed.

Keywords Adrenocorticotropic hormone • ACTH-producing adenoma • Cortisol • Pituitary adenoma • Glucocorticoid

Introduction

Cushing's disease is best treated with surgical removal of the ACTH-producing adenoma [1]. The optimal outcome is a decline in serum cortisol to subnormal, ideally to <1 μg/dl, immediately after surgery. Postoperative management is dependent on several factors including the size of the pituitary adenoma, the amount of normal pituitary gland removed, steroid administration at the time of surgery and afterward, and the skill and expertise of the neurosurgeon. Classical management and an "ideal" situation are discussed. There is no one best way to manage patients in the postoperative period, and there are different methods of assessing "cure" or remission.

M.L. Vance (✉)
Department of Medicine, University of Virginia Health System,
P.O. Box 800601, Charlottesville, VA 22908, USA
e-mail: mlv@virginia.edu

The usual discussion of postoperative management focuses on assessment of cortisol production after surgery, medical treatment with a glucocorticoid, dose and duration of treatment, methods to assess recovery of the hypothalamic–pituitary–adrenal (HPA) axis and need for other hormone replacement therapy or therapies. While these are important, a unique aspect of recovery from Cushing's disease that is rarely discussed is the delay in recovery from the effects of the disease, despite prompt biochemical remission. Ongoing symptoms may include fatigue, new onset myalgias, arthralgias, persistent muscle weakness, and neuropsychological difficulties such as problems with memory and concentration, and persistent depression. This consequence of successful treatment is not simple to either quantify or treat, particularly because of the variability among patients' symptoms and severity of disease. Although there are no specific tests or treatments for these conditions (caution patients not to go to a "pain clinic" where a steroid injection is the usual practice), the physician should inform the patient of these possibilities before surgery and provide support when these symptoms occur. After successful surgery, the patient should be reminded that these symptoms are expected and they will improve gradually over time. Many patients report that it takes 6–12 months or more to return to normal functioning. It is likely that the time to recovery and degree of recovery is dependent upon the duration of disease, the severity of disease and the comorbidities (hypertension, diabetes mellitus, osteoporosis, myopathy), but there are no prospective studies to support this opinion. For additional discussion of these issues, see Chap. 18.

Factors Influencing Postoperative Management

Preoperative Adenoma Size

The majority of patients with Cushing's disease have a microadenoma (<10 mm), and often a tumor is not visible on the MRI study. This may require surgical exploration of the entire gland. In this situation, the ideal is removal of the adenoma with removal of a minimal amount of normal pituitary tissue. Surgical expertise is variable, and it is not possible to know how much normal functioning pituitary remains after surgery; this is usually assessed 6–8 weeks later. In the less common situation of a macroadenoma, complete resection is ideal, but if the tumor has invaded the dura or cavernous sinus or sinuses, complete resection and remission is less likely. If there is obvious cavernous sinus invasion, the patient should be informed before the operation, that additional treatment may be required after the bulk of the tumor is removed.

Postoperative Steroid Replacement

If the patient is not given a steroid at the time of surgery, serial serum cortisol measurements (every 6 h) are useful to determine the outcome of surgery and whether the patient requires steroid replacement on discharge from the hospital. If glucocorticoid is administered at the time of surgery and afterward, assessment of the response to surgery will be delayed. However, since many patients are discharged within 24–48 h, serial inpatient sampling may not be possible, and coverage with steroids is necessary to avoid symptomatic and potentially dangerous hypoadrenalism in the outpatient setting. Some endocrinologists choose low-dose dexamethasone for a few days so that outpatient assessment of remission can proceed without interrupting steroid replacement; for a discussion of this approach see Chap. 9.

Amount of Normal Pituitary Tissue Removed

If no obvious tumor is seen at operation, some neurosurgeons recommend removal of one-half of the pituitary gland (hemihypophysectomy), based on lateralization from the preoperative inferior petrosal sinus sampling. In some circumstances, the entire pituitary is removed. In these situations the risk of postoperative diabetes insipidus and anterior pituitary hormone deficiencies is increased and should be anticipated. In addition to the potential need for steroid replacement, patients should be followed carefully for postoperative polyuria and polydipsia with measurement of serum and urine osmolality and given desmopressin as indicated by the results. Because thyroid hormone is protein-bound, the decline in the serum thyroid hormone level is slow and serum Free T4 should be measured 6–8 weeks after surgery. Assessment of gonadal function can also be performed at this time, by measurement of testosterone in men and obtaining a postoperative menstrual history in premenopausal women. Delayed decline in serum IGF-1 also occurs and evaluation of growth hormone production should be delayed for 6–8 weeks. If other axes are deficient, growth hormone testing is postponed until the patient is on adequate replacement.

Definition of Remission from Cushing's Disease

Clinical improvement is an important part of assessing remission after surgery. However, because the degree of improvement is highly variable and often slow, particularly weight loss, this cannot be the main criterion for remission. Remission is defined in biochemical terms.

The biochemical criteria for remission are several; there is no one best test to recommend. There are no comparative studies in patients with Cushing's disease that determine which test is the most accurate [2–7]. Table 10.1 lists the most commonly used tests to determine if the patient is in remission and if the patient requires continued glucocorticoid replacement.

Some centers test for remission and assess the need for glucocorticoid replacement off all steroid replacement. Considering the half-life of glucocorticoid preparations,

Table 10.1 Remission: postoperative tests of hypothalamic–pituitary–adrenal (HPA) function[a]

Test	Result	Utility/interpretation
Serum cortisol	<2 µg/dl, <1 µg/dl	Remission; need for steroid replacement
Plasma ACTH	Low or normal	Questionable remission; interdeterminate
1 mg overnight dexamethasone	Cortisol: <1.8 µg/dl	Remission
Morning, 11 p.m. serum cortisol (inpatient)	Normal circadian rhythm	Remission; discontinue steroid replacement
24 h urine free cortisol	Normal	Best to assess cortisol overproduction; if undetectable may be suggestive of remission
ACTH stimulation test	Subnormal cortisol (<18 µg/dl)	Remission; continue steroid replacement
ACTH stimulation test	Normal cortisol (18 µg/dl or greater)	Discontinue steroid replacement
Insulin hypoglycemia test (ITT)[a]	Subnormal cortisol (<18 µg/dl)	Remission; continue steroid replacement
Insulin hypoglycemia test (ITT)[a]	Normal cortisol (18 µg/dl or greater)	Discontinue steroid replacement

[a]Usually performed off glucocorticoid replacement, or on nonsuppressive doses of dexamethasone

2–3 days off of hydrocortisone, 3–4 days off of prednisone and 4–5 days off of dexamethasone is usually adequate. While patients may feel fatigued during this time, hypotension and hyponatremia do not usually occur because aldosterone secretion is preserved. Other centers prefer to continue low-dose dexamethasone in the immediate postoperative period during assessment for remission, as discussed in Chap. 9.

Since elevated preoperative cortisol levels have usually suppressed normal ACTH producing cells (with a variable time to recovery), after removal of the adenoma an undetectable serum cortisol indicates removal of the tumor and physiologic suppression of the normal ACTH cells: remission. Some investigators have considered remission after surgery as a serum cortisol of <1 or 2 µg/dl (off of glucocorticoid for an adequate time) in conjunction with a normal or low plasma ACTH level. Some investigators perform a 1 mg overnight dexamethasone test several weeks after surgery to document a subnormal cortisol level (<2.8, 2.5 or <1 µg/dl). Early morning and 11 p.m. or midnight serum cortisol levels have been used to determine if there is a normal circadian rhythm of cortisol secretion. This test usually requires hospitalization and is not practical in most settings. Absence of a cortisol response to exogenous ACTH, most commonly 250 µg intravenously, with measurement of cortisol before administration, and 30 and 60 min later is usually indicative of remission. If this test is performed immediately after surgery, the hyperplastic adrenal glands are likely to respond. Therefore, this test is best performed 6–8 weeks after the operation. Measurement of 24 h urine free cortisol (UFC) concentration has been used to assess remission. This may be problematic because partial removal of an adenoma may reduce 24 h UFC to the normal range, yet the patient still has residual tumor. Additionally, this test is best used to assess cortisol overproduction

10 Postoperative Management and Assessment of Cure

and many normal subjects have a low 24 h UFC. However, undetectable or extremely low levels may be suggestive of remission, especially when combined with other test results. Because about 5% of patients may have a delayed decline in cortisol after surgery, continued testing for a longer period of time than usual is advised if there is a progressive decrease in levels following surgery [8]. Remission criteria as employed in the major surgical series are reviewed in Chap. 9, Table 9.3.

Achievement of remission, by any criterion or criteria, is not always predictive of continued remission. There is always a risk of recurrence, as occurs with all types of pituitary adenomas, emphasizing the need for long term follow up.

Postoperative Management

Classical Postoperative Management

In many centers, a patient with Cushing's disease is given a steroid (hydrocortisone, dexamethasone) at the time of surgery and afterward. Determination of the outcome of surgery and need for continued steroid replacement is usually delayed until several weeks after the operation. This is a safe method to protect the patient from secondary adrenal insufficiency and avoids symptoms associated with a precipitous decline in the cortisol level. It may also delay assessment of the outcome of surgery and may prolong recovery. There is no one best steroid regimen, but at our institution dexamethasone is avoided because of the long biological effect (up to 3 days) that may lead to an overlap of drug when given daily and prolongation of recovery. Intravenous hydrocortisone, 50 or 100 mg, can be given at the time of surgery and every 6 or 8 h afterward for 24–48 h, followed by oral hydrocortisone upon discharge from the hospital; its use as replacement requires discontinuation to assess remission. If the patient suffers severe steroid withdrawal symptoms, a supraphysiologic dose of hydrocortisone, 40 mg on awakening and 20 mg at 6 p.m., can be given for 1–2 weeks, with reduction to 20 mg on awakening and 10 mg at 6 p.m. until the postoperative outpatient evaluation. Six to eight weeks after surgery, the patient is asked to stop the hydrocortisone for 2–3 days for the postoperative assessment (discussed below). Other centers begin low-dose dexamethasone on the first postoperative day after a fasting cortisol level has been obtained. For a discussion of this alternative approach, see Chap. 9.

Ideal Situation

The patient has a visible microadenoma on MRI, the neurosurgeon is an expert in pituitary operations, the patient is not given steroid coverage at the time of surgery, the hospital laboratory provides a rapid turnaround time (1–2 h) for serum cortisol measurements and the nursing personnel are experienced in postoperative care and recognition of symptoms and signs of adrenal insufficiency. If these requirements are not realistic or possible, the following recommendations are not safe for the patient.

In the assessment algorithm as currently practiced at our institution, no steroid is administered before or after surgery, and serum cortisol is measured every 6 h after the operation (with cortisol results available within 1–2 h) to assess the outcome of the operation. With successful tumor removal, the serum cortisol usually declines over 24–48 h in most patients [9]. During this decline in serum cortisol, the patient often reports headache, malaise, and nausea. When the serum cortisol declines to 2 µg/dl or lower, an intravenous dose of hydrocortisone, 50 or 100 mg, is administered, and oral hydrocortisone is instituted (recommend: 40 mg on awakening, 20 mg at 6 p.m. initially). The patient is discharged on this supraphysiologic dose for 1–2 weeks with a decrease to 20 mg on awakening and 10 mg at 6 p.m. until the postoperative clinic visit (usually 6–8 weeks after surgery). Two to three days before the postoperative clinic visit, the patient is instructed to hold the hydrocortisone for measurement of ACTH and cortisol levels. If the cortisol level remains low, the hydrocortisone is restarted at a dose of 15 mg on awakening and 5 mg at 6 pm (physiologic replacement) and the patient is retested (off of hydrocortisone for 2–3 days) about 2 months later. The cycle is repeated if the cortisol is again low. Most patients can discontinue hydrocortisone 3–6 months after successful surgery (presuming adequate normal pituitary tissue remains). This is a general observation, not a rule, and some patients may take a year or more to recover, if ever (depending on the amount of normal pituitary gland removed). While this is one approach, it is important to emphasize that there are few data about the optimal postoperative management, and many centers use other steroid preparations and other algorithms. The goal is to provide the lowest glucocorticoid dose that the patient will tolerate, both to allow resolution of Cushingoid features as well as to allow recovery of the HPA axis. Other assessments 6–8 weeks after surgery should include measurement of serum Free T4, IGF-1, testosterone (men) and assessment of menstrual function in pre-menopausal women. These assessments provide valuable information regarding residual pituitary function. In the case of premenopausal women, return of menses may take 3–6 months.

Need for Continued Glucocorticoid Replacement

Measurement of serum cortisol and ACTH levels after discontinuation of glucocorticoid for several days may be all that is necessary to determine if glucocorticoid replacement needs to be continued. At our center, we discontinue glucocorticoid replacement if the serum cortisol level is normal (e.g. >10 µg/dl) and the ACTH is not suppressed, although other centers require a higher threshold (see Chap. 9 for additional discussion and criteria as described in the literature.) These baseline measurements do not assess ACTH reserve during times of stress (intercurrent illness) and administration of ACTH can also used to determine the continued need for glucocorticoid replacement. One caveat regarding the ACTH stimulation test is that it only tests adrenal responsiveness to ACTH with the *presumption* that a normal cortisol response indicates sufficient endogenous ACTH secretion to maintain adrenal responsiveness. It is not known exactly how much ACTH secretion is needed to maintain adrenal responsiveness or how much is required during times of stress. A subnormal cortisol response to exogenous ACTH indicates need for continued glucocorticoid therapy. The most rigorous test of HPA function is insulin-induced hypoglycemia (insulin tolerance test, ITT), which stimulates the entire HPA axis. This test is also the most rigorous test to determine if the patient has growth hormone deficiency. The ITT must be conducted with a physician present and is contraindicated in patients with coronary artery disease, seizure disorder or generalized debility.

Conclusion

Successful treatment of Cushing's disease results in the lowering of cortisol production to subnormal or undetectable levels requiring glucocorticoid replacement. Because it is not possible to predict how long glucocorticoid replacement is needed, patients should be tested 6–8 weeks after surgery and every 2–3 months thereafter. While biochemical recovery may be prompt, the physical and emotional recovery from Cushing's disease is usually prolonged.

References

1. Arnaldi G, Angeli A, Atkinson AB, et al. Diagnosis and complications of Cushing's syndrome: aconsensus statement. J Clin Endocrinol Metab. 2003;88:5593–602.
2. Chen JC, Amar AP, Choi S, Singer P, Couldwell WT, Weiss MH. Transsphenoidal microsurgical treatment of Cushing disease: postoperative assessment of surgical efficacy by application on a overnight low-dose dexamethasone suppression test. J Neurosurg. 2003;98:967–73.
3. Czepielewski MA, Rollin GA, Casagrande A, Ferreira NP. Criteria of cure and remission in Cushing's disease: an update. Arq Bras Endocrinol Metab. 2007;51:1362–72.
4. Estrada J, Garcia-Uria J, Lamas C, et al. The complete normalization of the adrenocortical function as the criterion of cure after transsphenoidal surgery for Cushing's disease. J Clin Endocrinol Metab. 2001;86:5695–9.
5. Imaki T, Tsushima T, Hizuka N, Odagiri E, Murata Y, Suda T, et al. Plasma cortisol levels predict long-term outcome in patients with Cushing's disease and determine which patients should be treated with pituitary irradiation after surgery. Endocr J. 2001;48:53–62.
6. McCance DR, Gordon DS, Fannin TF, et al. Assessment of endocrine function after transsphenoidal surgery for Cushing's disease. Clin Endocrinol (Oxf). 1993;38:79–86.
7. Yap LB, Turner HE, Adams CB, Wass JA. Undetectable postoperative cortisol does not always predict long-term remission in Cushing's disease: a single centre audit. Clin Endocrinol (Oxf). 2002;56:19–21.
8. Valassi E, Biller BM, Swearingen B, PecoriGiraldi F, Losa M, Mortini P, et al. Delayed remission after transsphenoidal surgery in patients with Cushing's disease. J Clin Endocrinol Metab. 2010;95(2):601–10. Epub 2010 Jan 15.
9. Simmons NE, Alden TD, Thorner MO, Laws ER. Serum cortisol response to transsphenoidal surgery for Cushing disease. J Neurosurg. 2001;95:1–8.

Chapter 11
Radiation Therapy in the Management of Cushing's Disease

Kevin S. Oh, Helen A. Shih, and Jay S. Loeffler

Abstract Radiation therapy is most commonly offered to patients with Cushing's disease who are incompletely treated after transsphenoidal surgery because of residual or recurrent disease. Retrospective data suggest that both fractionated External Beam Radiation Therapy (EBRT) and single-fraction Stereotactic Radiosurgery (SRS) offer biochemical remission rates of 50–80%. SRS appears to normalize hormonal levels more rapidly than fractionated EBRT and should be offered when technically feasible. Hypopituitarism is common and expected after pituitary irradiation. Other late side effects are uncommon.

Keywords Adrenocorticotropic hormone • Fractionation schedules • Radiation therapy • Fractionated external beam radiation therapy • Stereotactic radiosurgery

Introduction

Pituitary irradiation in the treatment of Cushing's disease has a long history as an effective strategy for biochemical normalization and local control, but is generally considered second-line therapy after transsphenoidal resection. Upfront resection has the advantage of providing immediate adrenocorticotropic hormone (ACTH) normalization in 70–90% of cases. However, relapse after initially successful resection occurs in 11–17% of cases [1–3]. Because of the serious implications of progressive disease on metabolism, and possibly vision, the most common indication for radiation therapy is persistent or recurrent Cushing's disease after surgery. Other indications for radiation therapy include invasive or subtotally resected

K.S. Oh (✉)
Department of Radiation Oncology, Massachusetts General Hospital,
100 Blossom Street, Cox 3, Boston, MA 02114, USA
e-mail: KOh2@partners.org

disease, medical contraindications to transsphenoidal surgery, and in some centers, prophylaxis of Nelson's syndrome after bilateral adrenalectomy. This chapter reviews the fractionation schedules, technology, remission rates, and late effects of radiation therapy for Cushing's disease.

Fractionation Schedules and Technology in Radiation Therapy

Fractionation refers to the number of radiation treatments (or "fractions") and the dose per fraction. Laboratory and clinical data suggest that higher dose per fraction increases the relative biological equivalence (RBE) for both tumor and normal tissues. RBE is used to compare the biologic effect for various types or schedules of radiation. For example, 10 Gy delivered in a single fraction would have a greater biologic effect than five fractions of 2 Gy each. The balance between maximizing tumor control and minimizing injury to normal surrounding tissue is the major determinant in selecting standard fractionation or stereotactic hypofractionated radiation therapy in the treatment of pituitary adenomas.

Fractionated External Beam Radiation Therapy

Standard fractionated external beam radiation therapy (EBRT) refers to the delivery of 1.8–2 Gy per day, generally 5 days per week. The total recommended dose for ACTH-producing pituitary adenomas is 45–50.4 Gy. The advantages of fractionated EBRT over stereotactic radiosurgery (SRS) include its widespread availability and theoretical reduction in the risk for late complications with smaller doses per fraction. Fractionated photon EBRT is delivered by a linear accelerator (Linac) and is considered the mainstay of all radiation therapy practices. Prior to treatment, a thermoplastic mesh mask is fitted to the patient's facial contour to immobilize the head and minimize localization uncertainty to within 3–5 mm.

Three-dimensional conformal radiation therapy (3D-CRT) refers to treatment planning based on axial imaging (such as CT or MRI) to delineate the tumor and normal tissues, visualize beam trajectory, and calculate dose in three-dimensional space. For 3D-CRT, CT simulation is performed in the treatment position and images acquired for treatment planning. IV contrast during image acquisition is not required, but often helpful for definition of both tumor and normal tissues, such as the optic chiasm in relation to the pituitary infundibulum and middle cerebral arteries. Fusion with previously obtained pituitary protocol MRI sequences is commonly performed. During simulation and treatment, the head is flexed toward the upper chest. The standard 3-field arrangement of beams consists of opposed laterals that enter the brain from left and right and an anterior superior oblique ("vertex") beam from above. The lateral fields are often modified using wedges, which are triangular metal pieces placed in front of the beam path to improve dose homogeneity. However, with this arrangement, unacceptable "hot spots" may still remain within the temporal lobes. The dose distribution may be improved by instead using unopposed superior lateral beams. Another common technique for small tumors involves bilateral coronal 110° arcs with wedges [4, 5]. For complex tumor shapes, inverse-planned intensity modulated radiation therapy (IMRT) may allow improved sparing of normal tissue. In contrast to 3D-CRT, inversed-planned IMRT relies on the physician inputting the goals of therapy into software that uses a continuous process of evaluation and iteration until an optimized pattern of beamlet intensities is achieved. However, in most pituitary adenoma cases, IMRT is not required because the target has a regular shape and the total dose does not exceed normal tissue tolerances. Beam energy should be 6–10 MV.

Stereotactic Radiosurgery

The term "stereotactic" describes a system that defines a target volume and uses a highly accurate and reproducible three-dimensional coordinate system for localization. The term "radiosurgery" refers to the delivery of radiation in a single treatment. Together, stereotactic radiosurgery (SRS) is the delivery of a high dose of radiation at a single sitting to a small target that can be safely given only within the confines of a fixed, accurate, and reproducible coordinate system. If the radiation dose is divided over several treatments using such a system, this is more appropriately termed "fractionated stereotactic radiation therapy" (FSRT). One universal requirement of stereotactic treatments is the creation of a steep gradient between high-dose regions (within the target) and low-dose regions (normal tissues) immediately adjacent to the target. Therefore, the volume of surrounding normal tissue irradiated is generally lower with SRS or FSRT compared to standard 3D-CRT. In many cases, pituitary adenomas are well suited for SRS because they are often small, well circumscribed, and spherical. There are several commercially available stereotactic systems, the most common of which are Gamma knife (GK; Elekta, Stockholm, Sweden) and linear accelerated-based systems.

Gamma Knife

Gamma knife was the first SRS system, devised in 1951 by Lars Leksell, MD, a Swedish neurosurgeon. After several years of development, the first GK facility opened in the late 1960s, initially for the treatment of functional lesions such as trigeminal neuralgia and later of benign conditions, such as arteriovenous malformations. Because of its favorable local control and side effect profile, the medical indications for GK quickly broadened to include other small volume intracranial targets including pituitary adenomas. With this long-history, GK-based SRS has the most widely published experience for the treatment of pituitary adenomas. The radioisotope within GK is cobalt-60, which has an average energy of 1.25 MV and half-life of 5.5 years. The patient's head is placed in a metal helmet used for immobilization and distancing from the sources. The treatment head is comprised of 201 cobalt-60 sources distributed in a hemispheric array behind bores, which are removable columns that can be systematically removed to allow beam arrays to converge at a spherical isocenter. In Linac-based treatments, the "isocenter" is the point around which the radiation treatment machine rotates. Because the GK contains multiple fixed cobalt-60 sources, the term "isocenter" refers to the target. The bores vary in diameter to modulate the width of the beams. Special "plugging" is used with GK treatment of adenomas to reduce the exposure to the optic apparatus. To conform to irregular-shaped targets, several adjacent or overlapping isocenters are required. For GK, the prescribed dose is typically 15–35 Gy × 1. The term "isodose" refers to the area in a radiation plan that receives equivalent dose. GK plans typically surround the tumor with and prescribe the intended dose to the 50% isodose line. This implies that portions of the tumor receive twice the prescribed dose. These areas of high dose above the prescribed dose are often referred to as "hot spots." As such, GK plans have the potential to be more conformal (i.e., closely shaped around the target), but less homogeneous than linac-based SRS.

Linear Accelerator-Based Stereotactic Radiosurgery

Linac-based SRS uses the standard linear accelerator that is widely available in radiation therapy practices, but requires special equipment to adapt the beam profile for use in treating small volumes, as well as formal commissioning prior to use. The radiation beam from a linac can be shaped either by circular cones or multileaf collimators (MLCs) located at the end of the beam path. Historically, submillimeter immobilization is achieved with a rigid stereotactic head frame that is surgically fixed to the calvarium under local anesthesia using four pins above the level of the brow. With the frame in place, a thin-cut CT scan is acquired for treatment planning. After pretreatment quality assurance, the same frame setup is used to position the patient on the treatment unit. MRI brain images are often fused with the CT scan to improve tumor definition. Treatment planning can use static fields, dynamic arcs, step-and-shoot pseudoarcs, or a combination of these strategies [6]. In static field plans, radiation is delivered through several fixed gantry positions. When using dynamic arcs, radiation is continuously delivered while the gantry is moving. Step-and-shoot pseudoarcs refer to an intermediate strategy of using multiple static fields in a pattern resembling an arc. Like most intracranial treatments, lower photon energies are preferable (~6 MV). Linac-based SRS plans are generally more homogeneous (lower hot spots) than those seen with GK. However, when using cones to treat irregularly shaped targets, the conformality may be inferior to MLC- or GK-based SRS. For linac-based therapy, the prescription dose is typically 12–20 Gy × 1 to the 80–90% isodose line.

Choosing Between Fractionated EBRT and SRS

When feasible, SRS is generally preferred to EBRT because of its convenience, ability to provide faster hormonal control of secretory adenomas [7], and favorable side-effect profile [8]. However, not all patients are candidates for SRS. The optimal tumor size for SRS is ≤3 cm, beyond which the dosimetric advantages rapidly diminish. In SRS for pituitary adenomas, the optic chiasm is the normal tissue of greatest concern because of its crucial function and proximity to the pituitary gland. As a rule of thumb, the target volume should be ≥5–10 mm from the optic chiasm to ensure adequate sparing. When delivered as a single fraction, dosage to the optic apparatus should be limited to 8–10 Gy in a single fraction [9]. If this requirement cannot be met, then standard fractionated EBRT should be used to reduce the risk of late complications. Using standard fractionation, the optic chiasm should be limited to ≤54 Gy, which is easily achieved with the recommended total dose for Cushing's disease.

Fractionated Stereotactic Radiotherapy

Fractionated stereotactic radiotherapy (FSRT) is an intermediate strategy that combines the submillimeter immobilization of SRS with the multifraction treatment schedule of standard fractionated EBRT. FSRT is indicated when rigid immobilization is beneficial, but large tumor size or intimate proximity to a critical normal tissue (e.g., optic chiasm) makes single-fraction SRS unsafe. Because of the protracted treatment schedule, a noninvasive frame is typically used. For example, at the Massachusetts General Hospital (MGH), immobilization is achieved with a dental mold fixed to a stereotactic frame. FSRT fractionation schedules for pituitary adenomas are most commonly 1.8–2 Gy per day over 5–6 weeks, but some have used hypofractionated schedules.

Proton Therapy

In recent years, proton and other heavy-charged-particle therapies have gained considerable interest because of their ability to minimize exit dose. Similar to photon therapy for pituitary adenomas, protons can be used to deliver standard fractionation, single-fraction stereotactic radiosurgery (PSRS), or fractionated stereotactic radiotherapy (PSRT), with the same concepts noted above. Unlike standard photon therapy, the energy transferred from protons increases to a maximum as the particles' velocity slow near the end of their range, thereby creating a "Bragg peak," which is a sharp falloff of dose. Because the radiation dose immediately past the Bragg peak is minimized, this may be used to improve target conformality and increase relative biological effectiveness. Radiation doses in proton therapy are often referred to as "Cobalt Gray Equivalents" (CGE), which are biologically equivalent to the term "gray" in photon therapy nomenclature. The elimination of exit dose reduces the integral low- and medium-doses to uninvolved brain tissue and, therefore, theoretically improves the risk of neurocognitive dysfunction and second tumor formation when compared to photon therapy. This dosimetric advantage is particularly important for larger volume pituitary adenomas that require treatment of the entire sella or extrasellar regions. It should be noted, however, that prospective clinical data is currently lacking. At the MGH proton facility, immobilization for PSRS and PSRT utilizes the MGH-modified Gill-Thomas-Cosman frame (Integra-Radionics Inc. Burlington, MA), which relies on integrated custom dental molds for precise setup. For patients with poor dentition or base of skull tumors, an alternative mask is used. At MGH, three fiducial markers are placed in the outer table of the skull prior to CT simulation to define the reference coordinates. The widespread use of proton therapy is limited by the expense and complexity of constructing and maintaining these centers, but a number are under construction nationwide.

Interstitial Brachytherapy

"Brachytherapy" refers to the use of implantable or indwelling radiation sources to deliver high radiation doses over a short distance. Transphenoidally implanted radioactive-labeled seeds have also been used with considerable success for ACTH-secreting adenomas. The most common isotopes used are yttrium-90 (Y-90) and gold-198 (Au-198). Sandler et al. published the largest series of 82 patients using both isotopes. The crude remission rate was 77% at a mean follow-up interval of 10.5 years [10]. A similar experience from Molinatti et al. reported complete remission in 57/76 (75%) with 100,000–150,000 rad. Brachytherapy is felt to induce remission much faster than other radiation approaches [10–12], but its widespread use is limited because of the invasive procedure and logistical challenges involved.

Target Definition

Approximately 90% of ACTH-producing adenomas are microadenomas that do not distort the sella turcica. Therefore, most cases are difficult to delineate by conventional plain films or CT. A pituitary protocol MRI is required to accurately define anatomy and may still not demonstrate the lesion. With T1-weighted images, the posterior lobe of the pituitary gland is usually high-signal, while the anterior lobe has signal similar to white matter. Pituitary adenomas are typically hypo- or isointense. Adenomas usually are hypoenhancing to non-enhancing after an appropriately timed gadolinium dose. The gross tumor volume (GTV) is volume of the pituitary adenoma as visualized by both CT and MRI. The clinical target volume (CTV) encompasses subclinical microscopic disease and often includes the entire sella or, for advanced lesions, any extension into the sphenoid sinus, cavernous sinus, or other intracranial regions. In standard fractionated photon EBRT, the planning target volume (PTV) includes an additional 3–5 mm expansion to account for setup uncertainty within the thermoplastic mask. In stereotactic treatments and proton therapy, the PTV expansion is often excluded. The organs at risk (OARs) include the globes, lenses, optic nerves, optic chiasm, brain stem, and temporal lobes.

Dose

The recommended fractionated dose for ACTH-producing adenoma is 45–50.4 Gy in 1.8–2 Gy fractions. Retrospective data from Zierhut et al., which included 139 patients with pituitary adenomas of various types, demonstrated a statistically significant dose response favoring ≥45 Gy with respect to disease recurrence (11% vs. 1%) [13]. A similar study described a dose threshold at 40 Gy [14]. A smaller study limited to Cushing's disease reported no difference in remission rates at a threshold of 50 Gy [15]. Low-dose radiation of 20 Gy in 2.5 Gy fractions has been attempted in Cushing's disease with the hopes of reducing the risk of hypopituitarism. However, while initial results were favorable, only 25% remained in remission with longer-term median follow-up of 93 months [16, 17]. For stereotactic radiosurgery, the range of doses used in clinical practice is highly variable. At high dose per fraction, the biological equivalent dose (BED) dramatically increases, such that 20 Gy × 1 is estimated to produce the equivalent clinical effect as 50–110 Gy with standard fractionation [18]. The prescribed marginal dose most commonly used for Cushing's disease and other functioning pituitary adenomas is 18–35 Gy × 1. The prescription isodose line ranges from 50% to 100% depending on whether GK or linac-based SRS is used, implying that there may be considerable hot spots within the target.

Remission After Radiation Therapy

Radiation therapy achieves biochemical control of Cushing's disease in approximately 50–80% of cases whether given as primary treatment or post-operatively. However, the published outcomes after radiation therapy in the treatment of Cushing's disease are limited by wide variability in defining "remission," variable case mix, use of concurrent medical therapy, and lack of prospective data. Most often, remission is considered normalization of urinary free cortisol and/or serum ACTH and cortisol within a specified time period, but does not always account for subsequent relapse. Results of larger retrospective series are summarized in Table 11.1.

Table 11.1 Series of radiation therapy for Cushing's disease

Modality	Year	N	Dose	Remission	Median/mean F/U (years)	Remission criteria
Fractionated photons						
Schteingart et al. [40]	1980	36	40/2 Gy	81%	NR	Clinical and biochemical remission by plasma cortisol, UFC, and plasma ACTH
Howlett et al. [20]	1989	21	45/1.8 Gy	57%	9.5	Mean plasma cortisol throughout day of 300–400 nmol/L
Littley et al. [17].	1990	24	20/2.5 Gy	46%	7.8	Clinical and biochemical remission by UFC and normal serum cortisol diurnal rhythm
Murayama et al. [15]	1992	20	Mean 53.9/1.5–2.5 Gy	55%	7	Clinical and biochemical remission by 24-h UFC and serum cortisol level
Hughes et al. [21]	1993	40	45–100 Gy/1.8–5 Gy	59% actuarial	10	Lack of clinical worsening, radiographic progression, and persistent biochemical abnormality
Tsang et al. [41]	1996	29	Median 50/2 Gy	53%	7.3	Radiographic stabilization and normal 24-h UFC
Estrada et al. [19]	1997	30	48–54/1.8–2 Gy	83%	3.5	Regression of clinical syndrome, normal 24-h UFC, and AM plasma cortisol <5 μg/dl after dex 1 mg
Fractionated protons						
Ronson et al. [30]	2006	4 Cushing's/23 total secretory	50.4–55.9/1.8–2 CGE	50/86%	3.9	Hormonal normalization
Helium-ion SRT						
Levy et al. [29]	1991	83	30–150 Gy/3–4 fractions	85%	NR	Normal basal cortisol and dexamethasone test results

Proton SRS						
Petit et al. [31]	2008	33	15–20 CGE × 1	52%	5.2	Normal 24-h UFC
Gamma knife SRS						
Laws and Vance [42]	1999	50	NR	58%	NR	Normal 24-h UFC
Sheehan et al. [25]	2000	43	20 Gy × 1 (median)	63%	3.7	Normal 24-h UFC
Hoybye et al. [33]	2001	18	30–50 Gy × 1	44% (SRS × 1), 83% (SRS × 1–4)	17	Normal 24-h UFC
Kobayashi et al. [43]	2002	20	29 Gy × 1	35%	5.3	ACTH <50 pg/ml; cortisol <10 μg/dl
Castinetti et al. [44]	2007	40	29.5 Gy × 1 (median)	42%	4	Normal 24-h UFC
Jagannathan et al. [45]	2007	90	25 Gy × 1 (median)	54%	3.8	Normal 24-h UFC
Linac-based SRS						
Mitsumori et al. [27]	1998	5	10–15 Gy	40%	3.9	Hormonal abnormality normalization or reduction by 25%

Abbreviations: *UFC* urine free cortisol, *NR* not reported, *CGE* cobalt gray equivalent

Fractionated EBRT

For fractionated EBRT, Estrada et al. reported that 25/30 (83%) cases of Cushing's disease treated with 48–54 Gy in 1.8–2 Gy daily fractions achieved remission, which was defined as meeting three criteria: regression of clinical Cushing's syndrome, normalized urine free cortisol (UFC), and normalized overnight dexamethasone suppression. Actuarial remission rates were 44% at 1 year and 83% at 3 years after radiation. None of these cases relapsed at a median follow-up of 42 months [19]. Howlett et al. described 21 patients uniformly treated to 45 Gy in 1.8 Gy fractions for Cushing's disease and found 57% clinical remission rate off all adrenal blocking therapy at a median follow-up of 9.5 years [20]. Hughes et al. reported outcomes of 40 patients with Cushing's disease treated with 45–100 Gy and found 59% actuarial 10-year progression-free survival, defined as lack of clinical, biochemical, and radiographic recurrence [21]. Childhood Cushing's disease appears to respond very favorably to fractionated EBRT with a response rate of approximately 80% and few late neuroendocrine effects [22–24].

Stereotactic Radiosurgery

After SRS the reported remission rate ranges from 35% to 63%, but the current literature has relatively short follow-up intervals (Table 11.1). One of the largest series was reported by Sheehan et al. and included 43 patients after failed transsphenoidal surgery who were treated with GK to a mean margin dose of 20 Gy (range 3.6–30 Gy). At median follow-up of 44 months, 63% achieved normal or below-normal 24-h urinary free cortisol. However, 3 of 27 patients experienced recurrence [25]. Devin et al. described 35 patients treated with linac-based SRS and reported 49% biochemical control. However, 4/17 patients experienced recurrence [26]. The efficacy of linac-based SRS is felt to be comparable with results from GK SRS for pituitary adenoma, but there are no prospective data on this subject [27, 28].

Heavy-Charged Particles

The pioneering experience of the Lawrence Berkeley Laboratory in treating the pituitary gland with heavy-charged particles was published by Levy et al. [29]. Of 840 patients in their entire series, 83 had Cushing's disease and were treated with helium ion FSRT to doses ranging from 30 to 150 Gy in three to four fractions. In adult patients, 85% (50/59) were considered biochemically cured. Ronson et al. reported the Loma Linda experience of 47 patients with pituitary adenomas treated with fractionated protons to 50.4–55.9 CGE in 1.8–2.0 CGE fractions [30].

Of these, 23 had secretory tumors. With median follow-up of 83 months, 86% achieved biochemical control. However, in the four patients with ACTH-secreting adenomas, two (50%) demonstrated disease progression despite therapy. The recent proton SRS experience of the MGH included 33 patients with Cushing's disease who failed or recurred after transsphenoidal surgery. The median dose was 20 CGE (range 15–20 CGE) prescribed to the 100% isodose line in all but one patient. At median follow-up of 62 months, 52% achieved a complete response, which was defined as radiographic stability and sustained (≥3 months) normalization of urinary free cortisol off medical therapy [31]. An additional 12 patients (36%) who were not "cured" did achieve stable and normalized UFC, but remained on medical therapy.

Latency Period

The latency period, or time until remission, is the primary drawback of radiation therapy compared to surgical resection. During this period, adrenal suppression with medication is typically required. In retrospective series of both standard fractionated EBRT and SRS, there is a wide variation in the reported latency period likely owing to differences in the biochemical criteria used to define remission [8]. After standard fractionation, most successful treatments will cause biochemical normalization within 1–2 years [15, 19]. For example, Estrada et al. reported a mean time to remission of 18 months (range 6–60 months), with 69% of cases within 2 years [19]. In general, SRS is felt to have a shorter time to remission when compared to fractionated EBRT. In a series from the University of Virginia, Sheehan et al. reported a median latency period of 7 months (range 3–48 months), with 78% achieving remission before 1 year [25]. The Joint Center for Radiation Therapy (JCRT) experience included 29 hormonally active adenomas treated with either SRS (10–15 Gy × 1) or FSRT (45 Gy in 25 fractions) and found that the average time to hormonal normalization was 8.5 vs. 18 months, respectively [27]. For this reason, SRS is often recommended over fractionated schedules when technically feasible.

Late Effects After Radiation Therapy

The risk of late complications after radiation therapy is related to the proximity of the sella turcica to adjacent normal tissues, including the uninvolved pituitary gland, optic chiasm and nerves, carotid vessels, and brain parenchyma. The incidences of late complications listed below are drawn from experiences of radiation therapy for various subtypes of pituitary adenomas, as their likelihood is related more to radiation dose than tumor histology. Advanced technologies including proton therapy, IMRT, and stereotactic immobilization are used to create a sharper and more reproducible dose penumbra between target and normal tissues to minimize these risks.

Hypopituitarism

Hypopituitarism, or the loss of one or more functions of the hypothalamic-pituitary axis, is the most common late sequela of pituitary irradiation. Many of these patients have preexisting hormonal deficiencies or have had surgical removal of a portion of their gland, which may predispose them to damage from radiation. The risk of new hypopituitarism in the literature ranges from 20% to 60% at 5 years for both fractionated and stereotactic radiation therapy. Estrada et al. reported that 57% of patients developed new growth hormone deficiency after 48–54 Gy in 1.8–2 Gy fractions, with the majority having more than one axis involved [19]. In 47 GH-secreting tumors, Minniti et al. reported new hypopituitarism in various axes in 57% at 5 years and 85% at 15 years after 45–50 Gy [32]. In the SRS literature, Sheehan et al. demonstrated encouraging results with only 16% new hormonal abnormalities after 20 Gy × 1 delivered by GK [25]. However, the median follow-up was less than 4 years. With longer follow-up of 17 years, Hoybye et al. reported 69% hypothyroidism and 100% GH insufficiency in evaluable patients who received SRS [33]. The JCRT experience compared 3-year freedom from newly initiated hormonal replacement after SRS vs. FSRT and found no significant difference (77% for SRS and 80% for FSRT) [27]. Because the pituitary gland itself is the radiation target, subsequent hypopituitarism is often impossible to avoid. However, several dosimetric studies suggest that mean dose to the pituitary [34], infundibulum [35], and hypothalamus [36] may be important predictors of endocrinologic sequelae.

Visual Deficits

The long-term risk of visual changes from fractionated RT alone is 1–2% using recommended total doses of 45–50 Gy [21, 24, 27, 37]. The Royal Marsden Hospital (RMH) experience included 411 patients with pituitary adenomas treated with 45–50 Gy in 25–30 fractions and found 1.5% incidence of visual deterioration at 20 years [37]. A systematic review of 11 series including 1,388 patients treated with fractionated RT concluded 1.7% risk of visual injury [24]. When fractionated radiation therapy was given in the post-operative setting, Hughes et al. reported 3% risk of long-term visual sequela [21]. SRS and fractionated RT seem to have comparable risks of visual deficits. A multicenter SRS experience was compiled by Sheehan et al. and included 1,621 patients within 35 series. Of these, 16 cases (1%) of visual deficits were documented [8]. The majority of these data are obtained from series including multiple types and sizes of pituitary adenomas. It is conceivable that, since the target volume in Cushing's disease is typically quite small, the risk of visual complications is considerably less.

Induction of Secondary Tumors After Radiation

The long-term risk of secondary tumors after fractionated RT for pituitary adenomas is 1–3%, most commonly sarcomas, gliomas, and meningiomas. However, the risk of carcinogenesis is heavily dependent on treatment volume, radiation dose, technique, and elapsed time. Becker et al. reported a secondary tumor rate of 0.8% in a review of 1,388 patients, but these series had relatively short median follow-up intervals (range 3–10.5 years) [24]. The RMH experience concluded a 20-year second tumor rate of 1.9% [37]. In 305 patients, Tsang et al. reported cumulative actuarial risk of secondary glioma of 1.7% at 10 years and 2.7% at 15 years [38]. However, these publications primarily comprised treatment delivered between the 1960s and 1980s when larger treatment volumes and two-dimensional treatment planning was utilized. In the SRS literature summarized by Sheehan et al., there were no reported cases of radiation-induced neoplasms among 1,621 patients [8]. In the modern era, with smaller treatment volumes and a more conformal dose distribution, lower secondary tumor risks may be expected, but insufficient time has elapsed for clinical confirmation.

Radionecrosis

Radionecrosis within the temporal lobes is an uncommon occurrence at the doses typically used for ACTH-secreting adenomas, and this is further minimized with the use of 3D-CRT to improve heterogeneity. In their systematic review of fractionated EBRT, Becker et al. reported a 0.2% risk of radionecrosis [24]. In the 35 series of SRS reviewed by Sheehan et al., there were 13 cases (0.8%) of radiation effect. However, 6 of these had received previous fractionated radiation therapy.

Cerebrovascular Accidents

The late vascular effects of pituitary irradiation are due to the proximity of the sella turcica to the internal carotid artery and its branches within the circle of Willis. Becker et al. reported a crude rate of 6.3% vascular changes in 1,388 patients over 11 series [24]. In one of these series, Brada et al. reported cerebrovascular accidents (CVA) risk of 4% at 5 years, 11% at 10 years, and 21% at 20 years [39]. When compared to the general population, the estimated relative risk was 4.1. However, this study did not include patient and disease-related factors to confirm the causal relationship between radiation and vascular events and lacked details of their clinical significance.

Conclusion

Radiation therapy offers long-term biochemical normalization and radiographic local control in the majority of patients with Cushing's disease for whom transsphenoidal surgery is insufficient. When compared to fractionated EBRT, SRS has the advantage of convenience and potential for shorter latency period to hormonal response. However, the proximity of the gross disease to the optic apparatus may limit the ability to safely offer radiosurgery, although Cushing's microadenomas are usually amenable to SRS. Hypopituitarism is a common and expected sequela of pituitary irradiation, but is correctable with close neuroendocrinologic follow-up. Other late effects of RT including visual deficits, second tumor development, radionecrosis, and CVA have been documented, but are very uncommon.

References

1. Bochicchio D, Losa M, Buchfelder M. Factors influencing the immediate and late outcome of Cushing's disease treated by transsphenoidal surgery: a retrospective study by the European Cushing's Disease Survey Group. J Clin Endocrinol Metab. 1995;80:3114–20.
2. Invitti C, Pecori Giraldi F, de Martin M, Cavagnini F. Diagnosis and management of Cushing's syndrome: results of an Italian multicentre study. Study Group of the Italian Society of Endocrinology on the Pathophysiology of the Hypothalamic-Pituitary-Adrenal Axis. J Clin Endocrinol Metab. 1999;84:440–8.
3. Knappe UJ, Ludecke DK. Persistent and recurrent hypercortisolism after transsphenoidal surgery for Cushing's disease. Acta Neurochir Suppl. 1996;65:31–4.
4. Hallberg F. Pituitary tumors. In: Liebel S, editor. Textbook of radiation oncology. Philadelphia: WB Saunders; 1998. p. 357.
5. Suh JH, Saxton JP. Conventional radiation therapy for skull base tumors: an overview. Neurosurg Clin N Am. 2000;11:575–86.
6. Kooy HM, Nedzi LA, Loeffler JS, et al. Treatment planning for stereotactic radiosurgery of intra-cranial lesions. Int J Radiat Oncol Biol Phys. 1991;21:683–93.
7. Landolt AM, Haller D, Lomax N, et al. Stereotactic radiosurgery for recurrent surgically treated acromegaly: comparison with fractionated radiotherapy. J Neurosurg. 1998;88:1002–8.
8. Sheehan JP, Niranjan A, Sheehan JM, et al. Stereotactic radiosurgery for pituitary adenomas: an intermediate review of its safety, efficacy, and role in the neurosurgical treatment armamentarium. J Neurosurg. 2005;102:678–91.
9. Tishler RB, Loeffler JS, Lunsford LD, et al. Tolerance of cranial nerves of the cavernous sinus to radiosurgery. Int J Radiat Oncol Biol Phys. 1993;27:215–21.
10. Sandler LM, Richards NT, Carr DH, Mashiter K, Joplin GF. Long term follow-up of patients with Cushing's disease treated by interstitial irradiation. J Clin Endocrinol Metab. 1987;65:441–7.
11. Cassar J, Doyle FH, Mashiter K, Joplin GF. Treatment of Cushing's disease in juveniles with interstitial pituitary irradiation. Clin Endocrinol (Oxf). 1979;11:313–21.
12. Molinatti GM, Limone P, Porta M. Treatment of Cushing's disease by interstitial pituitary irradiation: short- and long-term follow-up. Panminerva Med. 1995;37:1–7.
13. Zierhut D, Flentje M, Adolph J, Erdmann J, Raue F, Wannenmacher M. External radiotherapy of pituitary adenomas. Int J Radiat Oncol Biol Phys. 1995;33:307–14.
14. Aristizabal S, Caldwell WL, Avila J. The relationship of time-dose fractionation factors to complications in the treatment of pituitary tumors by irradiation. Int J Radiat Oncol Biol Phys. 1977;2:667–73.

15. Murayama M, Yasuda K, Minamori Y, Mercado-Asis LB, Yamakita N, Miura K. Long term follow-up of Cushing's disease treated with reserpine and pituitary irradiation. J Clin Endocrinol Metab. 1992;75:935–42.
16. Ahmed SR, Shalet SM, Beardwell CG, Sutton ML. Treatment of Cushing's disease with low dose radiation therapy. Br Med J (Clin Res Ed). 1984;289:643–6.
17. Littley MD, Shalet SM, Beardwell CG, Ahmed SR, Sutton ML. Long-term follow-up of low-dose external pituitary irradiation for Cushing's disease. Clin Endocrinol (Oxf). 1990;33:445–55.
18. Marks LB. Conventional fractionated radiation therapy vs. radiosurgery for selected benign intracranial lesions (arteriovenous malformations, pituitary adenomas, and acoustic neuromas). J Neurooncol. 1993;17:223–30.
19. Estrada J, Boronat M, Mielgo M, et al. The long-term outcome of pituitary irradiation after unsuccessful transsphenoidal surgery in Cushing's disease. N Engl J Med. 1997;336:172–7.
20. Howlett TA, Plowman PN, Wass JA, Rees LH, Jones AE, Besser GM. Megavoltage pituitary irradiation in the management of Cushing's disease and Nelson's syndrome: long-term follow-up. Clin Endocrinol (Oxf). 1989;31:309–23.
21. Hughes MN, Llamas KJ, Yelland ME, Tripcony LB. Pituitary adenomas: long-term results for radiotherapy alone and post-operative radiotherapy. Int J Radiat Oncol Biol Phys. 1993;27:1035–43.
22. Jennings AS, Liddle GW, Orth DN. Results of treating childhood Cushing's disease with pituitary irradiation. N Engl J Med. 1977;297:957–62.
23. Ross WM, Evered DC, Hunter P, Benaim M, Cook D, Hall R. Treatment of Cushing's disease with adrenal blocking drugs and megavoltage therapy to the pituitary. Clin Radiol. 1979;30:149–53.
24. Becker G, Kocher M, Kortmann RD, et al. Radiation therapy in the multimodal treatment approach of pituitary adenoma. Strahlenther Onkol. 2002;178:173–86.
25. Sheehan JM, Vance ML, Sheehan JP, Ellegala DB, Laws Jr ER. Radiosurgery for Cushing's disease after failed transsphenoidal surgery. J Neurosurg. 2000;93:738–42.
26. Devin JK, Allen GS, Cmelak AJ, Duggan DM, Blevins LS. The efficacy of linear accelerator radiosurgery in the management of patients with Cushing's disease. Stereotact Funct Neurosurg. 2004;82:254–62.
27. Mitsumori M, Shrieve DC, Alexander 3rd E, et al. Initial clinical results of LINAC-based stereotactic radiosurgery and stereotactic radiotherapy for pituitary adenomas. Int J Radiat Oncol Biol Phys. 1998;42:573–80.
28. Yoon SC, Suh TS, Jang HS, et al. Clinical results of 24 pituitary macroadenomas with linac-based stereotactic radiosurgery. Int J Radiat Oncol Biol Phys. 1998;41:849–53.
29. Levy RP, Fabrikant JI, Frankel KA, et al. Heavy-charged-particle radiosurgery of the pituitary gland: clinical results of 840 patients. Stereotact Funct Neurosurg. 1991;57:22–35.
30. Ronson BB, Schulte RW, Han KP, Loredo LN, Slater JM, Slater JD. Fractionated proton beam irradiation of pituitary adenomas. Int J Radiat Oncol Biol Phys. 2006;64:425–34.
31. Petit JH, Biller BM, Yock TI, et al. Proton stereotactic radiotherapy for persistent adrenocorticotropin-producing adenomas. J Clin Endocrinol Metab. 2008;93:393–9.
32. Minniti G, Osti M, Jaffrain-Rea ML, Esposito V, Cantore G, Maurizi Enrici R. Long-term follow-up results of postoperative radiation therapy for Cushing's disease. J Neurooncol. 2007;84:79–84.
33. Hoybye C, Grenback E, Rahn T, Degerblad M, Thoren M, Hulting AL. Adrenocorticotropic hormone-producing pituitary tumors: 12- to 22-year follow-up after treatment with stereotactic radiosurgery. Neurosurgery. 2001;49:284–91. discussion 91–2.
34. Vladyka V, Liscak R, Novotny Jr J, Marek J, Jezkova J. Radiation tolerance of functioning pituitary tissue in gamma knife surgery for pituitary adenomas. Neurosurgery. 2003;52:309–16. discussion 16–7.
35. Feigl GC, Bonelli CM, Berghold A, Mokry M. Effects of gamma knife radiosurgery of pituitary adenomas on pituitary function. J Neurosurg. 2002;97:415–21.

36. Pai HH, Thornton A, Katznelson L, et al. Hypothalamic/pituitary function following high-dose conformal radiotherapy to the base of skull: demonstration of a dose-effect relationship using dose-volume histogram analysis. Int J Radiat Oncol Biol Phys. 2001;49:1079–92.
37. Brada M, Rajan B, Traish D, et al. The long-term efficacy of conservative surgery and radiotherapy in the control of pituitary adenomas. Clin Endocrinol (Oxf). 1993;38:571–8.
38. Tsang RW, Laperriere NJ, Simpson WJ, Brierley J, Panzarella T, Smyth HS. Glioma arising after radiation therapy for pituitary adenoma. A report of four patients and estimation of risk. Cancer. 1993;72:2227–33.
39. Brada M, Burchell L, Ashley S, Traish D. The incidence of cerebrovascular accidents in patients with pituitary adenoma. Int J Radiat Oncol Biol Phys. 1999;45:693–8.
40. Schteingart DE, Tsao HS, Taylor CI, McKenzie A, Victoria R, Therrien BA. Sustained remission of Cushing's disease with mitotane and pituitary irradiation. Ann Intern Med. 1980;92:613–9.
41. Tsang RW, Brierley JD, Panzarella T, Gospodarowicz MK, Sutcliffe SB, Simpson WJ. Role of radiation therapy in clinical hormonally-active pituitary adenomas. Radiother Oncol. 1996;41:45–53.
42. Laws Jr ER, Vance ML. Radiosurgery for pituitary tumors and craniopharyngiomas. Neurosurg Clin N Am. 1999;10:327–36.
43. Kobayashi T, Kida Y, Mori Y. Gamma knife radiosurgery in the treatment of Cushing disease: long-term results. J Neurosurg. 2002;97:422–8.
44. Castinetti F, Nagai M, Dufour H, et al. Gamma knife radiosurgery is a successful adjunctive treatment in Cushing's disease. Eur J Endocrinol. 2007;156:91–8.
45. Jagannathan J, Sheehan JP, Pouratian N, Laws ER, Steiner L, Vance ML. Gamma knife surgery for Cushing's disease. J Neurosurg. 2007;106:980–7.

Chapter 12
Medical Management of Cushing's Disease

Stephan Petersenn

Abstract Because established therapies for Cushing's disease – surgery and radiation – are not consistently successful and have clear limitations with respect to efficacy and side effects, there is a need for an effective medical treatment. The most commonly used drugs act by inhibition of steroidogenesis in the adrenals, with the greatest experience available for ketoconazole and metyrapone. Although effective, access to these compounds is limited in many countries, long-term experience is scarce, and side effects are significant. When choosing between these agents, metyrapone may be preferable to ketoconazole in males, and vice versa in women, because of their association with hirsutism and hypogonadism, respectively. Recent proof-of-concept studies suggest a role for a pituitary-directed therapy, applying new multireceptor ligand somatostatin analogs such as pasireotide or second-generation dopamine agonists. However, larger multicenter studies are required to establish their long-term efficacy and safety. The glucocorticoid receptor antagonist mifepristone offers an alternative approach, but thus far experience is very limited, and dosing needs to be titrated with respect to clinical improvements rather than conventional hormonal assays, as there is no biochemical assay to monitor efficacy. Hopefully, currently ongoing studies of these different approaches will increase the possibilities for medical treatment of this fascinating, but sometimes dreadful, disease.

Keywords Steroidogenesis • Hirsutism • Hypogonadism • Adrenal-directed therapy • Pituitary-directed therapy • Multireceptor ligand somatostatin

S. Petersenn (✉)
ENDOC Center for Endocrine Tumors, Altonaer Str. 59, 20357 Hamburg, Germany

University of Duisburg-Essen, Essen, Germany
e-mail: stephan.petersenn@endoc-med.de

Introduction

Cushing's disease is associated with significant morbidity and mortality and, therefore, requires early intervention and effective treatment. Transsphenoidal surgery is clearly the first-line therapy, with remission rates between 65 and 90% in microadenomas, although somewhat lower rates (<65%) in macroadenomas [1]. Radiotherapy is an alternative in patients with residual or recurrent disease after surgery, but may take months to years to achieve biochemical normalization. There is, therefore, an urgent need for medical therapy to reverse clinical features and normalize biochemical parameters in Cushing's disease, both acutely and during chronic treatment. Although minimally-invasive bilateral adrenalectomy is an effective alternative which can be performed with minimal complications, growth of the underlying corticotroph adenoma may eventually progress to Nelson's disease, and life-long substitution with glucocorticoids and mineralocorticoids may itself be associated with significant morbidity from recurrent adrenal crises during later life.

Although there is currently no licensed medical treatment available, several compounds have demonstrated efficacy in decreasing cortisol excess in Cushing's disease [2]. They can be divided by their therapeutic target: the most commonly used drugs reduce cortisol levels via inhibition of steroidogenesis in the adrenal glands, whereas more recently investigated compounds potentially target ACTH-secretion at the pituitary level, possibly also inhibiting corticotroph proliferation (Fig. 12.1). A third group includes agents which antagonize the effect of glucocorticoids at their specific receptors.

The interpretation of currently available data on the efficacy and safety of drug therapy in Cushing's disease is difficult for various reasons. The study design in published reports varies considerably, with very few prospective, controlled, randomized studies available, potentially presenting a publication bias, with few

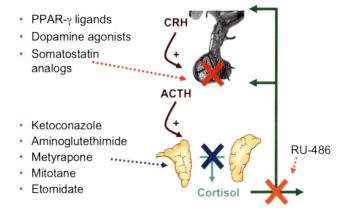

Fig. 12.1 Current approaches to medical therapy in Cushing's disease, with compounds listed with their main level of action. RU-486=mifepristone

consecutive series published. There is a large variation in biochemical parameters used for the primary end point (UFC, serum cortisol, plasma ACTH), and reference values derived from a sufficiently large population are mostly lacking especially for some of the newer assays. Cushing's disease may not be conclusively proven in all patients, due to the difficulties in diagnostic testing, and biochemical activity may undergo spontaneous variability, which may confound assessment of response. Finally, the criteria to define response to treatment and control of disease are insufficiently established.

Adrenal-Directed Therapy

The principle of pharmacologic inhibition of steroidogenesis originated in the 1950s with studies of amphenone B [3]. Because of its limited efficacy and tolerability, however, this compound is no longer employed [4]. Currently used agents include metyrapone and ketoconazole, which are generally more effective and better tolerated than other steroidogenesis inhibitors.

Metyrapone was studied in humans soon after the discovery of its steroidogenesis blocking effects in animals [5]. It acts primarily by inhibiting 11ß-hydroxylase and to a lesser extent 17α, 18-, and 19-hydroxylase activities [6]. Because of this, aldosterone biosynthesis is more severely affected than that of cortisol [7]. The initial dose usually consists of 250 mg qid, which is adjusted during treatment to a total daily dose of 500–6,000 mg [1]. In patients with Cushing's disease, a significant drop in cortisol levels is usually seen within 2 h after the first dose [8]. When followed on short-term metyrapone therapy (1–16 weeks) prior to other, more definitive treatment, biochemical control of Cushing's disease as assessed by means of a cortisol day profile was observed in 75% of patients on a median metyrapone dose of 2,250 mg/day (range 750–6,000), and was associated with clinical improvement in the majority of patients. When given long term (median: 27 months, range 3–140), adequate control of hypercortisolaemia was seen in 83%. Of note, all of the latter subjects had received pituitary irradiation in addition to their medical treatment, and ACTH levels started to decrease after 1 year, reflecting the effects of radiotherapy. Another study reported biochemical control in 13 patients with Cushing's disease for up to 66 months, of whom nine had also received pituitary irradiation [9]. Increased ACTH secretion may override steroidogenic blockade in some patients with Cushing's disease [10]. However, although ACTH levels increased significantly in one of the largest studies on metyrapone, this effect occurred predominantly in the first 4–6 weeks after initiation of therapy, after which no further increase was seen [8].

Side effects include acne and hirsutism (19%) due to increased androgens, and infrequently hypokalemia (6%), edema (8%) and hypertension due to increased 11-deoxycorticosterone levels [8]. Although worsening hirsutism or persistent acne was observed in approximately 70% of women treated for 6 months or longer in another study, these effects were mild [9]. The association of metyrapone with hirsutism may make ketoconazole a better choice in women. When used without sufficient glucocorticoid replacement, symptoms of adrenal insufficiency have been observed in 13% of patients treated with metyrapone [8]. Other adverse reactions included cutaneous rash (4%), which may be transient, effects on the central nervous system such as lethargy and dizziness (15%), and gastrointestinal complaints (5%). Although successful treatment of Cushing's syndrome in pregnancy with metyrapone has been described [11], it was associated with a hypertensive crisis in another patient [12]. Metyrapone is not available in many countries (e.g., Germany, United States), but can be ordered through an international drugstore or by contacting the manufacturer (Novartis) directly.

Ketoconazole was licensed as an antifungal agent, but was soon demonstrated to lower cortisol [13] and testosterone [14] levels by inhibition of a variety of cytochrome P450 enzymes (side-chain cleavage complex, 17,20-lyase, 11ß-hydroxylase, and 17α-hydroxylase) [15, 16]. The most sensitive site of action seems to be the 17,20-lyase involved in the synthesis of sex steroids, explaining the greater suppression of testosterone compared with cortisol [7]. Additional effects on the HPA axis by inhibition of ACTH secretion at the pituitary level, or action as a glucocorticoid receptor antagonist, have been described in cell models, but lack clear evidence in humans [1, 10]. Treatment may be initiated with 200 mg bid [1], and effective doses range from 200 to 1,200 mg/day, with most studies reporting biochemical response at 600–800 mg/day administered twice daily [10]. Ketoconazole is effective in Cushing's disease, as demonstrated in a meta-analysis of 12 studies treating 85 patients, with normalization of urinary steroids observed in 81% [10]. Following initiation of treatment, a rapid improvement in clinical symptoms of hypercortisolism may be observed, with regression of diabetes mellitus, hypokalemia, hypertension, hirsutism, and depression [7]. After long-term treatment, a recent retrospective analysis with a mean follow-up of 23 months (range 6–72 months) found normalization of urinary free cortisol in 45% of patients [17]. However, in patients without pituitary irradiation, escape from pharmacological control may occur [18]. Owing to its widespread inhibition of cytochrome P450 enzymes in several organs (adrenal gland, testis, ovary, liver, kidney), ketoconazole may reduce cholesterol [19] and vitamin D levels [20]. Combination treatment with metyrapone should be avoided, with both compounds leading to the accumulation of 11ß/18-hydroxylase precursors followed by the development of mineralocorticoid-induced hypertension. The availability of ketoconazole is limited in many countries. However, fluconazole appears to have similar effects [21], and it normalized urinary free cortisol levels in the author's limited experience of two patients who were treated with fluconazole 100 mg bid.

Side effects of ketoconazole are dose dependent, and include gynecomastia in 13% of males, gastrointestinal symptoms in 8%, edema in 6%, and skin rash in 2% [10]. Owing to the possible development of hypogonadism in males with ketoconazole, metyrapone may be preferred in this population. Mild and transient elevations in liver enzymes up to threefold normal are not a contraindication for further treatment, but liver function should be monitored carefully and more severe abnormalities require discontinuation [1]. Severe hepatic injury is estimated to occur in 1/15,000 cases [22]. The typical onset of ketoconazole-induced hepatitis is reported to occur within 60 days after initiation of treatment and to resolve within 3 months after discontinuation [23].

Aminoglutethimide was introduced as an antiseizure medication but soon was shown to lower cortisol secretion. It inhibits a variety of steroidogenic enzymes including the side-chain cleavage complex, 21-hydroxylase, 17α-hydroxylase, 11ß-hydroxylase, aromatase, 17,20-lyase, and 18-hydroxylase [10]. The inhibition of the aromatizing system results in reduced conversion of androgens to estrogens in extraglandular tissues such as fat, muscle, liver, and breast [7]. Aminoglutethimide appears to be somehow more effective in patients with autonomous adrenal hyperfunction or ectopic ACTH production than in patients with Cushing's disease, possibly due to ACTH stimulation overriding the adrenal blockade in the latter group. Daily doses range from 0.75 to 2 mg/day [10], with a reported response rate of 46% [24]. Side effects are more pronounced than with ketoconazole or metyrapone and include sedation (30%), nausea or anorexia (12%), and transient rash (18%) [10]. Impairment of T4 release, possibly due to interference with iodine incorporation, may lead to TSH increase and development of goiter [25]. Aminoglutethimide appeared especially effective in combination with metyrapone or irradiation. However, the compound is currently not available worldwide.

Mitotane (o,p'-DDD) is a derivative of the pesticide DDT that specifically inhibits cells of the adrenal cortex. Its effects are most pronounced in the zona fasciculata and zona reticulata of the adrenal cortex, with little effects in the zona glomerulosa [26]. It is highly effective in the treatment of hypercortisolism, with a normalization rate of 83% reported in a study of 46 patients treated for 3–34 months [27]. As 30% of patients maintained remission during a follow-up period of 37 months after withdrawal, its effects may be long-lasting, potentially due to an adrenolytic action. When combined with pituitary irradiation, mitotane led to clinical and biochemical remission in 81–100% of patients [27, 28]. However, its onset of action is slow, and due to the initial accumulation in fat tissue careful monitoring of drug levels is required. Saturation is to be expected 2–3 months after initiation of therapy, requiring more frequent measurements of drug levels to recognize this and reduce the dose accordingly. In contrast to its use in adrenal carcinoma, specific target ranges for drug concentrations in Cushing's disease have not been established. Significant and frequent side effects include disturbances of the GI tract (72%) and the central nervous system (impaired mentation and dizziness, 45%), as well as gynecomastia, rash, increases in liver enzymes, and hypercholesterinemia [10]. Because mitotane induces hepatic enzymes, there is accelerated metabolism of exogenous steroids, especially of hydrocortisone, and replacement doses must be increased to avoid adrenal crises [29, 30]. Its use should, therefore, be limited to centers with special expertise. When comparing the dosages as reported in the literature, special note should be given to the preparation used, as they demonstrate variable activity. Recently, a defined preparation has been licensed in Europe (Lysodren).

The nonopioid anesthetic etomidate induces adrenocortical suppression by dose-dependent inhibition of 11ß-hydroxylase and desmolase. Although it needs to be administered as a continuous infusion, it may be helpful in situations where rapid control of hypercortisolism is required or oral therapy is problematic. An initial bolus of 0.03 mg/kg body weight is followed by an infusion of 0.03–

0.3 mg/kg/h. With this, significant suppression of serum cortisol levels is observed within 5 h, with a maximum effect at 11 h [31]. Its efficient short-term control of hypercortisolism has also been demonstrated in pediatric patients with severe Cushing's disease [32]. Limitations include severe fatigue and the need for intravenous infusion.

Pituitary-Directed Therapy

Pituitary-targeted therapy, by acting on the underlying corticotroph adenoma, represents an alternative approach in the therapy of Cushing's disease. Although various substances have been tried for many years with limited efficacy, the success of recent agents may eventually lead to medical treatment of selected patients with Cushing's disease. Currently, three classes of drugs are under investigation in humans: PPARγ ligands, dopamine agonists, and somatostatin analogs.

PPARγ (peroxisome proliferator-activated receptor-γ) is a member of the nuclear receptor superfamily, and functions as a transcription factor. PPARγ ligands have been shown to inhibit the growth of many tumors, including breast, colon, and prostate cancer cells. Furthermore, PPARγ ligands demonstrated antiproliferative and apoptotic effects in a cell model of corticotropic adenoma cells, and inhibited POMC transcription [33]. However, very little PPARγ protein was found in pituitary adenomas, and the antiproliferative effects of PPARγ ligands were only seen with very high doses of rosiglitazone, without significant reversal by a PPARγ antagonist [34]. Additional actions in Cushing's disease may include suppression of steroidogenesis in the adrenals by inhibition of P450c17 and 3ßHSD [35]. Clinical experience with PPARγ ligands for the treatment of Cushing's disease is limited thus far. In an initial study on rosiglitazone (8–16 mg) in 14 patients treated for 1–7 months, normalization of urinary free cortisol was observed in 42.9%, with mild improvements of clinical features [36]. A subsequent study in ten patients treated for 1–8 months with 4–16 mg rosiglitazone demonstrated normalization in 30% of patients, but none of those patients normalized were willing to reenter the treatment protocol [37]. Side effects, at least in the latter study, were significant and included edema, hypertension, weight gain of several kilograms, somnolence, increased hirsutism, and worsening of bruisability. The efficacy of rosiglitazone may not be long lasting, as a recent study reported an initial significant drop of ACTH and cortisol levels, but subsequent increase after 28 weeks of therapy, despite dose increases up to 28 mg [38]. Furthermore, the efficacy may vary for different PPARγ ligands. In a study of five patients treated with pioglitazone 45 mg for 1 month, none responded with a significant drop in ACTH or cortisol secretion [39]. A recent consensus conference concluded that, based on current evidence and the panel's experience, the routine clinical use of PPARγ ligands in Cushing's disease is not advised [1].

The successful use of dopamine agonists in patients with prolactin and growth hormone secreting pituitary adenomas has also led to trials in patients with Cushing's disease. Dopamine subtype 2 receptors are expressed in corticotrope pituitary adenomas [40], and in vitro studies demonstrated inhibition of ACTH secretion by the dopamine agonist bromocriptine [41]. Furthermore, bromocriptine was shown to induce apoptosis in an ACTH-secreting mouse cell line [42]. In a meta-analysis of earlier small studies and case reports, including 23 patients followed for 3–180 weeks, bromocriptine in doses of 1.25–30 mg/day allowed normalization of steroid secretion in 48% (adapted from [10]). It should be noted, however, that this cohort may present a positive selection bias, and the primary end point varied significantly between the studies including plasma cortisol, cortisol secretion rate, and 24-h urinary glucocorticoid assessment. Subsequent consecutively treated series demonstrated lower response rates of 4% [43] and 23% [44] with bromocriptine treatment. Newer dopamine agonists may be more effective. In a recent single center study of ten patients treated with cabergoline 1–3 mg/week for 3 months, a normalization rate of 40% for urinary free cortisol was observed [45]. Moreover, the same authors confirmed the long-term efficacy of cabergoline in Cushing's disease in a subsequent study, in which normalized urinary free cortisol was maintained in 40% of 20 patients with at least 12 months follow-up [46]. The dose of 1–7 mg/week (median 3.5 mg) was well tolerated, except by two patients with hypotension and severe asthenia, who stopped treatment after 12 and 18 months, respectively. It is currently unclear whether recently documented cardiac valve changes in patients with Parkinson's disease who received much higher doses of cabergoline [47, 48] also translate to the lower doses used in this cohort. Of note, no development of cardiac valve insufficiency or worsening of previously diagnosed valve insufficiency was documented by Pivonello et al. [46], except in one patient who had a mild tricuspid regurgitation at baseline and a moderate tricuspid regurgitation with normal pulmonary pressure after 2 years treatment. Therefore, the use of a second generation dopamine agonist such as cabergoline may present an interesting option for the medical treatment of Cushing's disease. However, this single center experience needs to be confirmed in larger multicenter studies looking both at efficacy and safety. As non-ergot-derived dopamine agonists such as quinagolide probably do not possess the same risk for inducing cardiac valve changes (possibly due to differences in the affinity for valvular $5-HT_{2B}$ receptors), studies on these second generation compounds may be of special interest.

Somatostatin receptor ligands may present another avenue for the medical treatment of Cushing's disease. Table 12.1 summarizes several studies investigating the expression of the five somatostatin receptor subtypes in corticotropic pituitary adenomas [49–55]. Although *sst1*, *sst2*, and *sst5* are widely expressed, the expression levels are low, except for *sst5* [52]. Interestingly, however, both *sst2* ligands and *sst5* ligands were found to inhibit CRH-stimulated ACTH secretion in vitro in a mouse corticotropic cell model [56]. Similar, native somatostatin binding to all five somatostatin receptor subtypes with high affinity is able to inhibit CRH-stimulated ACTH release in normal rat pituitary cells, but only when incubated in serum-deprived conditions or after pretreatment with a glucocorticoid-receptor blocking agent [57]. Stalla et al. demonstrated clear efficacy of the *sst2* ligand octreotide in primary cell culture of corticotropic pituitary tumors [58]. This effect,

Table 12.1 Somatostatin receptor subtype expression in corticotropic pituitary adenomas (predominant expression levels in brackets, where available)

Reference	Method	sst1	sst2	sst3	sst4	sst5
Greenman [50, 51]	RPA, RT-PCR	1/3	0/3	1/2	0/1	1/1
Miller [53]	RT-PCR	3/5	5/5	0/5	0/5	4/5
Nielsen [53]	RT-PCR	0/1	0/1	1/1	1/1	0/1
Panetta [55]	RT-PCR	1/1	1/1	1/1	0/1	0/1
Batista [49]	Real-time RT-PCR	12/13 (high)	9/13 (low)	0/13 (−)	5/13 (?)	13/13 (high)
Hofland [52]	Real-time RT-PCR	1/6 (low)	6/6 (low)	2/6 (low)	2/6 (low)	6/6 (high)
Author's data	Real-time RT-PCR	7/10 (l-h)	8/10 (l-h)	3/10 (med)	4/10 (high)	7/10 (l-h)
Total		25/39	29/39	8/38	12/37	31/37
%		64	74	21	32	84

RPA RNA protection assay, *RT-PCR* reverse transcriptase polymerase chain reaction, *l-h* low to high

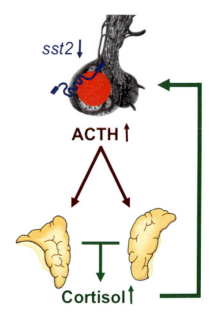

Fig. 12.2 Downregulation of *sst2* in the corticotropic pituitary adenomas due to transcriptional inhibition by systemic glucocorticoids

however, was abolished by pretreatment with glucocorticoids, which may be explained by downregulation of *sst2* by glucocorticoids (Fig. 12.2). Our studies of a transient transfection system suggested a negative glucocorticoid responsive element in the sst2 promoter [59], indicating transcriptional inhibition of *sst2* by glucocorticoids. Assuming inhibition of *sst2* expression in the corticotropic pituitary tumor by continuously elevated systemic cortisol levels, *sst2* ligands would be largely ineffective in vivo. Indeed, although the clinical experience is limited, single injections of octreotide 100 µg did not demonstrate any effect on ACTH levels in several studies of patients with hypercortisolism (Table 12.2, [58, 60, 61]). Furthermore, short-term treatment of patients with Cushing's disease

Table 12.2 Efficacy of single subcutaneous injection of octreotide (*upper half*) and continuous subcutaneous treatment with octreotide (*lower half*) in ACTH levels

Reference	Compound	Effects on ACTH
Ambrosi [60]	Oct (100 μg)	0/9 CD
Lamberts [61]	Oct (100 μg)	0/3 CD
Stalla [58]	Oct (100 μg)	0/5 CD
Total		0/17
Invitti [62]	Oct (400–1,200 μg)	1/3 CD 24–49 day
Woodhouse [63]	Oct (3 × 100–500 μg)	0/2 CD 24 h
Total		1/5

Number of patients with relevant inhibition in relation to the total number of patients investigated for the respective dose and duration of octreotide is shown
Oct octreotide, *CD* Cushing's disease

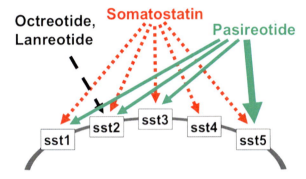

Fig. 12.3 Preferential affinities of somatostatin, the currently licensed somatostatin analogs octreotide and lanreotide, and the new multireceptor ligand somatostatin analog pasireotide for the five known somatostatin receptor subtypes *sst1–sst5*

with repeated subcutaneous injections of octreotide proved to be largely ineffective (Table 12.2, [62, 63]).

To facilitate treatment of patients with Cushing's disease with octreotide or lanreotide, one could envision pretreatment with steroidogenesis inhibitors to lower cortisol levels, with subsequent treatment with *sst2* ligands following enhanced *sst2* expression to control the pituitary tumor. However, this concept may even require induction of hypocortisolism. Physiological concentrations of cortisol may already suppress *sst2* expression, as ACTH secretion in normal individuals is not affected by infusion of octreotide [64]. On the other hand, octreotide induced significant suppression of ACTH levels in patients with Nelson's syndrome, despite regular glucocorticoid replacement [61, 65, 66].

An alternative approach may be to use *sst5* ligands, considering the high expression of *sst5* in corticotropic adenomas. Pasireotide (SOM230) is a recently developed multireceptor ligand somatostatin analog. Whereas octreotide and lanreotide have high affinity for *sst2* and modest affinity for *sst5*, pasireotide demonstrates high binding affinity for *sst1,2,3*, and *5*, and has a 40-fold higher affinity for *sst5* than octreotide (Fig. 12.3, [67, 68]). Pasireotide was highly effective in lowering ACTH secretion in a mouse cell model. Of note, dexamethasone pretreatment did not influence the sensitivity of the cells to the inhibitory effect of pasireotide, suggesting that *sst5* is relatively resistant to negative control by glucocorticoids [52]. Indeed, quantitative PCR analysis showed that *sst5* mRNA levels were not significantly affected by dexamethasone treatment, whereas dexamethasone lowered *sst2* mRNA expression significantly [69]. In primary cultures of corticotropic pituitary adenomas, pasireotide inhibited ACTH secretion in 3/5 [52] and 5/6 [49] tumors, respectively. In addition, significant suppression of cell proliferation was observed in all tumors cultured in the latter study. The strong inhibition of the HPA axis by pasireotide was confirmed in an animal model. Pasireotide suppressed both CRH-induced ACTH release and corticosterone secretion in rats [70]. By overexpression of either sst2 or sst5 in a mouse cell model, it was clearly shown that the suppressive effects of pasireotide in corticotropic cells are determined by sst5, whereas the ligand action on sst2 is negligible [71]. In a phase II, proof-of-concept, open-label, single-arm, multi-center study, the in vivo efficacy of pasireotide was evaluated in patients with either de novo or with persistent or recurrent Cushing's disease [72]. After a short treatment period of 15 days with pasireotide 600 µg given subcutaneously twice daily, the mean UFC level decreased significantly by 45%. Normalization of UFC was found in 17% of patients, with 76% of patients demonstrating a reduction in UFC levels. Serum cortisol levels and plasma ACTH levels were also reduced. Reported side effects with a frequency of at least 10% included GI tract symptoms (diarrhea (44%), nausea (23%), abdominal pain (18%)), asthenia (13%), fatigue (10%), hyperglycemia (36%), headache (18%), and hypotension (13%). These very much resemble the side effects observed with currently licensed somatostatin analogs. In a recent case report, a dramatic drop of elevated UFC levels in a patient treated with pasireotide 600 µg bid was observed, leading to symptomatic and biochemical hypocortisolism [73]. Prior to pasireotide, the patient demonstrated UFC levels approximately 1.5–2-fold above normal, despite three surgical attempts and radiotherapy. After 10 months of reduced pasireotide therapy at 300 µg bid, improved mood, stable weight, and normal UFC levels were noted. An ongoing phase III study will determine the long-term efficacy and safety of pasireotide in Cushing's disease.

The observation of a high co-expression of somatostatin and dopamine subtype 2 receptors in the majority of human corticotropic pituitary adenomas suggests the combined use of their specific ligands [74]. Interestingly, a chimeric molecule BIM23A760 has recently been developed, with high sst2 and D2 activity and moderate sst5 activity [75–77]. Interaction between those receptors may allow for even greater suppression of ACTH. However, a clinical evaluation in patients with Cushing's disease has not yet been published.

Glucocorticoid Receptor Antagonists

Glucocorticoid receptor antagonists present another approach to the medical therapy of Cushing's disease. However, their use is hindered by the difficulties in determining the efficacy of the treatment, without a clear cut biochemical marker correlating with the treatment response, since cortisol levels do not decrease. Mifepristone is the only available glucocorticoid receptor antagonist [78–80], and there are very limited data published concerning its use in hypercortisolism [81, 82]. Only five patients with Cushing's disease treated with mifepristone have been described thus far. Chu et al. presented a case report on an extremely ill patient with an ACTH-secreting pituitary macroadenoma, without sufficient response to transsphenoidal surgery, radiotherapy, and medical treatment with mitotane [83]. Ketoconazole was not tolerated because of severe side effects. As the patient was considered too ill for bilateral adrenalectomy, he was treated with mifepristone starting with 6 mg/kg/day up to a maximum of 25 mg/kg/day. A dramatic improvement in clinical symptoms was reported, and when radiation eventually became effective, treatment with mifepristone was stopped after 18 months. During treatment the patient developed severe hypokalemia that was attributed to excessive cortisol activation of the mineralocorticoid receptor, and which responded to spironolactone administration. In a retrospective report on the use of mifepristone in patients with hypercortisolism in seven European centers, four additional patients with Cushing's disease were presented [82]. Clinical signs improved in three of them during treatment for 3–24 months. The fourth patient was treated for 0.5 months, during which time he demonstrated rapid improvement in psychiatric symptoms, before undergoing surgery. One of the four patients in this series developed severe hypertension and hypokalemia. Although mifepristone may present an effective treatment, clearly more experience in clinical trials is needed to standardize dosing and monitoring of side effects such as hypokalemia and hypertension, as well as to enable early recognition of adrenal insufficiency.

Conclusions

Cushing's disease is potentially life threatening and, therefore, requires rapid and effective treatment. Because surgery and radiation therapy are not always effective, medical therapy presents a useful addition for a multimodality approach to these patients. Most currently used medications inhibit adrenal steroidogenesis. Although they appear to be effective, there is little data from controlled studies regarding their use, and efficacy data may be influenced by a publication bias. There is little experience with long-term use of these compounds, and relevant side effects limit their therapeutic use. Furthermore, they do not target the underlying pituitary tumor, and escape of ACTH secretion may require dose adjustments to maintain efficacy. Pituitary-targeted therapies may allow both an antisecretory and antiproliferative treatment. Both new multireceptor ligand somatostatin analogs and dopamine agonists have demonstrated some efficacy in small proof-of-concept studies, which support further investigation in larger multicenter trials. If proven effective and safe, they may be potentially useful either as short-term therapy bridging the interval before surgery becomes available or radiation effective, or as a long-term alternative to current treatment options. Similarly, the glucocorticoid receptor antagonist needs further evaluation, with special emphasis on the development of criteria for the adjustment of dosage and treatment of potential side effects. Hopefully, these therapies may eventually provide a viable medical alternative to currently available treatment of this fascinating, but sometimes dreadful, disease.

References

1. Biller BM, Grossman AB, Stewart PM, et al. Treatment of adrenocorticotropin-dependent Cushing's syndrome: a consensus statement. J Clin Endocrinol Metab. 2008;93:2454–62.
2. Stewart PM, Petersenn S. Rationale for treatment and therapeutic options in Cushing's disease. Best Pract Res Clin Endocrinol Metab. 2009;23 Suppl 1:S15–22.
3. Thorn GW, Renold AE, Goldfien A, et al. Inhibition of corticosteroid secretion by amphenone in a patient with adrenocortical carcinoma. N Engl J Med. 1956;254:547–51.
4. Hertz R, Pittman JA, Graff MM. Amphenone: toxicity and effects on adrenal and thyroid function in man. J Clin Endocrinol Metab. 1956;16:705–23.
5. Liddle GW, Island D, Lance EM, et al. Alterations of adrenal steroid patterns in man resulting from treatment with a chemical inhibitor of 11 beta-hydroxylation. J Clin Endocrinol Metab. 1958;18:906–12.
6. Gower DB. Modifiers of steroid-hormone metabolism: a review of their chemistry, biochemistry and clinical applications. J Steroid Biochem. 1974;5:501–23.
7. Sonino N, Boscaro M. Medical therapy for Cushing's disease. Endocrinol Metab Clin North Am. 1999;28:211–22.
8. Verhelst JA, Trainer PJ, Howlett TA, et al. Short and long-term responses to metyrapone in the medical management of 91 patients with Cushing's syndrome. Clin Endocrinol (Oxf). 1991;35:169–78.
9. Jeffcoate WJ, Rees LH, Tomlin S, et al. Metyrapone in long-term management of Cushing's disease. Br Med J. 1977;2:215–7.
10. Miller JW, Crapo L. The medical treatment of Cushing's syndrome. Endocr Rev. 1993;14:443–58.
11. Aron DC, Schnall AM, Sheeler LR. Cushing's syndrome and pregnancy. Am J Obstet Gynecol. 1990;162:244–52.
12. Connell JM, Cordiner J, Davies DL, et al. Pregnancy complicated by Cushing's syndrome: potential hazard of metyrapone therapy. Case report. Br J Obstet Gynaecol. 1985;92:1192–5.
13. Pont A, Williams PL, Loose DS, et al. Ketoconazole blocks adrenal steroid synthesis. Ann Intern Med. 1982;97:370–2.
14. Pont A, Williams PL, Azhar S, et al. Ketoconazole blocks testosterone synthesis. Arch Intern Med. 1982;142:2137–40.
15. Feldman D. Ketoconazole and other imidazole derivatives as inhibitors of steroidogenesis. Endocr Rev. 1986;7:409–20.
16. Sonino N. The use of ketoconazole as an inhibitor of steroid production. N Engl J Med. 1987;317:812–8.
17. Castinetti F, Morange I, Jaquet P, et al. Ketoconazole revisited: a preoperative or postoperative treatment in Cushing's disease. Eur J Endocrinol. 2008;158:91–9.
18. Sonino N, Boscaro M, Paoletta A, et al. Ketoconazole treatment in Cushing's syndrome: experience in 34 patients. Clin Endocrinol (Oxf). 1991;35:347–52.
19. Miettinen TA. Cholesterol metabolism during ketoconazole treatment in man. J Lipid Res. 1988;29:43–51.
20. Glass AR, Eil C. Ketoconazole-induced reduction in serum 1,25-dihydroxyvitamin D. J Clin Endocrinol Metab. 1986;63:766–9.

21. Riedl M, Maier C, Zettinig G, et al. Long term control of hypercortisolism with fluconazole: case report and in vitro studies. Eur J Endocrinol. 2006;154:519–24.
22. Lewis JH, Zimmerman HJ, Benson GD, et al. Hepatic injury associated with ketoconazole therapy. Analysis of 33 cases. Gastroenterology. 1984;86:503–13.
23. Lake-Bakaar G, Scheuer PJ, Sherlock S. Hepatic reactions associated with ketoconazole in the United Kingdom. Br Med J (Clin Res Ed). 1987;294:419–22.
24. Misbin RI, Canary J, Willard D. Aminoglutethimide in the treatment of Cushing's syndrome. J Clin Pharmacol. 1976;16:645–51.
25. Rallison ML, Kumagai LF, Tyler FH. Goitrous hypothyroidism induced by amino-glutethimide, anticonvulsant drug. J Clin Endocrinol Metab. 1967;27:265–72.
26. Kaminsky N, Luse S, Hartroft P. Ultrastructure of adrenal cortex of the dog during treatment with DDD. J Natl Cancer Inst. 1962;29:127–59.
27. Luton JP, Mahoudeau JA, Bouchard P, et al. Treatment of Cushings disease by O,p'DDD. Survey of 62 cases. N Engl J Med. 1979;300:459–64.
28. Schteingart DE, Tsao HS, Taylor CI, et al. Sustained remission of Cushing's disease with mitotane and pituitary irradiation. Ann Intern Med. 1980;92:613–9.
29. Hague RV, May W, Cullen DR. Hepatic microsomal enzyme induction and adrenal crisis due to o,p'DDD therapy for metastatic adrenocortical carcinoma. Clin Endocrinol (Oxf). 1989;31:51–7.
30. Robinson BG, Hales IB, Henniker AJ, et al. The effect of o,p'-DDD on adrenal steroid replacement therapy requirements. Clin Endocrinol (Oxf). 1987;27:437–44.
31. Schulte HM, Benker G, Reinwein D, et al. Infusion of low dose etomidate: correction of hypercortisolemia in patients with Cushing's syndrome and dose-response relationship in normal subjects. J Clin Endocrinol Metab. 1990;70:1426–30.
32. Greening JE, Brain CE, Perry LA, et al. Efficient short-term control of hypercortisolaemia by low-dose etomidate in severe paediatric Cushing's disease. Horm Res. 2005;64:140–3.
33. Heaney AP, Fernando M, Yong WH, et al. Functional PPAR-gamma receptor is a novel therapeutic target for ACTH-secreting pituitary adenomas. Nat Med. 2002;8:1281–7.
34. Emery MN, Leontiou C, Bonner SE, et al. PPAR-gamma expression in pituitary tumours and the functional activity of the glitazones: evidence that any anti-proliferative effect of the glitazones is independent of the PPAR-gamma receptor. Clin Endocrinol (Oxf). 2006;65:389–95.
35. Heaney AP. PPAR-gamma in Cushing's disease. Pituitary. 2004;7:265–9.
36. Ambrosi B, Dall'Asta C, Cannavo S, et al. Effects of chronic administration of PPAR-gamma ligand rosiglitazone in Cushing's disease. Eur J Endocrinol. 2004;151:173–8.
37. Pecori Giraldi F, Scaroni C, Arvat E, et al. Effect of protracted treatment with rosiglitazone, a PPARgamma agonist, in patients with Cushing's disease. Clin Endocrinol (Oxf). 2006; 64:219–24.
38. Morcos M, Fohr B, Tafel J, et al. Long-term treatment of central Cushing's syndrome with rosiglitazone. Exp Clin Endocrinol Diab. 2007;115:292–7.
39. Suri D, Weiss RE. Effect of pioglitazone on adrenocorticotropic hormone and cortisol secretion in Cushing's disease. J Clin Endocrinol Metab. 2005;90:1340–6.
40. Stefaneanu L, Kovacs K, Horvath E, et al. Dopamine D2 receptor gene expression in human adenohypophysial adenomas. Endocr. 2001;14:329–36.
41. Adams EF, Ashby MJ, Brown SM, et al. Bromocriptine suppresses ACTH secretion from human pituitary tumour cells in culture by a dopaminergic mechanism. Clin Endocrinol (Oxf). 1981;15:479–84.
42. Yin D, Kondo S, Takeuchi J, et al. Induction of apoptosis in murine ACTH-secreting pituitary adenoma cells by bromocriptine. FEBS Lett. 1994;339:73–5.
43. Hale AC, Coates PJ, Doniach I, et al. A bromocriptine-responsive corticotroph adenoma secreting alpha-MSH in a patient with Cushing's disease. Clin Endocrinol (Oxf). 1988;28:215–23.
44. Koppeschaar HP, Croughs RJ, Thijssen JH, et al. Response to neurotransmitter modulating drugs in patients with Cushing's disease. Clin Endocrinol (Oxf). 1986;25:661–7.

45. Pivonello R, Ferone D, de Herder WW, et al. Dopamine receptor expression and function in corticotroph pituitary tumors. J Clin Endocrinol Metab. 2004;89:2452–62.
46. Pivonello R, De Martino MC, Cappabianca P, et al. The medical treatment of Cushing's disease: effectiveness of chronic treatment with the dopamine agonist cabergoline in patients unsuccessfully treated by surgery. J Clin Endocrinol Metab. 2009;94:223–30.
47. Schade R, Andersohn F, Suissa S, et al. Dopamine agonists and the risk of cardiac-valve regurgitation. N Engl J Med. 2007;356:29–38.
48. Zanettini R, Antonini A, Gatto G, et al. Valvular heart disease and the use of dopamine agonists for Parkinson's disease. N Engl J Med. 2007;356:39–46.
49. Batista DL, Zhang X, Gejman R, et al. The effects of SOM230 on cell proliferation and adrenocorticotropin secretion in human corticotroph pituitary adenomas. J Clin Endocrinol Metab. 2006;91:4482–8.
50. Greenman Y, Melmed S. Expression of three somatostatin receptor subtypes in pituitary adenomas: evidence for preferential SSTR5 expression in the mammosomatotroph lineage. J Clin Endocrinol Metab. 1994;79:724–9.
51. Greenman Y, Melmed S. Heterogeneous expression of two somatostatin receptor subtypes in pituitary tumors. J Clin Endocrinol Metab. 1994;78:398–403.
52. Hofland LJ, van der Hoek J, Feelders R, et al. The multi-ligand somatostatin analogue SOM230 inhibits ACTH secretion by cultured human corticotroph adenomas via somatostatin receptor type 5. Eur J Endocrinol. 2005;152:645–54.
53. Miller GM, Alexander JM, Bikkal HA, et al. Somatostatin receptor subtype gene expression in pituitary adenomas. J Clin Endocrinol Metab. 1995;80:1386–92.
54. Nielsen S, Mellemkjaer S, Rasmussen LM, et al. Gene transcription of receptors for growth hormone-releasing peptide and somatostatin in human pituitary adenomas. J Clin Endocrinol Metab. 1998;83:2997–3000.
55. Panetta R, Patel YC. Expression of mRNA for all five human somatostatin receptors (hSSTR1-5) in pituitary tumors. Life Sci. 1995;56:333–42.
56. Strowski MZ, Dashkevicz MP, Parmar RM, et al. Somatostatin receptor subtypes 2 and 5 inhibit corticotropin-releasing hormone-stimulated adrenocorticotropin secretion from AtT-20 cells. Neuroendocrinology. 2002;75:339–46.
57. Lamberts SW, Zuyderwijk J, den Holder F, et al. Studies on the conditions determining the inhibitory effect of somatostatin on adrenocorticotropin, prolactin and thyrotropin release by cultured rat pituitary cells. Neuroendocrinology. 1989;50:44–50.
58. Stalla GK, Brockmeier SJ, Renner U, et al. Octreotide exerts different effects in vivo and in vitro in Cushing's disease. Eur J Endocrinol. 1994;130:125–31.
59. Petersenn S, Rasch AC, Presch S, et al. Genomic structure and transcriptional regulation of the human somatostatin receptor type 2. Mol Cell Endocrinol. 1999;157:75–85.
60. Ambrosi B, Bochicchio D, Fadin C, et al. Failure of somatostatin and octreotide to acutely affect the hypothalamic-pituitary-adrenal function in patients with corticotropin hypersecretion. J Endocrinol Invest. 1990;13:257–61.
61. Lamberts SW, Uitterlinden P, Klijn JM. The effect of the long-acting somatostatin analogue SMS 201–995 on ACTH secretion in Nelson's syndrome and Cushing's disease. Acta Endocrinol (Copenh). 1989;120:760–6.
62. Invitti C, de Martin M, Brunani A, et al. Treatment of Cushing's syndrome with the long-acting somatostatin analogue SMS 201–995 (sandostatin). Clin Endocrinol (Oxf). 1990;32:275–81.
63. Woodhouse NJ, Dagogo-Jack S, Ahmed M, et al. Acute and long-term effects of octreotide in patients with ACTH-dependent Cushing's syndrome. Am J Med. 1993;95:305–8.
64. Invitti C, Pecori Giraldi F, Dubini A, et al. Effect of sandostatin on CRF-stimulated secretion of ACTH, beta-lipotropin and beta-endorphin. Horm Metab Res. 1991;23:233–5.
65. Petrini L, Gasperi M, Pilosu R, et al. Long-term treatment of Nelson's syndrome by octreotide: a case report. J Endocrinol Invest. 1994;17:135–9.
66. Kelestimur F, Utas C, Ozbakir O, et al. The effects of octreotide in a patient with Nelson's syndrome. Postgrad Med J. 1996;72:53–4.

67. Bruns C, Lewis I, Briner U, et al. SOM230: a novel somatostatin peptidomimetic with broad somatotropin release inhibiting factor (SRIF) receptor binding and a unique antisecretory profile. Eur J Endocrinol. 2002;146:707–16.
68. Schmid HA, Schoeffter P. Functional activity of the multiligand analog SOM230 at human recombinant somatostatin receptor subtypes supports its usefulness in neuroendocrine tumors. Neuroendocrinology. 2004;80 Suppl 1:47–50.
69. van der Hoek J, Waaijers M, van Koetsveld PM, et al. Distinct functional properties of native somatostatin receptor subtype 5 compared with subtype 2 in the regulation of ACTH release by corticotroph tumor cells. Am J Physiol Endocrinol Metab. 2005;289:E278–87.
70. Silva AP, Bethmann K, Raulf F, et al. Regulation of ghrelin secretion by somatostatin analogs in rats. Eur J Endocrinol. 2005;152:887–94.
71. Ben-Shlomo A, Schmid H, Wawrowsky K, et al. Differential ligand-mediated pituitary somatostatin receptor subtype signaling: implications for corticotroph tumor therapy. J Clin Endocrinol Metab. 2009;94:4342–50.
72. Boscaro M, Ludlam WH, Atkinson B, et al. Treatment of pituitary-dependent Cushing's disease with the multireceptor ligand somatostatin analog pasireotide (SOM230): a multicenter, phase II trial. J Clin Endocrinol Metab. 2009;94:115–22.
73. Cukier K, Tewari R, Kurth F, et al. Significant response to pasireotide (SOM230) in the treatment of a patient with persistent, refractory Cushing's disease. Clin Endocrinol (Oxf). 2009;71:305–7.
74. de Bruin C, Pereira AM, Feelders RA, et al. Coexpression of dopamine and somatostatin receptor subtypes in corticotroph adenomas. J Clin Endocrinol Metab. 2009;94:1118–24.
75. Jaquet P, Gunz G, Saveanu A, et al. BIM-23A760, a chimeric molecule directed towards somatostatin and dopamine receptors, vs universal somatostatin receptors ligands in GH-secreting pituitary adenomas partial responders to octreotide. J Endocrinol Invest. 2005;28:21–7.
76. Florio T, Barbieri F, Spaziante R, et al. Efficacy of a dopamine-somatostatin chimeric molecule, BIM-23A760, in the control of cell growth from primary cultures of human non-functioning pituitary adenomas: a multi-center study. Endocr Relat Cancer. 2008;15:583–96.
77. Peverelli E, Olgiati L, Locatelli M, et al. The dopamine-somatostatin chimeric compound BIM-23A760 exerts antiproliferative and cytotoxic effects in human non-functioning pituitary tumors by activating ERK1/2 and p38 pathways. Cancer Lett. 2010;288:170–6.
78. Gaillard RC, Riondel A, Muller AF, et al. RU 486: a steroid with antiglucocorticosteroid activity that only disinhibits the human pituitary-adrenal system at a specific time of day. Proc Natl Acad Sci USA. 1984;81:3879–82.
79. Gaillard RC, Poffet D, Riondel AM, et al. RU 486 inhibits peripheral effects of glucocorticoids in humans. J Clin Endocrinol Metab. 1985;61:1009–11.
80. Bertagna X, Bertagna C, Laudat MH, et al. Pituitary-adrenal response to the antiglucocorticoid action of RU 486 in Cushing's syndrome. J Clin Endocrinol Metab. 1986;63:639–43.
81. Johanssen S, Allolio B. Mifepristone (RU 486) in Cushing's syndrome. Eur J Endocrinol. 2007;157:561–9.
82. Castinetti F, Fassnacht M, Johanssen S, et al. Merits and pitfalls of mifepristone in Cushing's syndrome. Eur J Endocrinol. 2009;160:1003–10.
83. Chu JW, Matthias DF, Belanoff J, et al. Successful long-term treatment of refractory Cushing's disease with high-dose mifepristone (RU 486). J Clin Endocrinol Metab. 2001;86:3568–73.

Chapter 13
Recurrent Cushing's Disease

Nancy McLaughlin, Amin Kassam, Daniel Prevedello, and Daniel Kelly

Abstract Remission of Cushing's disease after successful transsphenoidal adenomectomy is characterized by a period of sustained hypocortisolemia for a period of at least 6–12 months post surgery. Recurrent Cushing's disease, defined as a return of ACTH-dependent hypercortisolemia beginning 6 months or more after initially successful surgery, occurs in 3–27% of patients. The management options for recurrent Cushing's disease include repeat surgery with either selective adenomectomy or hemihypophysectomy or total hypophysectomy. Other options include radiosurgery or stereotactic radiotherapy, bilateral adrenalectomy, adrenolytic medical therapy, or a combination of these treatments. In the majority of patients, given that the recurrence is typically at the site of the original adenoma, repeat transsphenoidal surgery by an experienced pituitary surgeon is recommended as the initial treatment of recurrent Cushing's disease prior to offering other adjuvant therapies. The surgical approach to such patients is discussed in detail including the use of the endoscope to help visualize and remove invasive adenomas that may extend into the cavernous sinus. Given that up to 50% of patients with recurrent Cushing's disease may not achieve remission with repeat transsphenoidal surgery, a multidisciplinary team involving endocrinologists, radiation oncologists, and neurosurgeons is recommended to offer the best possible treatment options.

Keywords Transsphenoidal adenomectomy • ACTH (adrenocorticotropic hormone) • ACTH-dependent hypercortisolemia • Hemihypophysectomy • Total hypophysectomy • Stereotactic radiotherapy

D. Kelly (✉)
Brain Tumor Center & Neuroscience Institute, John Wayne Cancer Institute
at Saint John's Health Center, 2121 Santa Monica Blvd, Santa Monica, CA 90404, USA
e-mail: KellyD@JWCI.org

Introduction

Cushing's disease is the most common cause of ACTH-dependent Cushing's syndrome [1]. If left untreated, the resultant chronically elevated cortisol levels significantly increase morbidity and mortality [2–6]. Therefore, initial treatment should aim for complete tumor removal with preservation of normal pituitary function. Following successful transsphenoidal adenomectomy, remission is characterized by a period of sustained hypocortisolemia that may last 4–18 months post surgery [7]. Recurrent Cushing's disease, defined as a return of ACTH-dependent hypercortisolemia beginning 6 months or more after initially successful surgery, occurs in 3–27% of patients [3, 7–14]. When Cushing's disease recurs after primary transsphenoidal surgery, the patient is again exposed to the harmful effects of elevated serum cortisol levels. Treatment options available for such patients include repeat surgery, radiosurgery or stereotactic radiotherapy, bilateral adrenalectomy, medical therapy, or a combination of these treatments. Repeat surgery is generally considered the preferred initial treatment of recurrent Cushing's disease prior to offering other adjuvant therapies, as it may lead to immediate and sustained remission of hypercortisolemia. A second surgery may include a selective adenomectomy, a hemihypophysectomy, or total hypophysectomy. This chapter reviews the overall management of recurrent Cushing's disease with special emphasis on the indications for repeat surgery and the operative techniques employed in reoperative surgery for such patients.

Surveillance of Patients in Remission After Initial Surgery

Following initial surgery, patients require close biochemical and clinical monitoring to determine whether remission was achieved. Once biochemical evidence of hypocortisolemia has been documented, glucocorticoid replacement is instated. In our practice, we withhold acute postoperative glucocorticoids until hypocortisolemia (serum cortisol ≤5 μg/dl) is documented, which typically occurs within 24–48 h of successful surgery [15]. Other centers prefer to administer low-dose dexamethasone postoperatively, which does not suppress the HPA-axis or interfere with cortisol assays, to prevent hypocortisolemia during the immediate postoperative period. Subsequent assessments of corticotroph function are performed at regular intervals, at least every 3 months as the glucocorticoid replacement (typically prednisone or hydrocortisone) is weaned off. Criteria for sustained remission include need for glucocorticoid replacement for at least 6 months and subsequent clinical and biochemical evidence of eucortisolemia (serum cortisol 8–25 μg/dl and normal 24 h urinary free cortisol) thereafter. Given the significant possibility of delayed recurrence of Cushing's disease after initially successful surgery, it is recommended patients be followed with 24 h urinary free cortisol levels and/or late evening or midnight salivary cortisol levels at 6 month intervals for the first 5 years post surgery and then at least annually [1].

Recurrent Cushing's Disease

Several studies with relatively long follow-up indicate recurrent Cushing's disease beginning more than 6 months after initial remission can occur in 3–27% of patients with the median interval from 2.3 to 7.2 years after surgery, and some rare cases as late as 10 years after surgery [3, 7, 8, 10–14, 16, 17]. Overall, factors associated with a lower probability of initial remission include ACTH-producing macroadenomas extending above the floor of the sella [13], cavernous sinus invasion [3, 18, 19], and dural invasion (which may be present even though no evidence of invasion is seen during surgery [3, 18, 20, 21]). In a recent series by Hammer, initial remission was 86% for microadenomas; 83% for macroadenomas contained within the sella; 63% if macroadenomas extended above the floor of the sella, and 65% if tumor extended to the cavernous sinus [3]. Not surprisingly, factors associated with lower chance of initial remission are also associated with a higher recurrence rate: recurrences are higher (12–45%) and occur sooner (mean of 16 vs. 49 months) in ACTH-secreting macroadenomas than in those with microadenomas [19, 21, 22].

Surgical Treatment of Recurrent Cushing's Disease

Since 1989, at least 12 studies have reported outcomes following repeat transsphenoidal surgery for recurrent Cushing's disease (Table 13.1) [9, 12, 18, 23–32]. The remission rate following repeat surgery using the conventional microscope technique for persistent and/or recurrent Cushing's disease varies from 37 to 87% [9, 12, 18, 23–32]. More recently, after fully endoscopic transsphenoidal surgery for recurrent Cushing's disease in eight patients, Wagenmaker et al. reported a remission rate of 87.5% (7/8) [28]. In this study, none of the patients that were in remission after repeat transsphenoidal surgery had a relapse during follow-up of mean 34 months [28]. These results in a small series compare favorably to those obtained with the conventional microsurgical technique. Therefore, it appears the majority of patients with recurrent Cushing's disease can achieve remission following repeat surgery using either a microsurgical, endoscopic-assisted approach or a purely endoscopic approach.

Complete adenoma resection during repeat transsphenoidal surgery is maximized by using the same methods that help tumor identification prior to the initial surgery. Although a high quality preoperative sellar MRI should be obtained on all patients, in many instances a definitive adenoma will not be seen; scar tissue and repair materials placed at the original surgery may also be misleading [27]. For patients with negative or ambiguous magnetic resonance imaging, inferior petrosal sinus sampling may help identify the side of the pituitary gland harboring the microadenoma, if it was not performed as part of the preoperative evaluation [17, 27]. However, this test is only 50% accurate in predicting microadenoma laterality during repeat transsphenoidal surgery [27]. This observation may be explained by the altered anatomy and scar tissue after initial surgery [27]. Perhaps the most important preoperative

Table 13.1 Studies of reoperation for recurrent or persistent Cushing's disease after failed transsphenoidal surgery

	N	Mean follow-up	Remission rate (%)	Relapse rate
Nakane et al. [23]	8R	N/R	87.5	N/R
Friedman et al. [29]	31P&R	11 months	71	13.6%
Ram et al. [26]	17P	34 months (range, 4–84)	71	25%
Knappe et al. [30]	16P	N/R	P:70.8	P:24%
	24R		R:56.3	R:22%
Shimon et al. [12]	13P&R	N/R	62	N/R
Locatelli et al. [32]	12P	27 months (range, 3–84)	67	0
Benveniste et al. [24]	12P, 30R	31 months	57	35%
Hofmann et al. [11]	16R	N/R	37	0
Hofmann et al. [25]	35P&R	N/R	37.1	N/R
Aghi et al. [9]	10P	N/R	P: 70	N/R
	13R		R: 77	
Patil et al. [31]	36R	36 months	61	9.1%
Wagenmakers et al. [28]	6P, 8R	34 months	71	0

N number of patients undergoing repeat surgery (include recurrent and persistent Cushing's disease), *N/R* not reported, *P* persistent Cushing's disease, *R* recurrent Cushing's disease

information to obtain is the location of tumor at the first surgery given that the majority of CD recurrences are local. In this regard, reviewing the original operative note, pathology, and the original preoperative MRI is extremely helpful.

Once the diagnosis of recurrent Cushing's disease is established, selective removal of the recurrent adenoma by transsphenoidal surgery is the preferred first treatment option as it is for newly diagnosed patients with CD. In some instances, a more aggressive removal of the gland may be indicated, including a hemihypophysectomy or possibly a total hypophysectomy [25, 27, 28, 31]. Repeat surgery for recurrent pituitary adenomas is in general more challenging than an initial operation given the presence of scar tissue and altered normal anatomy. Adhesions of soft tissues may render access to the sphenoid sinus and sella more difficult. If bony closure of the operated sella is encountered, careful reopening of the sellar face is required. The extent of bony removal can be adapted to the presumed location of the recurrent adenoma, but in general a wide exposure is essential. As such, a wide and tall sphenoidotomy should be performed to provide full access to the entire sella. Bone removal over the sellar face should extend laterally beyond the medial portions of the cavernous sinus (CS), superiorly to the planum–tuberculum junction and inferiorly to the sellar floor. As discussed below, this exposure over the cavernous sinus is particularly important in cases of recurrences that occur in patients whose original tumor was in the lateral aspect of the gland or sella. Altered anatomic conditions in revision surgery require particular precautions to identify key neurovascular structures, in particular the cavernous carotid arteries. Surgical navigation and the Doppler probe are highly recommended for localizing and confirming the cavernous ICA positions and regional anatomy [33, 34].

Once the sella is reached, the first step of repeat surgery should be a thorough reexploration of the original resection site given that several studies indicate the great majority of recurrences occur locally and that a selective adenomectomy is typically possible [18, 23, 27, 30]. In the study by Patil et al. of 36 patients with recurrent CD, 67% underwent selective adenomectomy and only 14% had a total hypophysectomy [31]. In Nakane's series of eight patients with recurrent Cushing's disease, all repeat surgeries found an adenoma in the same location as at the initial surgery [23]. In Hofmann's series, 13 of the 16 patients operated for recurrent Cushing's disease had recurrent adenoma found in the original tumor bed [27]. In Dickerman and Oldfield's series, of 68 patients with recurrent CD, in all 43 patients in whom tumor was found at the first surgery, recurrent tumor was encountered at the same site or immediately contiguous to the original tumor site [18]. Most importantly, dural invasion by tumor was identified in 62% of 68 patients, including all 11 macroadenomas and 54% of microadenomas [18]. Of these 42 invasive adenomas, 93% involved the cavernous sinus [18].

Given these observations, it appears the origin of recurrent tumor is typically in the original tumor bed within the pituitary gland or in the adjacent cavernous sinus, presumably resulting from growth of microscopic tumor rests left behind during the original surgery [27]. Therefore, for patients in whom the original tumor site was known to be in the lateral sella, even in instances with a negative MRI, a wide exploration of the lateral sellar area and clear visualization of the medial cavernous sinus wall are essential. Once the tumor is encountered, a selective extracapsular dissection should be attempted; however, because of scarring related to the prior surgery, this may not be feasible [25, 35]. Working medially from the recurrent tumor site, the tumor–gland interface may be ill-defined, and therefore, it is reasonable to include a margin of presumably normal appearing gland to maximize chances of remission. Taking a thin rim of normal gland is generally safe with a low risk of new hypopituitarism [36].

Adhesions may be present between the tumor wall and the cavernous sinus. Given the high frequency of dural invasion in recurrent tumors, adequate exposure of the medial cavernous sinus and sellar floor dura is essential in repeat surgeries for CD [18]. Safe and effective access to this region has improved over the last two decades with enhanced anatomical knowledge of the parasellar area, surgical navigation systems, and high definition endoscopy [37–39]. After sellar tumor removal, zero degree and angled endoscopes can be used to visualize the lateral sella and medial cavernous sinus. Although the medial cavernous sinus can often be visualized with the purely microscopic view, the more panoramic view afforded by the endoscope is typically superior and may thus allow a more complete removal of cavernous sinus tumor. If tumor extends into the cavernous sinus through a defect of the medial CS wall, this dura can be incised under direct endoscopic or microscopic visualization. Tumor within the medial CS can be removed using gentle suction and ring curettes. Abnormal appearing medial CS wall dura should also be removed and dural edges should be lightly cauterized. However, great care must be taken to avoid cavernous carotid artery injury. Despite this more aggressive technique, in experienced hands, surgical management of pituitary adenomas invading the cavernous sinus did not result in permanent cranial nerve palsy or ICA injury, including recent reports in Cushing's disease [18, 40]. Therefore, careful exploration of the medial cavernous sinus using a fully endoscopic or endoscope-assisted technique may become an important component of repeat surgery for recurrent Cushing's disease. Although cavernous sinus exploration is safe and effective when performed by experienced and dedicated pituitary surgeons, the overall safety and efficacy of this technique remains to be validated in larger series.

If no tumor is visualized on preoperative MRI, sequential vertical incisions in the gland are performed [35]. A bilateral periglandular inspection with visualization of the medial wall of both cavernous sinuses and of the diaphragm is also performed to identify tumoral tissue. Hemihypophysectomy or total hypophysectomy are performed more frequently in repeat surgery than at initial surgery [41]. The role of total hypophysectomy for patients with Cushing's disease remains controversial. The remission rate following total hypophysectomy ranges from 0 to 100% [31, 42]. This variable success rate is accompanied by a greater chance of developing hypopituitarism [43]. In cases in which complete removal of invasive tumor is not possible or no definitive tumor is identified, one possible maneuver to reduce the risk of postradiosurgery hypopituitarism is to mobilize the residual gland away from the invasive site and place an intervening fat graft, enabling safer targeting of the residual invasive adenoma with a reduced risk of hypopituitarism [43]. This presumes that margin of residual gland does not harbor residual invasive adenomatous cells. The efficacy of increasing the distance between the normal pituitary gland and the residual tumor within the cavernous sinus to reduce radiation exposure to the normal pituitary gland still needs to be validated in large series [43]. Finally, if no tumor is found in the anterior lobe, the interface between anterior and posterior lobes should be carefully explored given that there is a small subset of patients who may harbor residual tumor in this region of the sella or within the posterior lobe itself. In order to gain access to the posterior lobe, a vertical incision is made in the anterior gland, exposing the gelatinous contents of the intermediate lobe and then the anterior surface of the posterior lobe [44]. Weil and colleagues described that ACTH-secreting adenomas within the posterior lobe generally have a pale gray-blue or gray-brown color visible on inspection of the neurohypophysis [44]. However, if the entire posterior lobe must removed in hopes of treating an invasive adenoma, the insertion of the infundibulum into the hypophysis should be sharply cut, avoiding traction to the stalk and minimizing the risks of permanent diabetes insipidus (personal communication Edward Laws).

Reoperations are associated with a higher rate of postoperative hypopituitarism [28]. The risk of postoperative hypopituitarism is in part related to the extent of pituitary tissue removed at repeat surgery [28]. Overall, the risk of new hormonal deficiencies after a repeat transsphenoidal operation varies between 2 and 50% mostly around 20% [26, 28, 29, 31, 43]. Importantly, the risk of hypopituitarism after repeat surgery appears to be lower than reported rates of hypopituitarism occurring several years after radiotherapy [43].

Postoperative CSF leaks have been reported to occur more frequently during repeat transsphenoidal surgery than during first-time surgery [26, 32, 45].

Chee et al. have reported a 46% rate of CSF leak in patients who underwent repeat transsphenoidal surgery vs. 13% in those who underwent initial transsphenoidal surgery [46]. However, in experienced hands, the risk of CSF leak following repeat endonasal transsphenoidal surgery may be minimal as recently reported by Patil et al. [31]. In our series, none of the patients developed a CSF leak or meningitis. However, given the relative challenges of altered anatomy and scarring associated with both persistent and recurrent Cushing's disease, as well as their relatively uncommon nature, it has been recommended that such patients be treated at specialized pituitary centers [28, 43].

Adjuvant Therapies for Recurrent Cushing's Disease

After repeat transsphenoidal surgery for CD, if biochemical remission is not achieved, adjuvant treatment is indicated. In the report by Patil et al. of 36 patients being treated for recurrent CD, 61% achieved remission with surgery alone; adjuvant therapy using radiosurgery, adrenalectomy, and/or ketoconazole therapy was effective in achieving remission in another 22% of patients for a total success rate of 83% [31]. In general, implementation of such adjuvant therapies should begin as soon as clear remission was not achieved.

Adjuvant Radiotherapy for Recurrent Cushing's Disease

Although radiation therapy was widely used as a first-line therapy for Cushing's disease from the 1940s to the early 1980s, it is typically used now as a secondary treatment after failed transsphenoidal surgery [7, 41, 43, 47, 48]. Conventional fractionated radiation therapy has historically been the primary radiation regimen used to treat Cushing's disease. Reported remission rates vary from 56 to 83%, with an average time to remission of 2 years [9, 49], but it may take many years in some patients. The incidence of hypopituitarism after fractionated radiation therapy ranges from 50 to 100% several years after treatment [50, 51]. Other less common complications related to fractionated radiotherapy include radiation necrosis, cerebral vasculopathy, damage to surrounding sellar structures, and development of a radiation-induced neoplasm [18, 52–55].

Few studies have specifically assessed the efficacy of fractionated stereotactic radiotherapy (SRT) in patients with Cushing's disease [56, 57]. Colin et al. presented the results of 12 patients treated with SRT. Nine patients (75%) achieved complete remission after a mean time of 29 months [56]. In this series, the toxicity was significantly lower for ACTH-secreting pituitary adenomas, with no radio-induced pituitary deficiency and no neurological or optic injury [56]. Theoretically, SRT focused to the target volume may be more suitable than conventional external radiotherapy. However, series with larger populations and longer follow-ups are required to assess for radiation-induced complications that may occur in a delayed fashion as well as biochemical recurrence.

Single-treatment stereotactic radiosurgery (SRS) has largely replaced conventional fractionated radiation therapy as the primary radiation modalities for persistent or recurrent Cushing's disease [43, 58]. The radiobiological effect of one high dose being delivered to slowly growing lesions is greater than that of multiple lower doses. In the three largest series of patients who underwent adjuvant radiosurgery using the Gamma Knife (single-fraction therapy), normalization of cortisol production was achieved in 63% at an average of 12.1 month [59]; 54% at an average of 13 months [60] and 43% at an average of 22 months [61]. Despite initial enthusiasm for the SRS with Gamma Knife, there is a relapse rate of up to 20% following treatment [59–62]. The incidence of new-onset hypopituitarism requiring replacement therapy after SRS varies between 16 and 55% with a median period of 50–60 months [60–63]. Overall, SRS seems to lead to faster normalization of hormone levels with lower risk of hypopituitarism and visual deterioration compared to fractionated radiotherapy [58, 60]. Since recurrences of Cushing's disease and hormonal deficiencies may arise years after therapy, long-term biochemical surveillance is indicated.

Recently, the results of proton-beam radiosurgery have been reported [64]. Proton-beam radiosurgery offers improved dose distributions as compared with photon beams [65]. Remission rates of 52% [64] at median follow-up of 62 months were obtained, similar to those obtained with Gamma Knife SRS. The toxic effects to the cranial nerve and disease recurrence rates appear slightly lower than for Gamma Knife [9]. However, the incidence of hypopituitarism may be slightly higher, at 50% at 24 months [64]. Larger series with longer follow-up are required to assess the advantages of proton beam radiosurgery over Gamma Knife as well as the occurrence of late radiation-related sequelae.

Adjuvant Medical Treatment for Recurrent Cushing's Disease

Medical therapy is discussed extensively in Chap. 12. In the setting of recurrent Cushing's disease, medical therapy may be used to transiently lower cortisol levels and thereby improve a patient's clinical condition before undergoing repeat transsphenoidal surgery, particularly in cases of advanced CD. It may also be needed in patients with recurrent CD who have undergone SRS or SRT in the interim period while awaiting the effect of radiation. Overall, medical treatment may be useful in up to one third of Cushing's disease patients [66]. The most commonly used drugs in USA for recurrent Cushing's disease are ketoconazole and metyrapone, which inhibit adrenal steroidogenesis [1, 7, 67]. Other agents currently under investigation include cortisol-receptor antagonists and drugs modulating ACTH release [7, 17, 43, 66, 67]. Medical treatment often requires prolonged administration and careful cortisol monitoring for periodic dose adjustment to keep cortisol levels in normal ranges. If administered as a bridging treatment after radiation treatment, it may be discontinued once remission has been achieved and documented.

Bilateral Adrenalectomy

Bilateral adrenalectomy, especially laparoscopic approaches, for persistent and recurrent Cushing's disease is currently associated with relatively low perioperative morbidity [48, 68]. Remission rates after bilateral adrenalectomy with rapid reversal of hypercortisolism range from 88 to 100% [41]. Adrenalectomy is indicated in patients who have had multiple surgeries, radiosurgery, or both, but have ultimately failed to achieve remission, as well as for those who are unable to obtain medical control of their hypercortisolism without adverse effects. Open adrenalectomy has been associated with 23% perioperative morbidity and 4% operative mortality [69]. More recently, laparoscopic adrenalectomy has been accepted as the standard approach for resection of most benign adrenal lesions [68]. Recent series have reported approximately 10% perioperative morbidity, 1% perioperative operative mortality, decreased postoperative pain, and shorter hospital stay [68, 70]. Although there are persistent quality-of-life deficits after biochemical remission of Cushing's disease, some studies have found an improvement in quality of life after bilateral adrenalectomy for persistent or recurrent Cushing's disease [68, 71]. Lifelong mineralo- and glucocorticoid replacement therapy are required after bilateral adrenalectomy with their unavoidable risk of acute adrenal insufficiency [1, 7]. Furthermore, up to 10% of cases may resume endogenous cortisol secretion many years after a bilateral adrenalectomy [1]. Adrenal rest that escapes adrenalectomy and accessory glands located in various sites can grow under the chronic stimulation of highly elevated ACTH levels and result in recurrent hypercortisolism [1].

Clinical, biochemical and radiological surveillance are necessary to monitor for adenoma growth and increased ACTH plasma levels following bilateral adrenalectomy [1, 48]. The risk of Nelson's syndrome and Corticotroph Tumor Progression (CTP) is discussed in detail in Chap. 17. ACTH plasma level measurement and pituitary MRI are advised 3–6 months after bilateral adrenalectomy and at regular intervals thereafter [48]. Over time, there is a significant risk of developing Nelson's Syndrome characterized by elevated serum ACTH, skin hyperpigmentation, and a progressively enlarging corticotroph adenoma. The adenomas associated with Nelson's syndrome can be aggressive, are often invasive and can develop into pituitary carcinomas [41, 72]. In patient series published since 1983 with adequate follow-up, the rate of Nelson's Syndrome ranged from 15 to 46% [73–82], though some of these series included cases of CTP as defined by radiographic progression, rather than the full-blown Nelson's syndrome. The average interval between bilateral adrenalectomy and development of Nelson syndrome is approximately 5–10 years but may be as short as 6 months and as long as 24 years [76, 79, 80, 83]. The only study that assessed the role of prophylactic radiation showed that prior radiation therapy reduced the risk and delayed the onset of developing Nelson's Syndrome [79]. However, the potential benefits of this practice are not well defined, and it is presently not recommended to perform prophylactic radiotherapy [7, 48]. Bilateral adrenalectomy can be life-saving in critically ill patients with severe Cushing's disease, but in the majority of patients it should only be considered when pituitary-directed treatments have failed or are contraindicated.

Conclusions

The management of recurrent Cushing disease remains a challenge for the pituitary neurosurgeon. When possible, repeat transsphenoidal surgery for selective adenomectomy should be the treatment of choice with exploration of the sella and medial walls of the cavernous sinuses for possible invasive tumor. In some instances, hemi- or total hypophysectomy may be indicated. When repeat surgery fails, other treatment options including SRS or SRT, medical treatment, and/or bilateral adrenalectomy may be indicated. Given the complexity of this disorder and the wide spectrum of treatment options, patients with recurrent Cushing's disease are best cared for by a multidisciplinary team comprising a neurosurgeon specialized in pituitary adenoma surgery, a pituitary endocrinologist, radiation oncologists, and general surgeons.

References

1. Bertagna X, Guignat L, Groussin L, Bertherat J. Cushing's disease. Best Pract Res Clin Endocrinol Metab. 2009;23:607–23.
2. Etxabe J, Vazquez JA. Morbidity and mortality in Cushing's disease: an epidemiological approach. Clin Endocrinol (Oxf). 1994;40:479–84.
3. Hammer GD, Tyrrell JB, Lamborn KR, et al. Transsphenoidal microsurgery for Cushing's disease: initial outcome and long-term results. J Clin Endocrinol Metab. 2004;89:6348–57.
4. Lindholm J, Juul S, Jorgensen JO, et al. Incidence and late prognosis of cushing's syndrome: a population-based study. J Clin Endocrinol Metab. 2001;86:117–23.
5. Pikkarainen L, Sane T, Reunanen A. The survival and well-being of patients treated for Cushing's syndrome. J Intern Med. 1999;245:463–8.
6. Mancini T, Kola B, Mantero F, Boscaro M, Arnaldi G. High cardiovascular risk in patients with Cushing's syndrome according to 1999 WHO/ISH guidelines. Clin Endocrinol (Oxf). 2004;61:768–77.
7. Beauregard C, Dickstein G, Lacroix A. Classic and recent etiologies of Cushing's syndrome: diagnosis and therapy. Treat Endocrinol. 2002;1:79–94.
8. Barbetta L, Dall'Asta C, Tomei G, Locatelli M, Giovanelli M, Ambrosi B. Assessment of cure and recurrence after pituitary surgery for Cushing's disease. Acta Neurochir (Wien). 2001;143:477–81. discussion 81–2.
9. Aghi MK, Petit J, Chapman P, et al. Management of recurrent and refractory Cushing's disease with reoperation and/or proton beam radiosurgery. Clin Neurosurg. 2008;55:141–4.
10. Bocchicchio D, Losa M, Buchfelder M. Factors influencing the immediate and late outcome of Cushing's disease treated by transsphenoidal surgery: a retrospective study by the European Cushing's Disease Survey Group. J Clin Endocrinol Metab. 1995;80:3114–20.
11. Hofmann BM, Fahlbusch R. Treatment of Cushing's disease: a retrospective clinical study of the latest 100 cases. Front Horm Res. 2006;34:158–84.

12. Shimon I, Ram Z, Cohen ZR, Hadani M. Transsphenoidal surgery for Cushing's disease: endocrinological follow-up monitoring of 82 patients. Neurosurgery. 2002;51:57–61. discussion 61–2.
13. Fomekong E, Maiter D, Grandin C, Raftopoulos C. Outcome of transsphenoidal surgery for Cushing's disease: a high remission rate in ACTH-secreting macroadenomas. Clin Neurol Neurosurg. 2009;111:442–9.
14. Atkinson AB, Kennedy A, Wiggam MI, McCance DR, Sheridan B. Long-term remission rates after pituitary surgery for Cushing's disease: the need for long-term surveillance. Clin Endocrinol (Oxf). 2005;63:549–59.
15. Esposito F, Kelly DF, Vinters HV, DeSalles AA, Sercarz J, Gorgulhos AA. Primary sphenoid sinus neoplasms: a report of four cases with common clinical presentation treated with transsphenoidal surgery and adjuvant therapies. J Neurooncol. 2006;76:299–306.
16. Pereira AM, van Aken MO, van Dulken H, et al. Long-term predictive value of postsurgical cortisol concentrations for cure and risk of recurrence in Cushing's disease. J Clin Endocrinol Metab. 2003;88:5858–64.
17. Aghi MK. Management of recurrent and refractory Cushing disease. Nat Clin Pract Endocrinol Metab. 2008;4:560–8.
18. Dickerman RD, Oldfield EH. Basis of persistent and recurrent Cushing disease: an analysis of findings at repeated pituitary surgery. J Neurosurg. 2002;97:1343–9.
19. Blevins Jr LS, Christy JH, Khajavi M, Tindall GT. Outcomes of therapy for Cushing's disease due to adrenocorticotropin-secreting pituitary macroadenomas. J Clin Endocrinol Metab. 1998;83:63–7.
20. Meij B, Voorhout G, Rijnberk A. Progress in transsphenoidal hypophysectomy for treatment of pituitary-dependent hyperadrenocorticism in dogs and cats. Mol Cell Endocrinol. 2002;197:89–96.
21. De Tommasi C, Vance ML, Okonkwo DO, Diallo A, Laws Jr ER. Surgical management of adrenocorticotropic hormone-secreting macroadenomas: outcome and challenges in patients with Cushing's disease or Nelson's syndrome. J Neurosurg. 2005;103:825–30.
22. Swearingen B, Biller BM, Barker 2nd FG, et al. Long-term mortality after transsphenoidal surgery for Cushing disease. Ann Intern Med. 1999;130:821–4.
23. Nakane T, Kuwayama A, Watanabe M, et al. Long term results of transsphenoidal adenomectomy in patients with Cushing's disease. Neurosurgery. 1987;21:218–22.
24. Benveniste RJ, King WA, Walsh J, Lee JS, Delman BN, Post KD. Repeated transsphenoidal surgery to treat recurrent or residual pituitary adenoma. J Neurosurg. 2005;102:1004–12.
25. Hofmann BM, Hlavac M, Martinez R, Buchfelder M, Muller OA, Fahlbusch R. Long-term results after microsurgery for Cushing disease: experience with 426 primary operations over 35 years. J Neurosurg. 2008;108:9–18.
26. Ram Z, Nieman LK, Cutler Jr GB, Chrousos GP, Doppman JL, Oldfield EH. Early repeat surgery for persistent Cushing's disease. J Neurosurg. 1994;80:37–45.
27. Hofmann BM, Hlavac M, Kreutzer J, Grabenbauer G, Fahlbusch R. Surgical treatment of recurrent Cushing's disease. Neurosurgery. 2006;58:1108–18. discussion 1108–18.
28. Wagenmakers MA, Netea-Maier RT, van Lindert EJ, Timmers HJ, Grotenhuis JA, Hermus AR. Repeated transsphenoidal pituitary surgery (TS) via the endoscopic technique: a good therapeutic option for recurrent or persistent Cushing's disease (CD). Clin Endocrinol (Oxf). 2009;70:274–80.
29. Friedman RB, Oldfield EH, Nieman LK, et al. Repeat transsphenoidal surgery for Cushing's disease. J Neurosurg. 1989;71:520–7.
30. Knappe UJ, Ludecke DK. Persistent and recurrent hypercortisolism after transsphenoidal surgery for Cushing's disease. Acta Neurochir Suppl. 1996;65:31–4.
31. Patil CG, Veeravagu A, Prevedello DM, Katznelson L, Vance ML, Laws Jr ER. Outcomes after repeat transsphenoidal surgery for recurrent Cushing's disease. Neurosurgery. 2008;63:266–70. discussion 70–1.
32. Locatelli M, Vance ML, Laws ER. Clinical review: the strategy of immediate reoperation for transsphenoidal surgery for Cushing's disease. J Clin Endocrinol Metab. 2005;90:5478–82.

33. Dusick JR, Esposito F, Malkasian D, Kelly DF. Avoidance of carotid artery injuries in transsphenoidal surgery with the Doppler probe and micro-hook blades. Neurosurgery. 2007;60:322–8. discussion 8–9.
34. Fatemi N, Dusick JR, de Paiva Neto MA, Kelly DF. The endonasal microscopic approach for pituitary adenomas and other parasellar tumors: a 10-year experience. Neurosurgery. 2008;63:244–56. discussion 256.
35. Jagannathan J, Smith R, DeVroom HL, et al. Outcome of using the histological pseudocapsule as a surgical capsule in Cushing disease. J Neurosurg. 2009;111:531–9.
36. Fatemi N, Dusick JR, Mattozo C, et al. Pituitary hormonal loss and recovery after transsphenoidal adenoma removal. Neurosurgery. 2008;63:709–18. discussion 718–9.
37. Cavallo LM, de Divitiis O, Aydin S, et al. Extended endoscopic endonasal transsphenoidal approach to the suprasellar area: anatomic considerations – part 1. Neurosurgery. 2007;61:24–33. discussion 33–4.
38. Kassam A, Snyderman CH, Mintz A, Gardner P, Carrau RL. Expanded endonasal approach: the rostrocaudal axis. Part II. Posterior clinoids to the foramen magnum. Neurosurg Focus. 2005;19:E4.
39. Kassam A, Snyderman CH, Mintz A, Gardner P, Carrau RL. Expanded endonasal approach: the rostrocaudal axis. Part I. Crista galli to the sella turcica. Neurosurg Focus. 2005;19:E3.
40. Kitano M, Taneda M, Shimono T, Nakao Y. Extended transsphenoidal approach for surgical management of pituitary adenomas invading the cavernous sinus. J Neurosurg. 2008;108:26–36.
41. Kelly DF. Transsphenoidal surgery for Cushing's disease: a review of success rates, remission predictors, management of failed surgery, and Nelson's syndrome. Neurosurg Focus. 2007;23:E5.
42. Hardy J. Presidential address: XVII Canadian Congress of Neurological Sciences. Cushing's disease: 50 years later. Can J Neurol Sci. 1982;9:375–80.
43. Liu JK, Fleseriu M, Delashaw Jr JB, Ciric IS, Couldwell WT. Treatment options for Cushing disease after unsuccessful transsphenoidal surgery. Neurosurg Focus. 2007;23:E8.
44. Weil RJ, Vortmeyer AO, Nieman LK, Devroom HL, Wanebo J, Oldfield EH. Surgical remission of pituitary adenomas confined to the neurohypophysis in Cushing's disease. J Clin Endocrinol Metab. 2006;91:2656–64.
45. Rudnik A, Zawadzki T, Galuszka-Ignasiak B, et al. Endoscopic transsphenoidal treatment in recurrent and residual pituitary adenomas – first experience. Minim Invasive Neurosurg. 2006;49:10–4.
46. Chee GH, Mathias DB, James RA, Kendall-Taylor P. Transsphenoidal pituitary surgery in Cushing's disease: can we predict outcome? Clin Endocrinol (Oxf). 2001;54:617–26.
47. Blevins Jr LS, Sanai N, Kunwar S, Devin JK. An approach to the management of patients with residual Cushing's disease. J Neurooncol. 2009;94:313–9.
48. Biller BM, Grossman AB, Stewart PM, et al. Treatment of adrenocorticotropin-dependent Cushing's syndrome: a consensus statement. J Clin Endocrinol Metab. 2008;93:2454–62.
49. Estrada J, Boronat M, Mielgo M, et al. The long-term outcome of pituitary irradiation after unsuccessful transsphenoidal surgery in Cushing's disease. N Engl J Med. 1997;336:172–7.
50. Becker G, Kocher M, Kortmann RD, et al. Radiation therapy in the multimodal treatment approach of pituitary adenoma. Strahlenther Onkol. 2002;178:173–86.
51. Zierhut D, Flentje M, Adolph J, Erdmann J, Raue F, Wannenmacher M. External radiotherapy of pituitary adenomas. Int J Radiat Oncol Biol Phys. 1995;33:307–14.
52. Brada M, Ford D, Ashley S, et al. Risk of second brain tumour after conservative surgery and radiotherapy for pituitary adenoma. BMJ. 1992;304:1343–6.
53. Simmons NE, Laws Jr ER. Glioma occurrence after sellar irradiation: case report and review. Neurosurgery. 1998;42:172–8.
54. Salinger DJ, Brady LW, Miyamoto CT. Radiation therapy in the treatment of pituitary adenomas. Am J Clin Oncol. 1992;15:467–73.
55. Constine LS, Woolf PD, Cann D, et al. Hypothalamic-pituitary dysfunction after radiation for brain tumors. N Engl J Med. 1993;328:87–94.

56. Colin P, Delemer B, Nakib I, et al. Unsuccessful surgery of Cushing's disease. Role and efficacy of fractionated stereotactic radiotherapy. Neurochirurgie. 2002;48:285–93.
57. Colin P, Jovenin N, Delemer B, et al. Treatment of pituitary adenomas by fractionated stereotactic radiotherapy: a prospective study of 110 patients. Int J Radiat Oncol Biol Phys. 2005;62:333–41.
58. Sheehan JP, Niranjan A, Sheehan JM, et al. Stereotactic radiosurgery for pituitary adenomas: an intermediate review of its safety, efficacy, and role in the neurosurgical treatment armamentarium. J Neurosurg. 2005;102:678–91.
59. Sheehan JM, Vance ML, Sheehan JP, Ellegala DB, Laws Jr ER. Radiosurgery for Cushing's disease after failed transsphenoidal surgery. J Neurosurg. 2000;93:738–42.
60. Jagannathan J, Sheehan JP, Pouratian N, Laws ER, Steiner L, Vance ML. Gamma knife surgery for Cushing's disease. J Neurosurg. 2007;106:980–7.
61. Castinetti F, Nagai M, Dufour H, et al. Gamma knife radiosurgery is a successful adjunctive treatment in Cushing's disease. Eur J Endocrinol. 2007;156:91–8.
62. Oyesiku NM. Stereotactic radiosurgery for Cushing disease: a review. Neurosurg Focus. 2007;23:E14.
63. Kobayashi T, Kida Y, Mori Y. Gamma knife radiosurgery in the treatment of Cushing disease: long-term results. J Neurosurg. 2002;97:422–8.
64. Petit JH, Biller BM, Yock TI, et al. Proton stereotactic radiotherapy for persistent adrenocorticotropin-producing adenomas. J Clin Endocrinol Metab. 2008;93:393–9.
65. Lyman JT, Phillips MH, Frankel KA, Levy RP, Fabrikant JI. Radiation physics for particle beam radiosurgery. Neurosurg Clin N Am. 1992;3:1–8.
66. Miller JW, Crapo L. The medical treatment of Cushing's syndrome. Endocr Rev. 1993;14:443–58.
67. Fleseriu M, Loriaux DL, Ludlam WH. Second-line treatment for Cushing's disease when initial pituitary surgery is unsuccessful. Curr Opin Endocrinol Diabetes Obes. 2007;14:323–8.
68. Smith PW, Turza KC, Carter CO, Vance ML, Laws ER, Hanks JB. Bilateral adrenalectomy for refractory Cushing disease: a safe and definitive therapy. J Am Coll Surg. 2009;208:1059–64.
69. O'Riordain DS, Farley DR, Young Jr WF, Grant CS, VanHeerden JA. Long-term outcome of bilateral adrenalectomy in patients with Cushing's syndrome. Surgery. 1994;116:1088–93. discussion 93–4.
70. Chow JT, Thompson GB, Grant CS, Farley DR, Richards ML, Young Jr WF. Bilateral laparoscopic adrenalectomy for corticotrophin-dependent Cushing's syndrome: a review of the Mayo Clinic experience. Clin Endocrinol (Oxf). 2008;68:513–9.
71. Thompson SK, Hayman AV, Ludlam WH, Deveney CW, Loriaux DL, Sheppard BC. Improved quality of life after bilateral laparoscopic adrenalectomy for Cushing's disease: a 10-year experience. Ann Surg. 2007;245:790–4.
72. Kemink SA, Wesseling P, Pieters GF, Verhofstad AA, Hermus AR, Smals AG. Progression of a Nelson's adenoma to pituitary carcinoma; a case report and review of the literature. J Endocrinol Invest. 1999;22:70–5.
73. Assie G, Bahurel H, Coste J, et al. Corticotroph tumor progression after adrenalectomy in Cushing's disease: a reappraisal of Nelson's syndrome. J Clin Endocrinol Metab. 2007;92:172–9.
74. Brunicardi FC, Rosman PM, Lesser KL, Andersen DK. Current status of adrenalectomy for Cushing's disease. Surgery. 1985;98:1127–34.
75. McCance DR, Russell CF, Kennedy TL, Hadden DR, Kennedy L, Atkinson AB. Bilateral adrenalectomy: low mortality and morbidity in Cushing's disease. Clin Endocrinol (Oxf). 1993;39:315–21.
76. Kasperlik-Zaluska A, Migdalska B, Jeske W, Wisniewska-Wozniak T, Sek S. The relationship between cortisol and ACTH in patients with Cushing's disease following neurosurgery or pharmacotherapy. Endokrynol Pol. 1989;40:63–7.
77. Sonino N, Zielezny M, Fava GA, Fallo F, Boscaro M. Risk factors and long-term outcome in pituitary-dependent Cushing's disease. J Clin Endocrinol Metab. 1996;81:2647–52.
78. Pereira MA, Halpern A, Salgado LR, et al. A study of patients with Nelson's syndrome. Clin Endocrinol (Oxf). 1998;49:533–9.

79. Nagesser SK, van Seters AP, Kievit J, Hermans J, Krans HM, van de Velde CJ. Long-term results of total adrenalectomy for Cushing's disease. World J Surg. 2000;24:108–13.
80. Invitti C, Giraldi FP, de Martin M, Cavagnini F. Diagnosis and management of Cushing's syndrome: results of an Italian multicentre study. Study Group of the Italian Society of Endocrinology on the Pathophysiology of the Hypothalamic-Pituitary-Adrenal Axis. J Clin Endocrinol Metab. 1999;84:440–8.
81. Favia G, Boscaro M, Lumachi F, D'Amico DF. Role of bilateral adrenalectomy in Cushing's disease. World J Surg. 1994;18:462–6.
82. Hardy JD, Moore DO, Langford HG. Cushing's disease today. Late follow-up of 17 adrenalectomy patients with emphasis on eight with adrenal autotransplants. Ann Surg. 1985;201:595–603.
83. Nagesser SK, van Seters AP, Kievit J, et al. Treatment of pituitary-dependent Cushing's syndrome: long-term results of unilateral adrenalectomy followed by external pituitary irradiation compared to transsphenoidal pituitary surgery. Clin Endocrinol (Oxf). 2000;52:427–35.

Chapter 14
Diagnosis and Treatment of Pediatric Cushing's Disease

Claire R. Hughes, Helen L. Storr, Ashley B. Grossman, and Martin O. Savage

Abstract Cushing's disease (CD), which is caused by an ACTH-secreting pituitary corticotroph adenoma, is the commonest cause of Cushing's syndrome in children over 5 years of age. However, it remains rare in the pediatric age range and may present a difficult diagnostic and therapeutic challenge. Key presenting features include weight gain associated with growth failure. Parents and general practitioners frequently fail to appreciate the nature of the pathology, significantly delaying diagnosis. Most pediatric endocrinologists have limited experience managing children or adolescents with CD and thus benefit from close consultation with adult colleagues. We describe a diagnostic protocol for investigation that broadly follows the model for adult patients. Treatment strategies for CD are examined and critically appraised. The management of pediatric CD patients after cure is also discussed, as it presents unique challenges for optimizing growth, bone health, reproduction, and body composition from childhood into and during adult life.

Keywords Cushing's disease • Cushing's syndrome • Pediatrics • Transsphenoidal surgery • Radiotherapy

Introduction

Cushing's syndrome (CS) is a clinical syndrome that comprises many symptoms and signs reflecting excessive circulating glucocorticoid (GC) concentrations. It is very rare in childhood and adolescence, compared to the more common pediatric

---

M.O. Savage (✉)
Department of Endocrinology, William Harvey Research Institute,
Barts and the London School of Medicine and Dentistry, John Vane Science Centre,
Charterhouse Square, London, EC1M 6BQ, UK
e-mail: m.o.savage@qmul.ac.uk

Table 14.1 Classification of pediatric Cushing's syndrome

ACTH-independent
1. Exogenous glucocorticoid administration (tablets, nose drops, inhalers, nasal spray, skin cream)
2. Adrenocortical tumor (adenoma or carcinoma)
3. Primary adrenocortical hyperplasia
   (a) Primary pigmented nodular adrenocortical disease (PPNAD)
   (b) Macronodular adrenal hyperplasia (AIMAH)
   (c) Mc-Cune Albright syndrome

ACTH-dependent
1. Cushing's disease (ACTH-secreting pituitary adenoma)
2. Ectopic ACTH syndrome

endocrine pathologies such as disorders of growth, puberty, and thyroid. CS within the pediatric age range can be classified into two groups of adrenocorticotrophic hormone (ACTH)-independent and ACTH-dependent causes (Table 14.1). Iatrogenic exogenous GC administration remains the most common cause in pediatric as well as adult CS patients. These patients are rarely referred for endocrine review, and therefore, the following data assumes exclusion of iatrogenic CS.

Cushing's disease (CD), which is caused by an ACTH-secreting pituitary corticotroph adenoma, is the commonest cause of CS in children over 5 years of age [1–3]. CD accounts for 75–80% of pediatric CS cases compared to 49–71% of adult cases [1, 4].

Most pediatric endocrinologists have limited experience in the diagnosis and treatment of children with CD and, therefore, should benefit from close consultation with adult colleagues. However, some aspects of pediatric CD do differ from those present in adults. Examples are the increased frequency in prepubertal males compared to females, the frequent absence of radiological evidence of a corticotroph adenoma on pituitary scanning and the higher incidence of lateralization of ACTH secretion demonstrated by inferior petrosal sinus sampling. Children also have a more exuberant cortisol response to IV CRH and a more rapid response to external beam pituitary radiotherapy compared to adults. Clinically children can present differently from adults, most notably with growth failure associated with weight gain. These features are discussed, together with other diagnostic and therapeutic aspects of pediatric CD.

Clinical and Diagnostic Aspects of Pediatric Cushing's Disease

Epidemiology

CS can occur throughout childhood and adolescence; however, different etiologies are more commonly associated with particular age groups (Fig. 14.1), with CD being the commonest cause after the preschool years [3]. The peak incidence of

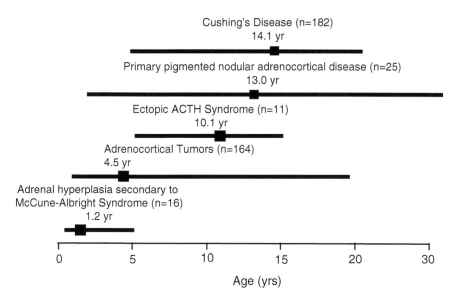

Fig. 14.1 Different etiologies of Pediatric Cushing's syndrome from the literature ($n=398$ cases) shown at ages of peak incidence (*boxes*)

pediatric CD is during adolescence; in 182 cases taken from the literature, the median age of presentation was 14.1 years. The youngest child in our series of 37 cases was aged 5.8 years at diagnosis.

Pediatric CD is almost always caused by a pituitary microadenoma with diameter <5 mm [5]. We have seen just one macroadenoma in 37 pediatric cases [6]. Children with macroadenomas are only rarely reported in the literature [7], and invasion of the cavernous sinus has been noted in one case [8]. Pituitary macroadenomas have been described as an early manifestation of MEN 1 [9] and, therefore, should alert the clinician to the possibility of this diagnosis in children.

In adults CD has a female preponderance [10]. We analyzed gender distribution in 50 CD patients aged from 6 to 30 years and found a significant predominance of males in the prepubertal patients (Fig. 14.2) [11]. The incidence in males and females during puberty was similar, with an increasing predominance of females in the postpubertal patients. In our current series of 37 cases aged from 5.8 to 17.8 years, there are 24 males and 13 females. Following this observation, the large series from the NIH [3] was examined and also revealed the same phenomenon of male predominance in young patients. No clear explanation for this exists, although a reasonable hypothesis would suggest that increasing estrogen levels during female puberty may be related to the relative increase in incidence in females during and following adolescence.

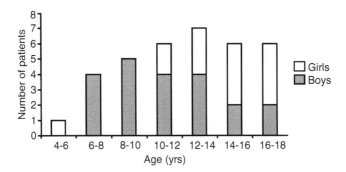

Fig. 14.2 Sex incidence and age of diagnosis in 36 pediatric patients with Cushing's disease (CD). There were 24 males (69%) and 12 females (31%). In a population of 126 adult CD patients, 31 (25%) were male and 95 (75%) were female

Clinical Features in CD

General Features

The early recognition of the salient features of CD is crucial to allow prompt diagnosis and effective treatment. Key presenting features include growth failure, weight gain, and a change in facial appearance. Most children and adolescents have a typical Cushingoid appearance. A subtle or subclinical presentation or even cyclical features are uncommon. Unfortunately, parents and general practitioners frequently fail to recognize the pathological nature of the change of the child's appearance, significantly delaying diagnosis. The mean length of symptoms prior to diagnosis in our 37 CD patients was 2.5 ± 1.7 years (range 0.3–6.6 years).

All of our patients complained of weight gain and a change in facial appearance. Striae were present in 50% of our patients, more frequently in the older patients. The young child with CD often presented with only obesity and growth failure, without the classical features of plethora, hirsutism, acne, and striae. Additional features noted in some children included emotional lability, hypertension, and fatigue. Muscle weakness and easy bruising were rare symptoms.

Characteristics of Growth and Auxological Parameters

Short stature (height less than −2.0 SD) was present in 43% of our patients, and growth velocity when available was subnormal. Growth failure has been attributed to growth hormone deficiency, resistance to insulin-like growth factor 1 (IGF-1) [12], and prolonged exposure to supraphysiological free circulating glucocorticoids [3, 13].

One of the most striking features in our cohort was the contrast between height SDS, which was almost always below the mean, and BMI SDS, which was consistently above it (Fig. 14.3), as has been previously reported [1]. One of the principal

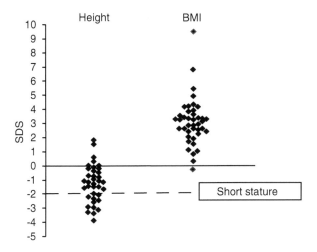

Fig. 14.3 Height and body mass index (BMI) SDS values in 37 pediatric patients with Cushing's disease. The *dotted line* indicates the SDS value below which patients are significantly shorter than average

features of CD, obesity, is now extremely common. However, there is an important difference in the growth pattern between obesity due to CD and simple obesity: CD is almost always associated with growth failure, while simple obesity is usually accompanied by advanced growth. We compared height and BMI SDS in 29 patients with CD and 44 age-matched patients with simple obesity. There was a significant difference in the ratio of these two variables between the two groups, height being increased in simple obesity and decreased in CD [14]. Bone age (BA) at diagnosis of CD was delayed in 15 of 17 patients (mean delay 2.0 year; range −0.5 to 4.1 year) and correlated negatively with height SDS ($r=-0.70$; $P<0.01$), duration of symptoms ($r=0.48$; $P=0.05$), and age at diagnosis ($r=0.48$; $P=0.05$) [15].

Pubertal Development

True precocious puberty in CD is unusual with very few cases reported in the literature. However, virilization with pseudoprecocious puberty is recognized as an important presenting feature [1, 3]. This was also demonstrated in our cohort. Abnormal virilization, defined as unusual advance of Tanner pubic hair stage compared to testicular volume or breast development, was identified in 12 of 27 patients [16]. In these patients, the values of serum androstenedione, DHEAS, (as previously reported [17]), and testosterone SDS were higher ($P=0.03$, 0.008, 0.03 respectively) than in subjects without abnormal virilization and SHBG SDS values were lower ($P=0.006$). Gonadotrophin levels were subnormal in the patients who had commenced true puberty, suggesting a suppressive effect of chronic hypercortisolemia.

Table 14.2 Scheme of investigation for patients with suspected Cushing's syndrome

Confirmation or exclusion of Cushing's syndrome
1. Urinary free cortisol excretion (24-h urine collection) daily for 3 days
2. Serum cortisol circadian rhythm study [0900 h, 1800 h, and midnight (sleeping)]
3. Low-dose dexamethosone suppression test (LDDST)
    (a) Dose 0.5 mg 6 hourly (0900, 1500, 2100, 0300 h) for 48 h
    (b) Dose for patients weighing <40 kg; 30 μg/kg/day
    (c) Serum cortisol measured at 0 and 48 h

Definition of etiology of Cushing's syndrome
1. Plasma ACTH (09.00 h)
2. CRH test (1.0 μg/kg IV)
3. Analysis of change in serum cortisol during LDDST
4. Adrenal or pituitary MRI scan
5. Bilateral inferior petrosal sinus sampling for ACTH (with CRH)

Investigation of CD

The investigation of patients with suspected CD has been extensively reviewed [18, 19] and guidelines for the diagnosis of pediatric CD have also been published [1]. A recent consensus statement advised that only those obese children who have demonstrated slowing of their growth velocity should be investigated, as a combined reduction in height velocity with increased weight was felt to have a high sensitivity and specificity for CD [20].

The algorithm for testing in children should be based on that performed in adults [18] and consists initially of confirmation or exclusion of the diagnosis of CS followed by investigations to determine the etiology. This scheme is listed in Table 14.2. The initial screening investigations shown have a high sensitivity; if the initial test results are normal, the patient is very unlikely to have CS. We have highlighted some aspects that we found helpful during the management of 37 CD patients over the past 27 years. Prior to embarking on biochemical evaluation, it is important to investigate the possible forms of glucocorticoid use detailed in Table 14.1, as exogenous CS is much more common than the endogenous form.

Confirmation or Exclusion of Cushing's Syndrome

Consistent with current recommendations [20], our initial screening test includes three consecutive 24-h urine collections for urinary free cortisol (UFC). This provides an integrated assessment of cortisol secretion over a 24-h period and measures only free, unbound hormone. If there is doubt about the interpretation of these values, we proceed to admit the child for measurement of serum cortisol at three time-points (09.00 h, 18.00 h, and midnight [sleeping]) to assess circadian rhythm. Determination of midnight cortisol in the sleeping child gives the highest sensitivity for the diagnosis of CS [21]. The value in normal subjects is <50 nmol/L (<1.8 μg/dl), although some young children may reach their cortisol nadir earlier than midnight. Midnight

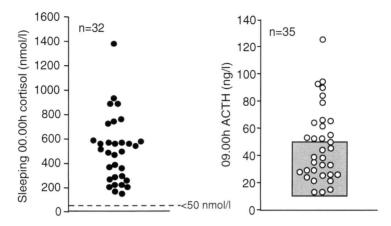

Fig. 14.4 Midnight cortisol was >50 nmol/L with detectable ACTH, ranging from 12 to 128 ng/L, in all patients with Cushing's disease

serum cortisol was measurable in all the patients with Cushing's syndrome who we have managed. Late-night salivary cortisol has also been evaluated as a screening test in the pediatric obese population to differentiate children with CS. A high sensitivity and specificity has been reported [22]; however, the influence of age has not been fully characterized. It can also be technically difficult to obtain a salivary sample in younger children; hence, our protocol uses midnight serum cortisol.

Following assessment of midnight cortisol, we perform a low-dose dexamethasone suppression test (LDDST), using the adult dose regimen of 0.5 mg every 6 h (at 0900, 1500, 2100 and 0300 h) for 48 h, unless the child weighs <40 kg when we use the NIH-recommended dose of 30 µg/kg/day [3]. In the LDDST, blood is taken for serum cortisol at 0 and at 48, 6 h after the last dose, when it is undetectable (<50 nmol/L, <1.8 µg/dl) in normal subjects. These tests performed individually, and particularly in combination, have a high sensitivity for CS and an even higher specificity for the exclusion of this diagnosis. The 1-mg overnight dexamethasone test has been used as a screening test in children, but there are no available data on its interpretation or reliability [20].

Confirmation of Cushing's Disease

Following confirmation of CS, the priority is to determine the cause of the hypercortisolism. CD is most easily confirmed by determination of basal plasma ACTH. In all of our patients with CD, ACTH was detectable, ranging from 12 to 128 ng/L (normal 10–50 ng/L) (Fig. 14.4). In ACTH-independent CS, ACTH is always low and usually undetectable.

We routinely perform a CRH test using human sequence CRH (1 µg/kg IV) and in 27 CD patients serum cortisol increased by >20% (range 106–554%). Ectopic ACTH syndrome is so rare in children that the need for a CRH test is questionable; however, we find that an increased cortisol response contributes to the diagnosis of CD.

Table 14.3 Pituitary imaging, surgical identification of microadenoma and cure by TSS

Total patients (n)	Adenoma CT/MRI image (n)	Concordance of image with surgery (n)	Cure by TSS (n)
36	19 (53%)	11 (31%)	23/34 (68%)

We no longer routinely perform a high dose dexamethasone suppression test (HDDST). This recent decision follows an analysis of serum cortisol suppression during L- and HDDST in our pediatric patients with CD [23]. In 24 patients, mean baseline serum cortisol values of 590.7 ± 168.8 nmol/L (21.4 ± 4.7 µg/dl) decreased to 337.4 ± 104.0 nmol/L (12.2 ± 3.8 µg/dl) at 48 h during LDDST ($P<0.05$; mean decrease, 45.1%) with 66% decreasing by >30%. Cortisol suppression during LDDST correlated with that during HDDST ($r=+0.45$, $P<0.05$). Consequently, decrease of cortisol during the LDDST strongly supports the diagnosis of CD and negates the need for a HDDST.

These results have also been demonstrated in adult patients with CD [23], as the change in cortisol during LDDST has been shown to distinguish between pituitary and ectopic ACTH secretion, again questioning the value of the HDDST.

Imaging Studies

Most ACTH-secreting pituitary tumors occurring in the pediatric age range are microadenomas with diameter <5 mm [5]. The majority of these have a hypointense signal on MRI, which fails to enhance with gadolinium [18]. In the large pediatric NIH series, approximately 50% of microadenomas were visible on pituitary MRI [3]. In our series, pituitary imaging was relatively unhelpful, showing a normal appearance in approximately half of the patients, with a low predictive value of the position of the adenoma as identified at surgery (Table 14.3) [6]. Therefore, although pituitary imaging using MRI is an important step toward the successful treatment of Cushing's disease by transsphenoidal surgery (TSS), results should be interpreted together with bilateral inferior petrosal sinus sampling (BIPSS) for ACTH (see below).

In some cases, the distinction between CD and ectopic ACTH syndrome may be in doubt. Here, a CT scan of the chest using 0.5-cm cuts will usually exclude a bronchial carcinoid tumor.

BIPSS for ACTH

BIPSS was initially piloted in adults at the NIH [24] to enable distinction between CD and ectopic ACTH syndrome and also to provide a method of identifying a lateral versus central source of pituitary ACTH secretion [18]. It has now become routine in adult practice unless the MRI unequivocally shows a pituitary adenoma.

In children, ectopic ACTH secretion is extremely rare and so the primary aim of BIPSS is to contribute to the localization of the microadenoma by demonstrating

14 Diagnosis and Treatment of Pediatric Cushing's Disease

Table 14.4 BIPSS results, surgical identification of adenoma, and cure by TSS

Total patients (n)	Lateralization (n)	Nonlateralization (n)	Concordance of BSIPSS result with surgery (n)	Cure by TSS (n)
28	22 (79%)	6 (21%)	23 (82%)	21 (75%)

lateral or midline ACTH secretion. The first pediatric data were reported in the large NIH series where a predictive value of lateralization was 75–80% [1, 3].

BIPSS is a highly specialized technique and in our unit is performed by the same radiologist who regularly studies adult patients. In the majority of cases, we do not use general anesthesia (GA) to avoid potential alteration of ACTH secretion. However, in two children aged 5.8 and 6.2 years, GA was used. The youngest patient we studied without GA was aged 8.4 year. We have now performed BIPSS in 28 pediatric CD patients without complications. Our results that are shown in Table 14.4 suggest that ACTH sampling gives a better prediction of the site of the microadenoma than pituitary imaging [6].

A more recent study from the NIH described their further experience of BIPSS in 94 pediatric patients and reported that localization of ACTH secretion concurred with the site of the adenoma at surgery in 58% of cases, concluding that the technique was not an essential part of a pediatric investigation protocol [25]. The percentage of predictive lateralization, however, increased to 70% (51/73) after exclusion of 18 centrally located and four bilateral lesions.

Treatment of Cushing's Disease

CD in childhood requires urgent evaluation, diagnosis, and prompt expert treatment to minimize the associated morbidity and maximize potential improvements in growth and body composition post cure. It is clear that curative treatment in patients with moderate to severe CS reduces morbidity and mortality. Furthermore, as there is a finite time available for normal growth, it could be argued that rapid diagnosis and treatment is even more important in children and may reduce the risk of residual morbidity post cure.

Treatment options have significantly advanced over the last 50 years. Initially bilateral adrenalectomy was widely practiced and while effective in lowering hypercortisolemia, had considerable consequences. The pituitary adenoma remained in situ and there was an appreciable risk of postadrenalectomy Nelson's syndrome [26, 27]. In addition, patients required lifelong glucocorticoid and mineralocorticoid replacement. In the management of 37 cases of CD, we have performed adrenalectomy twice, only when necessary as the patients were extremely unwell and not fit to undergo pituitary surgery. In one of these patients, the hypercortisolemia was uncontrollable by oral metyrapone, and treatment was given with IV etomidate, which successfully controlled the cortisol levels prior to adrenalectomy [28].

Medical therapy to lower cortisol using metyrapone or ketoconazole is a useful short-term option prior to surgery or radiotherapy but cannot be recommended as a long-term definitive therapy for CD.

Transsphenoidal Surgery

Definitive cure of CD can be achieved by transsphenoidal pituitary surgery (TSS) or radiotherapy. TSS is regarded as a safe and effective procedure in children [29–32] and is now considered first-line therapy, as it involves selective removal of the adenoma maximizing the potential for normal pituitary tissue to remain in situ. Low rates of postoperative hypopituitarism have been reported in several large studies [30, 33]. However, selective microadenomectomy can be technically very difficult in children. As discussed above, the microadenomas may be very small, and an appreciable rate of failure exists even in the hands of the most experienced transsphenoidal surgeons.

We recently analyzed our experience over the past 25 years and considered the factors that contributed to successful surgical therapy [6]. Clearly, the variable surgical success rates reported depend on which definition of cure is adopted in that unit. We define successful treatment, i.e., cure, as undetectable postoperative serum cortisol (<50 nmol/L, <1.8 μg/dl), which is consistent with our adult endocrine unit [34]. The overall cure rate from TSS in 33 pediatric patients with microadenomas treated by TSS from 1982 to 2008 was 61%. Since 1986, the cure rate has been 75% in the 28 of these patients who were treated since routine BIPSS was introduced as preoperative preparation (Table 14.4). We, therefore, feel that the ability of BIPSS to correctly identify the lateral or central position of the adenoma has contributed to an increased rate of surgical success [12]. Other pediatric series report cure rates varying from 45 to 78% [33, 35–37], but very few report rates of >90% [3, 5]. We have not seen recurrence of CD after cure by TSS, but as many patients are referred from other centers, this has not been formally studied.

Pituitary Radiotherapy

Pituitary radiotherapy (RT) has been considered a therapeutic option for pediatric CD for many years. In our center, external beam RT is used as second-line therapy, following unsuccessful TSS. We usually proceed to RT within 2–4 weeks of TSS, when it is clear from circulating cortisol levels that complete cure has not been achieved [38]. The RT protocol we follow consists of delivering 45 Gy in 25 fractions over 35 days [39] reflecting evidence demonstrating children with CD respond more rapidly than adults [40, 41]. We have treated 13 patients during the past 26 years with a successful cure rate of 85%, which occurred at a mean interval of 0.8 year (range 0.3–2.9) following completion of therapy. We have seen recurrence in one patient previously categorized as cured after RT.

Postcure Growth and Development and Pituitary Function

Growth failure and resultant short stature are almost always seen at diagnosis in pediatric patients with CD [1, 42]. Virilization may lead to acceleration of bone age and further compromise growth potential [43]. A key article from the NIH described the abnormalities of height and GH secretion [12] together with a poor outcome for posttreatment catch-up growth and adult height [13]. We also reported disappointing postcure catch-up, which we attributed to continuing GH deficiency, occurring either from TSS, pituitary RT or the long-standing effects of chronic hypercortisolemia on pituitary and growth plate physiology [42]. The challenge is to reverse these problems and maximize growth potential so as to achieve acceptable adult height and body composition.

Our approach now is to test for GH deficiency 3 months after TSS or completion of RT. If GH therapy is required, we start GH at a dose of 0.025 mg/kg/day (standard UK dose for pediatric growth hormone deficiency). GnRH analogue therapy may be added to delay puberty and epiphyseal closure. Results demonstrate that this regime usually enables adequate catch-up growth and adult height within range of target height for the majority of patients [44].

Normal body composition is more difficult to achieve. Many patients remain obese and BMI SDS was elevated ($P<0.01$) at a mean interval of 3.9 years after cure in 14 patients [44]. A long-term follow-up study of childhood and adolescent CD showed that total body fat and the ratio of visceral to subcutaneous fat were abnormally high in the majority of patients studied 7 years after cure [45]. The implications of chronic excess visceral fat in terms of risk for adult metabolic syndrome deserve future study. Bone mineral density (BMD) was closer to normal, a finding which we also reported, together with some patients having normal BMD at diagnosis [46].

We have recently analyzed pituitary function in six patients at intervals of 6.6 to 16.5 years after receiving RT and have shown that although GH deficiency was frequent initially, some recovery may occur in adult life [47]. Gonadotrophin secretion was generally preserved with normal or early puberty; the latter is a well-recognized complication of cranial radiotherapy. TSH and ACTH deficiency was minimal [47]. It is important to note that the risk of hypopituitarism may continue to increase in the years after radiation. We have not studied cognitive function following pituitary RT.

Studies of adult patients with CS have reported brain atrophy, cognitive impairment, and psychopathology, most commonly depression, associated with excess endogenous circulating glucocorticoids [48]. A study from the NIH [49] also found significant cerebral atrophy in children with CD at diagnosis; however, there was no difference in IQ scores between patients and controls. Interestingly, they found an almost complete reversal of the cerebral atrophy but a significant decline in cognitive function 1 year after cure with TSS. This is in contrast to adult studies, which report reversible cognitive impairment and reversible loss of brain volume associated with eucortisolaemia [49, 50]. In a more recent article, the NIH group reported that children with CD have impaired health-related quality of life (HRQL), which has not fully resolved 1 year post treatment [51].

Summary

Pediatric CD manifests a number of characteristic features distinct from adult CD, most notably the significant impact on linear growth. Early diagnosis remains a challenge because of the frequent lack of appreciation of the nature of the pathology by parents and general practitioners. Once suspected, the patient requires investigation using a formal protocol, and the choice and interpretation of tests is most productively discussed with an adult specialist with experience of CD. Referral should be considered to a center combining pediatric and adult endocrinology, TSS, and pituitary RT. In addition, choosing a neurosurgeon experienced in TSS in children is likely to significantly improve the chance of effective and curative therapy. The prognosis for cure is good in the majority of children and adolescents, and full recovery of the hypothalamic-pituitary-adrenal axis is possible. However, posttreatment management frequently presents challenges for optimization of growth, puberty, and body composition.

References

1. Magiakou MA, Chrousos GP. Cushing's syndrome in children and adolescents: current diagnostic and therapeutic strategies. J Endocrinol Invest. 2002;25(2):181–94.
2. Savage MO, Besser GM. Cushing's disease in childhood. Trends Endocrinol Metab. 1996;7(6):213–6.
3. Magiakou MA et al. Cushing's syndrome in children and adolescents. Presentation, diagnosis, and therapy. N Engl J Med. 1994;331(10):629–36.
4. Weber A et al. Investigation, management and therapeutic outcome in 12 cases of childhood and adolescent Cushing's syndrome. Clin Endocrinol (Oxf). 1995;43(1):19–28.
5. Fahlbusch R. Neurosurgical management of Cushing's disease in children. In: Savage MO, Bourguignon J-P, Grossman AB, editors. Frontiers of pediatric neuroendocrinology. Oxford: Blackwell Scientific; 1995. p. 68–72.
6. Storr HL et al. Factors influencing cure by transsphenoidal selective adenomectomy in paediatric Cushing's disease. Eur J Endocrinol. 2005;152(6):825–33.
7. Khadilkar VV, Khadilkar AV, Navrange JR. Cushing's disease in an 11-month-old child. Indian Pediatr. 2004;41(3):274–6.
8. Damiani D et al. Pituitary macroadenoma and Cushing's disease in pediatric patients: patient report and review of the literature. J Pediatr Endocrinol Metab. 1998;11(5):665–9.
9. Stratakis CA et al. Pituitary macroadenoma in a 5-year-old: an early expression of multiple endocrine neoplasia type 1. J Clin Endocrinol Metab. 2000;85(12):4776–80.
10. Besser G, Trainer PJ. Cushing's syndrome. In: Besser GM, Thorner MO, editors. Comprehensive clinical endocrinology. 3rd ed. Edinburgh: Mosby; 2002.
11. Storr HL et al. Prepubertal Cushing's disease is more common in males, but there is no increase in severity at diagnosis. J Clin Endocrinol Metab. 2004;89(8):3818–20.

12. Magiakou MA et al. Suppressed spontaneous and stimulated growth hormone secretion in patients with Cushing's disease before and after surgical cure. J Clin Endocrinol Metab. 1994;78(1):131–7.
13. Magiakou MA, Mastorakos G, Chrousos GP. Final stature in patients with endogenous Cushing's syndrome. J Clin Endocrinol Metab. 1994;79(4):1082–5.
14. Greening JE et al. Linear growth and body mass index in pediatric patients with Cushing's disease or simple obesity. J Endocrinol Invest. 2006;29(10):885–7.
15. Peters CJ et al. Factors influencing skeletal maturation at diagnosis of paediatric Cushing's disease. Horm Res. 2007;68(5):231–5.
16. Dupuis CC et al. Abnormal puberty in paediatric Cushing's disease: relationship with adrenal androgen, sex hormone binding globulin and gonadotrophin concentrations. Clin Endocrinol (Oxf). 2007;66(6):838–43.
17. Hauffa BP, Kaplan SL, Grumbach MM. Dissociation between plasma adrenal androgens and cortisol in Cushing's disease and ectopic ACTH-producing tumour: relation to adrenarche. Lancet. 1984;1(8391):1373–6.
18. Newell-Price J et al. The diagnosis and differential diagnosis of Cushing's syndrome and pseudo-Cushing's states. Endocr Rev. 1998;19(5):647–72.
19. Arnaldi G et al. Diagnosis and complications of Cushing's syndrome: a consensus statement. J Clin Endocrinol Metab. 2003;88(12):5593–602.
20. Nieman LK et al. The diagnosis of Cushing's syndrome: an endocrine society clinical practice guideline. J Clin Endocrinol Metab. 2008;93:1526–40.
21. Batista DL et al. Diagnostic tests for children who are referred for the investigation of Cushing syndrome. Pediatrics. 2007;120(3):e575–86.
22. Martinelli Jr CE et al. Salivary cortisol for screening of Cushing's syndrome in children. Clin Endocrinol (Oxf). 1999;51(1):67–71.
23. Dias R et al. The discriminatory value of the low-dose dexamethasone suppression test in the investigation of paediatric Cushing's syndrome. Horm Res. 2006;65(3):159–62.
24. Oldfield EH et al. Petrosal sinus sampling with and without corticotropin-releasing hormone for the differential diagnosis of Cushing's syndrome. N Engl J Med. 1991;325(13):897–905.
25. Batista D et al. An assessment of petrosal sinus sampling for localization of pituitary microadenomas in children with Cushing disease. J Clin Endocrinol Metab. 2006;91(1):221–4.
26. Hopwood NJ, Kenny FM. Incidence of Nelson's syndrome after adrenalectomy for Cushing's disease in children: results of a nationwide survey. Am J Dis Child. 1977;131(12):1353–6.
27. McArthur RG, Hayles AB, Salassa RM. Childhood Cushing disease: results of bilateral adrenalectomy. J Pediatr. 1979;95(2):214–9.
28. Greening JE et al. Efficient short-term control of hypercortisolaemia by low-dose etomidate in severe paediatric Cushing's disease. Horm Res. 2005;64(3):140–3.
29. Massoud AF et al. Transsphenoidal surgery for pituitary tumours. Arch Dis Child. 1997;76(5):398–404.
30. Knappe UJ, Ludecke DK. Transnasal microsurgery in children and adolescents with Cushing's disease. Neurosurgery. 1996;39(3):484–92. discussion 492–3.
31. Kanter AS et al. Single-center experience with pediatric Cushing's disease. J Neurosurg. 2005;103(5 Suppl):413–20.
32. Joshi SM et al. Cushing's disease in children and adolescents: 20 years of experience in a single neurosurgical center. Neurosurgery. 2005;57(2):281–5. discussion 281–5.
33. Linglart A, Visot A. Cushing's disease in children and adolescents. Neurochirurgie. 2002;48(2–3 Pt 2):271–80.
34. Trainer PJ et al. Transsphenoidal resection in Cushing's disease: undetectable serum cortisol as the definition of successful treatment. Clin Endocrinol (Oxf). 1993;38(1):73–8.
35. Leinung MC et al. Long term follow-up of transsphenoidal surgery for the treatment of Cushing's disease in childhood. J Clin Endocrinol Metab. 1995;80(8):2475–9.
36. Devoe DJ et al. Long-term outcome in children and adolescents after transsphenoidal surgery for Cushing's disease. J Clin Endocrinol Metab. 1997;82(10):3196–202.

37. Styne DM et al. Treatment of Cushing's disease in childhood and adolescence by transsphenoidal microadenomectomy. N Engl J Med. 1984;310(14):889–93.
38. Storr HL et al. Clinical and endocrine responses to pituitary radiotherapy in pediatric Cushing's disease: an effective second-line treatment. J Clin Endocrinol Metab. 2003;88(1):34–7.
39. Plowman PN. Pituitary radiotherapy: techniques and potential complications. In: Jenkins PJ, Wass JAH, Sheaves R, editors. Clinical endocrine oncology. Oxford: Blackwell Science Publications; 1997. p. 185–8.
40. Jennings AS, Liddle GW, Orth DN. Results of treating childhood Cushing's disease with pituitary irradiation. N Engl J Med. 1977;297(18):957–62.
41. Thoren M et al. Treatment of Cushing's disease in childhood and adolescence by stereotactic pituitary irradiation. Acta Paediatr Scand. 1986;75(3):388–95.
42. Lebrethon MC et al. Linear growth and final height after treatment for Cushing's disease in childhood. J Clin Endocrinol Metab. 2000;85(9):3262–5.
43. Hayles AB et al. Hormone-secreting tumors of the adrenal cortex in children. Pediatrics. 1966;37(1):19–25.
44. Davies JH et al. Final adult height and body mass index after cure of paediatric Cushing's disease. Clin Endocrinol (Oxf). 2005;62(4):466–72.
45. Leong GM et al. Effects of child- and adolescent-onset endogenous Cushing syndrome on bone mass, body composition, and growth: a 7-year prospective study into young adulthood. J Bone Miner Res. 2007;22(1):110–8.
46. Scommegna S et al. Bone mineral density at diagnosis and following successful treatment of pediatric Cushing's disease. J Endocrinol Invest. 2005;28(3):231–5.
47. Chan LF et al. Long-term anterior pituitary function in patients with paediatric Cushing's disease treated with pituitary radiotherapy. Eur J Endocrinol. 2007;156(4):477–82.
48. Dorn LD et al. The longitudinal course of psychopathology in Cushing's syndrome after correction of hypercortisolism. J Clin Endocrinol Metab. 1997;82(3):912–9.
49. Merke DP et al. Children experience cognitive decline despite reversal of brain atrophy one year after resolution of Cushing syndrome. J Clin Endocrinol Metab. 2005;90(5):2531–6.
50. McEwen BS. Cortisol, Cushing's syndrome, and a shrinking brain-new evidence for reversibility. J Clin Endocrinol Metab. 2002;87(5):1947–8.
51. Keil MF et al. Quality of life in children and adolescents 1-year after cure of Cushing syndrome: a prospective study. Clin Endocrinol (Oxf). 2009;71(3):326–33.

Chapter 15
Silent Corticotroph Adenomas

Kalpana Kaushal and Stephen M. Shalet

Abstract Silent corticotroph adenomas (SCAs) are a subtype of non-functioning pituitary adenomas (NFPA) demonstrating positive immunoreactivity for ACTH, but without clinical or biochemical features of hypercortisolism. A number of mechanisms have been proposed to explain the "silence" of these tumors. SCAs typically present as macroadenomas, with symptoms related to local mass effect as a result of extension outside the pituitary fossa. Recognition of SCAs is important because there may be a degree of dysregulation of the pituitary adrenal axis in some patients, necessitating a more prolonged course of peri-operative steroids, as is the case for patients with Cushing's disease. Furthermore, when these tumors recur, they demonstrate a more aggressive phenotype, often with multiple recurrences refractory to standard therapies. It is, therefore, imperative that closer surveillance is instigated following recurrence. Adjuvant radiotherapy following pituitary surgery appears to be as effective at reducing recurrence of SCAs as it is for other NFPAs. The benefit of pharmacological therapies for SCAs has yet to be elucidated.

Keywords Non-functioning pituitary adenomas • Adrenocorticotropic hormone (ACTH) • Hypercortisolism • Macroadenomas • Radiotherapy

Introduction

Silent corticotroph adenomas (SCAs) are a subtype of non-functioning pituitary tumors which demonstrate immunoreactivity for ACTH in the absence of any clinical evidence of hypercortisolism. Strictly speaking, the presence of cortisol excess should have been ruled out biochemically before a tumor can be labelled as an SCA;

S.M. Shalet (✉)
Department of Endocrinology, Christie Hospital,
Wilmslow Road, Manchester, M20 4BX, UK
e-mail: Stephen.m.shalet@man.ac.uk

in practice, screening tests for Cushing's are not usually performed if the patient exhibits no phenotypic features of hypercortisolism. The diagnosis of an SCA is, therefore, somewhat arbitrary, and one cannot exclude the possibility that some of the individuals included in published series of SCAs may in fact have had subclinical Cushing's disease. These rare tumors were originally described by Horvath et al. in 1980 [1]; the authors reported an overall frequency of 5.6% of all pituitary adenomas. A more recent study identified SCAs in only 1.1% of pituitary adenomas [2]. SCAs constitute 17–22% of all ACTH-immunoreactive pituitary tumors [2, 3].

Nearly one third of anterior pituitary tumors are non-functioning [4]. Immunohistochemistry often reveals evidence of hormone synthesis, but since there is no clinical evidence of hormone excess, these tumors are termed silent pituitary adenomas. The majority of these silent tumors are of gonadotroph origin, with SCAs making up the second largest subgroup [5], accounting for 12–13.4% of non-functioning pituitary adenomas (NFPAs) [6, 7].

Classification

SCAs are classified according to histopathological characteristics as subtypes I or II. Subtype 1 is morphologically indistinguishable from functioning corticotroph adenomas causing Cushing's disease [3, 8]. Type 1 SCAs are basophilic on haematoxylin and eosin staining and are densely granulated, and a large percentage of adenoma cells stain positively for ACTH [9]. They are usually moderately to strongly periodic acid-Schiff (PAS)-positive. By contrast, SCAs of subtype 2 are chromophobic on haematoxylin and eosin staining, stain more patchily for ACTH, with only 30–50% of cells immunoreactive for ACTH. In subtype 2 tumors PAS staining is usually weak. Co-expression of prolactin has been reported in a proportion of SCAs [2, 3, 8]. Lopez et al. found that 8 of the 12 SCAs they described contained occasional cells exhibiting positive immunoreactivity for prolactin [3].

A diagnosis of an SCA can only be made post-operatively, with close collaboration between the reporting pathologist who identifies the positive ACTH immunoreactivity on immunohistochemical staining and an endocrinologist who is able to link these findings with the absence of biochemical and clinical cortisol excess preoperatively.

Reasons for "Silence" of SCAs

The question remains as to whether SCAs are truly "silent". It is possible that in some cases sensitive diagnostic testing might have revealed subtle evidence of cortisol excess [5]. The majority of patients in the published series of SCAs did not undergo formal biochemical testing for Cushing's syndrome such as 24-h urinary free cortisol measurements or dexamethasone suppression testing, since it was not felt to be clinically indicated preoperatively [2, 3, 7, 8, 10–12]. One study comparing 6 SCAs with 24 NFPAs reported more extensive testing in all patients, comprising diurnal plasma ACTH/cortisol levels "and/or overnight 0.5 mg dexamethasone suppression". However, it is not stated what proportion of patients had suppression testing [13]. Histologically, Crooke's hyaline change, an indicator of cortisol excess, has been reported, albeit rarely, in SCAs and lends further support to the hypothesis that not all these tumors are completely silent [9].

In addition, Lopez et al. found that 2 of the 12 patients in their cohort with SCAs developed features consistent with post-operative hypoadrenalism and required glucocorticoid replacement for a period of time [3]. Although both patients, in fact, had normal 24 h urinary free cortisol measurements preoperatively, the development of transient hypocortisolism after removal of their pituitary tumors would suggest some degree of functional ACTH excess before surgery. Although ACTH levels in patients with SCAs are usually normal, elevations in ACTH preoperatively have been reported in some cases. However, because the patients did not appear Cushingoid clinically, the high ACTH levels were thought possibly to be due to stress [3, 8]. An alternative explanation proposed was that the type of ACTH being secreted was perhaps structurally abnormal and, therefore, biologically inactive. Other explanations for the "silence" of SCAs include cyclical secretion of ACTH or, alternatively, continuous secretion of very low levels of ACTH, [8] such that clinical features of Cushing's do not become apparent. It has also been suggested that in some of these cases the adrenal gland is less responsive to ACTH [12].

It is likely that specific defects in enzymes involved in pro-opiomelanocortin (POMC) processing in SCAs result in the production of abnormal non-functioning peptides rather than biologically active ACTH. One such enzyme is prohormone convertase 1/3, a proteolytic enzyme responsible for cleavage of POMC into smaller fragments including mature functioning ACTH. Some studies have demonstrated that expression of this enzyme is significantly reduced in SCAs compared with adenomas from patients with Cushing's disease (CDA) [13, 14]. Other genes coding for enzymes related to POMC transcription and processing, as well as ACTH secretion and glucocorticoid metabolism, may be differentially expressed in SCAs and CDAs, contributing to the clinical silence of SCAs [5, 15]. It may be that ACTH secretion in SCAs is not excessive due to inadequate development of the Golgi complex, or increased intracellular degradation [9].

It is also recognised that hypercortisolemia may develop later in the course of the disease process, being absent at initial presentation [11, 12, 16]. Baldeweg et al. found that 26.6% of their cohort of patients with SCAs developed clinical and biochemical evidence of Cushing's during a mean follow-up of 4.8 years [12]. This would tend to support the hypothesis of very low but continuous secretion of active ACTH, such that biochemical features of Cushing's are absent at initial presentation but develop over time.

Clinical Features of SCAs

As with other NFPAs, the lack of an associated clinical syndrome with an SCA results in diagnosis only when the tumor has enlarged significantly. SCAs, therefore, typically present as macroadenomas, with symptoms related to local mass

Table 15.1 Clinical characteristics of patients with SCAs in published series

	Scheithauer et al. [8]	Webb et al. [11]	Bradley et al. [10]	Lopez et al. [3]	Baldeweg et al. [12]	Cho et al. [7]
Number of cases	23	27	28	12	15	28
Male:female	16:7	8:19	16:12	3:9	10:5	Ratio 1:2.1
Mean age (years)	48	49.3	51.3	50.1	50.8	44
Duration of follow-up	Median 4.9 years	Median 60 months	Mean 7.4 years	–	Mean 4.8 years	Mean 5.2 years
Tumor size	All macroadenomas: mean diameter 2.4 cm	All macroadenomas	All macroadenomas	11/12 macroadenomas	All macroadenomas: mean maximum diameter 19 mm	All macroadenomas: mean 2.8 cm
Suprasellar (SS) extension	87%	48% – SS only 36% – SS and CS	–	–	100%	–
Sphenoid/cavernous sinus (CS) invasion	30%	16% – CS only	32%	–	40% – CS	39.3%
Headaches	50%	70.4%	–	8.3%	13%	56%
Visual field defects	61%	52% – visual field deficits, 55.6% – "visual disturbance"	78.6%	41.7% – "visual complaints"	86.7% – "visual deficits"	92.6% – "visual deficits"
Extraocular muscle palsies	13%	–	–	–	–	–
Hypopituitarism preoperatively	26% (35% "complete or partial anterior pituitary insufficiency")	–	–	33.3%	–	40.9% – Gonadotropin deficiency, 16% – TSH deficiency
Pituitary apoplexy	8.7%	33%	–	16.7% (clinical), 25% (radiological/histological)	40% (radiological)	25%
Post-operative radiotherapy	48%	33% overall (3 after initial surgery, 6 after reoperation)	39% overall (5 after initial surgery, 6 after reoperation)	–	40%	33.3%
Post-operative tumor recurrence	54% (persistence or recurrence)	37%	32%	0 (although 6 cases in series had <2 years follow-up)	33.3%	25%
Mean time to tumor regrowth	–	49.6 months	5.8 years	–	–	5.6 years

effects as a result of extension outside the pituitary fossa. Headaches, visual field deficits and hypopituitarism are the most common manifestations. By contrast, ACTH-secreting pituitary adenomas associated with Cushing's disease are typically microadenomas and patients present with features of cortisol excess rather than the consequences of local mass effect.

A number of published series of SCAs have provided valuable information about the clinical features and natural history of these tumors [2, 3, 7, 8, 10–13]. Two of these were large single-centre studies providing useful comparative data for SCAs vs. other NFPAs [7, 10]. Headaches have been reported to be a feature in 50–70.4% of patients in the larger series of SCAs [7, 8, 11]. Visual deficits were present in 41.7–92.6% of patients [3, 7, 8, 10–12]. Bradley et al., comparing 28 patients with SCAs with historical departmental data from 60 ACTH immunonegative NFPAs, found no significant difference in the incidence of visual field abnormalities at baseline in the two groups (78.6% SCAs vs. 68.3% ACTH immunonegative) [10, 17]. By contrast, Cho et al., who compared 28 SCAs and 134 non-SCAs (NFPAs without ACTH immunoreactivity) found visual deficits to be significantly more common in SCAs (92.6%) vs. non-SCAs (72.4%) despite similar tumor size in the two groups (2.8 cm vs. 3 cm) [7]. Secondary hypogonadism and secondary hypothyroidism were present at diagnosis in 40.9 and 16% of patients with SCAs, similar to the prevalences in patients with non-SCAs [7]. Other studies have reported the prevalence of preoperative hypopituitarism as 26–35% [3, 8]. Table 15.1 summarises the clinical features of patients with SCAs within the larger published series.

SCAs may be associated with a greater propensity to haemorrhage; pituitary apoplexy was described in 33% of patients in one series of 27 patients [11]. Radiological evidence of apoplexy may be evident in as many as 40% of SCAs [12]. Cho et al. found that pituitary apoplexy was three times as common in SCAs vs. non-SCAs (25% vs. 7.8%) and postulated that this may indicate that SCAs grew more rapidly than non-SCAs [7]. If so, this finding may also in part explain why visual deficits were more common in the SCA group.

Yamada et al. examined the frequency of cavernous sinus invasion amongst the various morphological subtypes of NFPA. SCAs constituted 12% of the 213 NFPAs included in the study. SCAs appeared to behave more aggressively than other NFPAs, with evidence of cavernous sinus invasion in 85%, compared to 11% of silent gonadotroph adenomas, 38% of null cell adenomas and 67% of subtype 3 adenomas [6].

The male–female ratio for SCAs is unclear, unlike adenomas associated with Cushing's disease which demonstrate a clear female preponderance [5]. In a recently published study, SCA patients were slightly younger at diagnosis compared to non-SCA patients (mean 44 years vs. 50 years) [7].

Post-operative Recurrence of SCAs

The main therapeutic option for SCAs is surgery. Several authors have reported that SCAs have a high recurrence rate following surgery [8, 11]. If this is the case, it provides valuable information about the natural history of SCAs, as distinct from other NFPAs, and can be used to devise appropriate post-operative follow-up regimens. The high post-operative recurrence rate of 54% reported by Scheithauer et al., however, included both persistent and recurrent SCAs, whereas Bradley et al., in their study, used the term "recurrence" only if there had been an increase in sellar tissue compared to the first post-operative scan [10]. Webb et al. reported a recurrence rate of 37% [11], but like Scheithauer et al., there were no comparative data available for NFPAs from the same centre. Comparing their results with historical data from other centres, Webb et al. concluded that the recurrence rate of SCAs was higher than that of NFPAs [18] but similar to that reported in a study of ACTH-secreting macroadenomas [19].

Bradley et al. found that the recurrence rate for SCAs was no higher than that of other non-functioning pituitary adenomas (NFPAs) (32% vs. 33%), although tumors that did recur demonstrated a more aggressive course, with multiple recurrences in two cases. By contrast, none of the ACTH immunonegative NFPAs demonstrated more than one episode of tumor regrowth. Mean time to tumor regrowth was similar between the two groups (5.8 years SCAs vs. 5.4 years) [10]. Cho et al. have recently confirmed these findings; in a direct comparison between 28 SCAs and 134 non-SCAs there was no significant difference in recurrence rates (25% vs. 26.9%) over a mean follow-up period of 4.4 years [7]. Similar to the findings of Bradley et al. [10], recurrences were associated with a more aggressive course; multiple recurrences were significantly more frequent in the SCA group compared with the non-SCA group. Multiple SCA recurrences occurred in younger patients and were refractory to standard therapies. Late recurrences (after more than 5 years) were also significantly more common for SCAs compared with non-SCAs [7]. In another study of 15 SCAs, 5 tumors recurred post-operatively (33.3%) during a mean follow-up of 4.8 years. In three of these cases, tissue was available for comparison with the initial tumor and showed either the appearance of frank malignancy (two cases) or increased mitoses (one case), indicating a change to a more aggressive tumor type [12].

Unfortunately, no definite predictors of SCA recurrence post-operatively have been identified to date. Recurrence rate appears not to be associated with tumor subtype, extension into the cavernous sinus, dural invasion, degree of tumor invasiveness, degree of ACTH immunoreactivity or Ki-67 index [7–12]. This means that a universal intensive programme of post-operative surveillance, incorporating pituitary imaging and visual field assessment, is required for all SCAs, regardless of initial tumor characteristics.

Non-surgical Management of SCAs

Although patients with SCAs, by definition, do not have cortisol excess, the possibility of some dysregulation of the pituitary adrenal axis cannot be ruled out in view of the findings of occasional elevated ACTH, transient hypocortisolism post-operatively and development of hypercortisolism later in the disease process

[3, 8, 11, 12]. It is, therefore, possible that some patients with SCAs could be at risk of some of the morbidity associated with Cushing's syndrome. For Cushing's disease patients, it has been demonstrated that even 5 years after biochemical cure they still have an adverse cardiovascular risk profile, [20] which appears related to the period of exposure to excess cortisol. This makes it imperative that the duration of hypercortisolism be kept as short as possible, usually by a combination of both medical and surgical therapies. For SCAs, the efficacy of non-surgical therapy needs to be examined, since it may be required in conjunction with surgery for residual/recurrent tumors. In addition to preventing complications from local mass effect resulting from tumor regrowth as with other NFPAs, such therapies for SCAs may also reduce the incidence of future endocrine complications.

Radiotherapy

For NFPAs it has been demonstrated that adjuvant radiotherapy within 12 months of initial surgery reduces the likelihood of tumor regrowth [21]. However, the indications for post-operative radiotherapy for NFPAs have changed such that routine radiotherapy is no longer offered automatically to all patients; now radiotherapy is administered on an individual basis. Criteria would generally include residual tumor post-operatively, particularly with suprasellar extension, parapituitary invasion or aggressive features histologically [10, 11]. It is important to determine whether SCAs, with their potential to behave more aggressively on recurrence, are more or less likely to benefit from post-operative radiotherapy. Webb et al., in their study of 27 SCAs, found a 41.7% recurrence rate in patients who received no post-operative radiotherapy, compared to an overall recurrence rate of 37%. The three patients who had radiotherapy after the first surgery had no tumor recurrence [11]. This raises the possibility of benefit from adjuvant radiotherapy for SCAs, although the numbers were too small for any statistical analysis. In their study, the authors stated that, due to the perceived high recurrence rate of SCAs, they tended to offer radiotherapy if residual tumor was evident post-operatively [11].

By contrast, Baldeweg et al. actually found an increased recurrence rate following radiotherapy in their study of 15 SCAs; tumor recurrence occurred in 66.7% of patients who received post-operative radiotherapy and 11.1% of those who had no radiotherapy [12]. The reason for this is not clear, although it is possible that the tumors requiring radiotherapy were more aggressive to begin with.

In the comparative study of SCA vs. non-SCAs carried out by Cho et al., similar percentages of patients in both groups required adjuvant radiotherapy/gamma knife surgery; even when these individuals were excluded, recurrence rates did not differ between the two groups [7]. Similarly, amongst patients who received adjuvant therapy, recurrence rates were similar between SCAs and non-SCAs, suggesting that the treatment has similar efficacy for both types of tumor [7]. On the basis of these results, it would seem reasonable to conclude that at the present time post-operative radiotherapy for SCAs should be considered based on the same criteria used for ACTH-immunonegative NFPAs.

Pharmacological Therapy

It is not clear whether existing drug therapies used for other subtypes of pituitary adenomas are likely to be more or less effective for SCAs. Whilst SCAs are a subtype of NFPA, undoubtedly they share some features with ACTH-secreting tumors. It, therefore, seems prudent to examine the evidence for effectiveness of pharmacological therapies both for NFPAs and ACTH-secreting tumors, and to infer from this the potential benefit for SCAs.

The two major classes of drugs that have been used to promote pituitary tumor shrinkage are dopamine agonists (DAs) and somatostatin analogues (SSAs). Their respective efficacy in prolactinomas and somatotroph adenomas is now well established. There is also a rationale for the use of these agents for shrinkage of NFPAs; the majority of these tumors express subtypes of dopamine and somatostatin receptors (D1-5 and SSTR1-5) [22]. Cumulative results to date, as summarised by Colao et al., have shown greater success with DAs than SSAs in inducing shrinkage of NFPAs (27.6% vs. 12%) [22]. It is likely that individual tumor response is determined by the receptor subtypes present. Indeed, one study, in which patients with residual NFPA post-operatively were treated with cabergoline for 12 months, demonstrated a 56% tumor shrinkage rate, and shrinkage was associated with the presence of D2 receptors [23]. The poorer response of NFPAs to existing SSA therapy may be due to the fact that both octreotide and lanreotide, with high affinity for SSTR 2 and 5, have a low affinity for SSTR3, the receptor subtype generally found in the highest amounts in NFPAs [24]. Newer SSAs such as SOM 230 (pasireotide), which binds SSTR1–3 and SSTR5, may prove more efficacious [25]. Combination therapy with SSAs and DAs may also have a role to play, due to a functional interaction between somatostatin and dopamine receptors [22].

There is some evidence that DA therapy may have a role in ACTH-secreting adenomas [26, 27]. Pivonello et al. have shown that approximately 80% of these tumors express functional D2 receptors [28]. Of a group of 20 patients with Cushing's disease unsuccessfully treated by surgery, 40% achieved control of cortisol secretion on cabergoline for the 24 month duration of the study [29]. Cabergoline resulted in an improvement in glucose intolerance and hypertension in the majority of subjects, regardless of whether cortisol levels normalised. Somatostatin receptor subtypes are also expressed in corticotroph adenomas, and SOM230 has been shown to reduce ACTH secretion in vitro [25].

A recent in vitro study compared mRNA levels for SSTR and DR subtypes between SCAs, ACTH-secreting pituitary adenomas and NFPAs [30]. SSTR2 mRNA expression in SCAs was similar to that in NFPAs, and fivefold higher than ACTH-secreting pituitary adenomas. SSTR1 expression in SCAs was 200-fold higher than in NFPAs and 17-fold higher than ACTH-secreting pituitary adenomas. This suggests that an SSA with high affinity for SSTRs 1 and 2 may be a useful therapeutic agent promoting shrinkage of SCAs. Tateno et al. found that DR2 mRNA expression in both SCAs and ACTH-secreting pituitary adenomas was markedly lower than in NFPAs, possibly indicating that DA therapy may be less efficacious for shrinkage of SCAs compared to NFPAs [30]. However, Petrossians et al. reported a patient with recurrence of an SCA 2 years post-operatively, in whom significant tumor shrinkage occurred following cabergoline therapy [31]. The tumor cells demonstrated high levels of D2 receptor mRNA. As with other pituitary tumors, receptor subtypes, amounts and activity are likely to vary greatly between SCAs, making responses to pharmacological therapy difficult to predict.

Conclusion

SCAs are a subtype of NFPA demonstrating positive immunoreactivity for ACTH, but without clinical or biochemical features of hypercortisolism. A number of mechanisms have been proposed to explain the "silence" of these tumors including secretion of endocrinologically inactive ACTH, intermittent or continuous low level secretion of ACTH and abnormal intracellular processing of ACTH [3]. The retrospective nature of the published series of SCAs has to be acknowledged when interpreting the data, particularly for the larger series with cases identified over a longer time period; in an individual centre, a number of different neurosurgeons, endocrinologists, radiotherapists and pathologists may have been involved in the management of these patients with SCAs. As such, there may well have been variability in surgical techniques and expertise, in the adequacy of screening tests for Cushing's, as well as in decisions regarding the need for adjuvant non-surgical therapies.

Recognition of SCAs is important because there may be a degree of dysregulation of the pituitary adrenal axis in some patients, necessitating a more prolonged course of peri-operative steroids as is the requirement for patients with Cushing's disease. Furthermore, it appears that when these tumors recur they demonstrate a more aggressive phenotype, often with multiple recurrences refractory to standard therapies. It is, therefore, imperative that closer surveillance is instigated following recurrence of an SCA. Adjuvant radiotherapy following the initial pituitary surgery appears to be as effective at reducing recurrence of SCAs as it is for other NFPAs. The benefit of pharmacological therapies for SCAs has yet to be elucidated.

References

1. Horvath E, Kovacs K, Killinger DW, et al. Silent corticotropic adenomas of the human pituitary gland: a histologic, immunocytologic, and ultrastructural study. Am J Pathol. 1980;98(3):617–38.
2. Sahli R, Christ ER, Seiler R, et al. Clinicopathologic correlations of silent corticotroph adenomas of the pituitary: report of four cases and literature review. Pathol Res Pract. 2006;202(6):457–64.
3. Lopez JA, Kleinschmidt-Demasters BB, Sze CI, et al. Silent corticotroph adenomas: further clinical and pathological observations. Hum Pathol. 2004;35(9):1137–47.
4. Harris PE. Biochemical markers for clinically non-functioning pituitary tumours. Clin Endocrinol (Oxf). 1998;49(2):163–4.

5. Korbonits M, Carlsen E. Recent clinical and pathophysiological advances in non-functioning pituitary adenomas. Horm Res. 2009;71 Suppl 2:123–30.
6. Yamada S, Ohyama K, Taguchi M, et al. A study of the correlation between morphological findings and biological activities in clinically nonfunctioning pituitary adenomas. Neurosurgery. 2007;61(3):580–4.
7. Cho HY, Cho SW, Kim SW, et al. Silent corticotroph adenomas have unique recurrence characteristics as compared with other non-functioning pituitary adenomas. Clin Endocrinol (Oxf). 2010;72(5):648–53.
8. Scheithauer BW, Jaap AJ, Horvath E, et al. Clinically silent corticotroph tumors of the pituitary gland. Neurosurgery. 2000;47(3):723–9.
9. Karavitaki N, Ansorge O, Wass JA. Silent corticotroph adenomas. Arq Bras Endocrinol Metabol. 2007;51(8):1314–8.
10. Bradley KJ, Wass JA, Turner HE. Non-functioning pituitary adenomas with positive immunoreactivity for ACTH behave more aggressively than ACTH immunonegative tumours but do not recur more frequently. Clin Endocrinol (Oxf). 2003;58(1):59–64.
11. Webb KM, Laurent JJ, Okonkwo DO, et al. Clinical characteristics of silent corticotrophic adenomas and creation of an internet-accessible database to facilitate their multi-institutional study. Neurosurgery. 2003;53(5):1076–84.
12. Baldeweg SE, Pollock JR, Powell M, et al. A spectrum of behaviour in silent corticotroph pituitary adenomas. Br J Neurosurg. 2005;19(1):38–42.
13. Tateno T, Izumiyama H, Doi M, et al. Defective expression of prohormone convertase 1/3 in silent corticotroph adenoma. Endocr J. 2007;54(5):777–82.
14. Ohta S, Nishizawa S, Oki Y, et al. Significance of absent prohormone convertase 1/3 in inducing clinically silent corticotroph pituitary adenoma of subtype I–immunohistochemical study. Pituitary. 2002;5(4):221–3.
15. Tateno T, Izumiyama H, Doi M, et al. Differential gene expression in ACTH-secreting and non-functioning pituitary tumors. Eur J Endocrinol. 2007;157(6):717–24.
16. Ambrosi B, Colombo P, Bochicchio D, et al. The silent corticotropinoma: is clinical diagnosis possible? J Endocrinol Invest. 1992;15(6):443–52.
17. Turner HE, Stratton IM, Byrne JV, et al. Audit of selected patients with nonfunctioning pituitary adenomas treated without irradiation – a follow-up study. Clin Endocrinol (Oxf). 1999;51(3):281–4.
18. Ebersold MJ, Quast LM, Laws Jr ER, et al. Long-term results in transsphenoidal removal of nonfunctioning pituitary adenomas. J Neurosurg. 1986;64(5):713–9.
19. Blevins Jr LS, Christy JH, Khajavi M, et al. Outcomes of therapy for Cushing's disease due to adrenocorticotropin-secreting pituitary macroadenomas. J Clin Endocrinol Metab. 1998;83(1):63–7.
20. Colao A, Pivonello R, Spiezia S, et al. Persistence of increased cardiovascular risk in patients with Cushing's disease after five years of successful cure. J Clin Endocrinol Metab. 1999;84(8):2664–72.
21. Gittoes NJ, Bates AS, Tse W, et al. Radiotherapy for non-function pituitary tumours. Clin Endocrinol (Oxf). 1998;48(3):331–7.
22. Colao A, Di SC, Pivonello R, et al. Medical therapy for clinically non-functioning pituitary adenomas. Endocr Relat Cancer. 2008;15(4):905–15.
23. Pivonello R, Matrone C, Filippella M, et al. Dopamine receptor expression and function in clinically nonfunctioning pituitary tumors: comparison with the effectiveness of cabergoline treatment. J Clin Endocrinol Metab. 2004;89(4):1674–83.
24. Taboada GF, Luque RM, Bastos W, et al. Quantitative analysis of somatostatin receptor subtype (SSTR1-5) gene expression levels in somatotropinomas and non-functioning pituitary adenomas. Eur J Endocrinol. 2007;156(1):65–74.
25. Batista DL, Zhang X, Gejman R, et al. The effects of SOM230 on cell proliferation and adrenocorticotropin secretion in human corticotroph pituitary adenomas. J Clin Endocrinol Metab. 2006;91(11):4482–8.

26. Colao A, Pivonello R, Di SC, et al. Medical therapy of pituitary adenomas: effects on tumor shrinkage. Rev Endocr Metab Disord. 2009;10(2):111–23.
27. Shalet S, Mukherjee A. Pharmacological treatment of hypercortisolism. Curr Opin Endocrinol Diabetes Obes. 2008;15(3):234–8.
28. Pivonello R, Ferone D, de Herder WW, et al. Dopamine receptor expression and function in corticotroph pituitary tumors. J Clin Endocrinol Metab. 2004;89(5):2452–62.
29. Pivonello R, De Martino MC, Cappabianca P, et al. The medical treatment of Cushing's disease: effectiveness of chronic treatment with the dopamine agonist cabergoline in patients unsuccessfully treated by surgery. J Clin Endocrinol Metab. 2009;94(1):223–30.
30. Tateno T, Kato M, Tani Y, et al. Differential expression of somatostatin and dopamine receptor subtype genes in adrenocorticotropin (ACTH)-secreting pituitary tumors and silent corticotroph adenomas. Endocr J. 2009;56(4):579–84.
31. Petrossians P, Ronci N, Valdes SH, et al. ACTH silent adenoma shrinking under cabergoline. Eur J Endocrinol. 2001;144(1):51–7.

Chapter 16
Cushing's Syndrome in Pregnancy

Frank McCarroll and John R. Lindsay

Abstract The maternal hypothalamic–pituitary–adrenal (HPA) axis is up-regulated in pregnancy leading to increased serum cortisol and adrenocorticotropin (ACTH) concentrations. Placental production of corticotropin-releasing hormone and ACTH, altered pituitary responsiveness to negative feedback of cortisol, or enhanced pituitary responses to corticotropin-releasing factors may all contribute to enhanced HPA activity in pregnancy. While physiological hypercortisolism is common during gestation, Cushing's syndrome occurs rarely in pregnancy. Its occurrence during gestation is associated with fetal morbidity and mortality and maternal complications including hypertension, hyperglycemia, and eclampsia. The clinical diagnosis may be overlooked due to overlapping features of weight gain, hypertension, fatigue, hyperglycemia, and emotional changes that occur in pregnancy. The biochemical diagnosis is more challenging than in the nonpregnant state due to the physiological hypercortisolism of pregnancy. Treatment appears to reduce but does not eliminate adverse outcomes. This chapter reviews the experience of diagnosis and management of Cushing's syndrome in pregnancy and explores caveats and special precautions required to safely diagnose and treat this challenging condition during pregnancy.

Keywords Pregnancy • Cushing's syndrome • Hypercortisolism • ACTH • CRH • Diagnosis • Morbidity • Transsphenoidal surgery

J.R. Lindsay (✉)
Altnagelvin Area Hospital, Western Health & Social Care Trust,
Glenshane Road, Londonderry, BT47 6SB, UK
e-mail: john.lindsay@westerntrust.hscni.net

Introduction

The challenge of diagnosis and treatment of patients with adrenocorticotropin (ACTH)-dependent Cushing's syndrome has been reviewed in earlier chapters. While Cushing's syndrome occurs rarely, this condition may present in pregnancy despite associated increased rates of amenorrhoea and subfertility. During pregnancy a delay in diagnosis may lead to similar complications as in the nonpregnant state, but with adverse consequences for both the mother and fetus. This chapter outlines the changes in normal physiology in pregnancy that make the diagnosis during pregnancy difficult and reviews testing and treatment strategies to optimize management. These observations represent the authors' opinion given the available evidence on management during pregnancy, as there are virtually no studies that would qualify to meet a high standard for evidence-based guidelines.

Normal Hypothalamic–Pituitary–Adrenal Axis in Pregnancy

Pregnancy is associated with increased HPA activity. There are elevations in plasma corticotropin-releasing hormone (CRH), ACTH, cortisol, cortisol binding globulin (CBG), and urine-free cortisol (UFC) [1–6]. Plasma CRH concentrations rise exponentially on the order of 1,000-fold [7], beginning at the end of the first trimester [8]. During the last 5 weeks before delivery there is a further sharp rise in CRH concentrations [3, 9], which normalizes rapidly by the end of the first postpartum day. CRH is present in fetal plasma, amniotic fluid [10, 11] and has been isolated from human placenta [12]. Systemic maternal effects of elevated CRH may be limited by binding to CRH-binding protein [CRH-BP] [13]. During the latter part of the third trimester CRH-BP concentrations fall by around 60%, leading to elevations in free CRH [14]. CRH appears to be an important mediator in determining the duration of normal gestation, the so-called placental clock [15]; conversely early activation of the placental CRH system is associated with premature onset of labor and delivery [16].

Plasma ACTH concentrations rise throughout gestation and attain maximal levels during labor and delivery [1, 17–19]. A range of factors, including placental synthesis and release of biologically active CRH and ACTH, pituitary desensitization to cortisol feedback, or enhanced pituitary responses to corticotropin-releasing factors may all contribute to elevated plasma ACTH concentrations. Circulating plasma ACTH and cortisol concentrations is highly correlated and shows diurnal variation [17, 18]. Rising estrogen concentrations during pregnancy stimulate the hepatic production of cortisol binding globulin (CBG), which remains elevated until at least the 12th postpartum day. Total and free serum cortisol concentrations rise in parallel across gestation, with serum cortisol elevated two- to threefold compared with nonpregnant controls [20]. Enhanced cortisol production is observed with a transient fall in free cortisol as CBG rises, probably from reduced negative feedback effects and increased ACTH production [19]. Serum cortisol concentrations in healthy pregnancy can reach values similar to those found in nonpregnant subjects with Cushing's syndrome. This increase occurs as early as the 11th week of gestation. It reaches a peak between the first and second trimesters and has a plateau in the third trimester [20]. Salivary cortisol increased more than twofolds as compared with nonpregnant controls in the third trimester [6]. Despite these changes, the circadian rhythm of serum and salivary cortisol is preserved but may be partly blunted [6]. UFC excretion parallels the rise in serum cortisol through the course of gestation. In healthy pregnant women, mean 24-h UFC is elevated at least 180% during gestation compared with nonpregnant concentrations [19].

Hypothalamic–pituitary responsiveness to exogenous glucocorticoids is blunted during pregnancy. In normal second–third trimester pregnancy, Odagiri observed suppression of serum cortisol following 1 mg dexamethasone to around 40%, compared to 87% in nongravid controls [21]. It is unclear whether the observed effects occur due to the previously discussed physiological changes during pregnancy or altered absorption of dexamethasone, as there are varying reports of changes in its bioavailability during gestation [22].

The fetus is protected in early gestation from the effects of maternal hypercortisolism by placental 11β-hydroxysteroid dehydrogenase 2 [11β-HSD2], which converts active glucocorticoids to their inactive 11-keto metabolites. This mechanism ensures that fetal cortisol exposure is much lower than maternal concentrations [23]. However, in late gestation there is a reversal of 11β-HSD 2 activity in favor of the active hormone in the uterus that may contribute to late fetal development including lung maturation [24].

The plasma concentrations of CRH, ACTH, and cortisol increase several fold with the onset of labor. Peak CRH concentrations occur within 48 h before delivery and fall during labor. In the immediate postpartum period, plasma CRH, ACTH, and cortisol concentrations decrease rapidly toward the nonpregnant range [8]. Both CRH and ACTH concentrations will return to normal within 2 h from delivery but serum cortisol concentrations will have a more protracted time course before normalization. Altered dynamics of exogenously administered corticosteroids persist into the early postpartum period until around the fifth postpartum week [25, 26].

Clinical Presentation

The clinical features of Cushing's syndrome in pregnancy are broadly similar to those in Cushing's syndrome in nonpregnant subjects (Chap. 4). However, typical features that may occur with Cushing's syndrome in pregnancy, including central weight gain, fatigue, hyperglycaemia, emotional change, hypertension, and striae, may be wrongly assumed to have arisen as a part of normal gestation [19, 27]. Evidence from the literature suggests that the diagnosis is often not made until the second trimester [19, 27]. Cushing's syndrome is rarely associated with pregnancy, probably because hypercortisolism prevents normal follicular development and ovulation [27]. The first description of Cushing's syndrome in pregnancy was reported by Hunt and McConahey in 1953 [28]. At least 150 pregnancies have been reported in the literature as single cases or in small series. Multiple pregnancies occurred in about 10% of the patients [19].

Maternal and Fetal Morbidity and Mortality

In order to improve outcomes in pregnancy it is important to consider hypercortisolism in individuals with relevant clinical features so that an early diagnosis can be made and appropriate treatment can be initiated. Around 70% of pregnant patients with Cushing's syndrome have associated maternal morbidity and, more rarely, mortality [19]. As in nonpregnant cases with Cushing's syndrome, the most common maternal complications were hypertension, diabetes, or impaired glucose tolerance [19]. Other risks include pre-eclampsia, wound infection and poor wound healing, osteoporosis, fracture, psychiatric complications, and maternal cardiac failure [29–33]. Despite these adverse events, in a series of 136 pregnancies complicated by Cushing's syndrome, we previously observed a high rate of live births in up to 80% of pregnancies [27]. Fetal complications included spontaneous abortion, premature birth, intrauterine growth retardation, hyaline membrane disease, intraventricular hemorrhage, and perinatal death [29–36]. Fetal adrenal insufficiency is rare, and signs of glucocorticoid excess have not been reported. This suggests that placental degradation of cortisol may protect the fetus. Congenital malformations are also uncommon [19].

Etiology

The etiology of Cushing's syndrome differs between the pregnant and nonpregnant state. In contrast to the nonpregnant population (see Chap. 4), Cushing's disease appears to be less common in pregnancy, with rates of 33% in reported series [29, 37–39] compared to 58–70% in the general population. In contrast, adrenal adenomas account for a disproportionately high proportion of Cushing's syndrome in pregnancy in up to 48% of cases compared with 15% in nonpregnant women. Adrenal carcinoma, pheochromocytoma, primary pigmented nodular adrenal disease, and ACTH-independent hyperplasia have also all been reported in pregnancy [37, 40]. The overall increased incidence of adrenal Cushing's syndrome suggests that anovulation may be less prevalent in adrenal cases. There have been a few reports of recurrent Cushing's syndrome during pregnancy that spontaneously remitted after delivery [41–43]. Cushing's syndrome induced by pregnancy seems to be caused by products of the feto-placental unit. Unrecognized illicit luteinizing hormone/human chorioic gonadotropin (LH/HCG) receptor expression is one potential mechanism for recurrent adrenal hypercortisolism and may account for a proportion of cases attributed to an adrenal adenoma [44–46]. In this latter setting, Cushing's syndrome would not be triggered until pregnancy is established. Cases with ectopic ACTH secretion in pregnancy are quite uncommon, probably as a result of severe hypercortisolism and amenorrhea [37, 40].

Diagnostic Strategies in Pregnancy

The diagnosis and differential diagnosis of Cushing's syndrome have been discussed in detail in earlier chapters. In this section, we explore how the physiological changes in pregnancy complicate this process. In individual cases standard screening tests have generally been employed, however, there has been limited or no validation of these techniques in pregnancy [37, 47, 48]. Several caveats should be observed in order to reliably interpret the results of testing during pregnancy.

Screening and Diagnosis

Mean morning serum total cortisol concentrations in Cushing's syndrome overlap concentrations seen in normal pregnancy [1]. Thus, as in the nonpregnant individual, random or morning serum cortisol concentrations are unhelpful as they are not discriminatory [19]. As the nocturnal nadir in serum cortisol is lost in Cushing's syndrome, but is preserved in healthy pregnancy, demonstration of loss of circadian rhythm by measuring a midnight serum cortisol may have utility for identifying individuals with Cushing's syndrome in pregnancy [1–3, 49–53]. However, this approach is practically challenging and there are no studies to determine whether testing in pregnancy is associated with the high levels of diagnostic accuracy observed in earlier studies of the nonpregnant population [54].

UFC excretion is normal in the first trimester of normal pregnancy and rises up to threefold the upper limit of normal during the second and third trimesters. A wide range in elevated UFC levels, between 2- and 22-fold of normal, was previously observed in pregnant Cushing's syndrome patients [27]. This overlap of UFC concentrations in pregnant women with and without Cushing's syndrome suggests that only UFC values in the late second and third trimester elevated to at least three times the upper limit of normal can be considered to be consistent with pathological hypercortisolism in Cushing's syndrome [46]. Measurement of UFC is recommended as an initial step in the diagnostic approach in conjunction with late-night salivary cortisol (Fig. 16.1).

Nighttime salivary cortisol testing is an easy and reliable screening test for nonpregnant subjects with Cushing's syndrome with high sensitivity and specificity [55]. Salivary cortisol concentrations reflect biologically unbound free serum cortisol reserve and represent around 3–6% of the total serum cortisol [55, 56]. In healthy pregnant subjects the diurnal rhythm of salivary cortisol is preserved, but at a higher level compared with nonpregnant subjects [56]. Twenty-four hour salivary cortisol

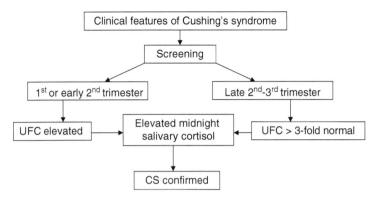

Fig. 16.1 Suggested diagnostic algorithm for Cushing's syndrome (CS) in pregnancy

levels correlate with total UFC concentrations and are elevated in pregnant individuals with Cushing's syndrome compared with healthy women at the same stage of pregnancy [57]. Salivary cortisol has been employed for screening of Cushing's syndrome in case series using standard criteria [57]. In pregnancy there has been insufficient validation of this test to make firm recommendations on a specific diagnostic cut-off level, however, a loss of circadian rhythm should prompt additional investigation (Fig. 16.1).

The overnight and 48 h low-dose dexamethasone-suppression tests are commonly employed for screening in Cushing's syndrome [58]. As discussed earlier (Chap. 4), a stringent criterion of suppression of serum cortisol to at least less than 1.8 μg/dL (50 nmol/L) is required to exclude Cushing's syndrome [59, 60]. In pregnancy however, suppression by dexamethasone of both serum and UFC is blunted in healthy subjects. For this reason, in our opinion, the 48 h and overnight dexamethasone suppression tests are not recommended as a first line screening test in pregnancy, due to the potential for increased risk of false-positive testing [61].

In summary, standard screening is likely to yield a higher proportion of false-positive diagnoses unless pregnancy specific cut-off points are developed for UFC, salivary cortisol, and low-dose dexamethasone suppression testing. A combination of UFC concentrations greater than threefold the upper range of normal and elevated midnight serum or salivary cortisol levels is suggested as a diagnostic strategy for Cushing's syndrome in pregnancy (Fig. 16.1) [46].

Tests for the Differential Diagnosis

As in the nonpregnant population, the first step in the differential diagnosis is to discriminate between ACTH-dependent and ACTH-independent hypercortisolism, which may be achieved by measuring plasma ACTH levels. In the nonpregnant population, plasma ACTH suppression (<5 pg/mL; 1.1 pmol/L) identifies

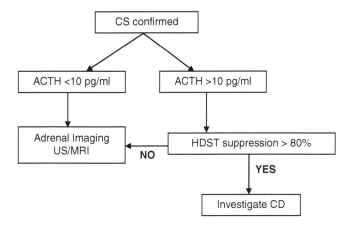

Fig. 16.2 Algorithm for the differential diagnosis of Cushing's syndrome. *UFC* urinary free cortisol, *CD* Cushing's disease, *ACTH* adrenocorticotropin, *US* ultrasound, *MRI* Magnetic resonance imaging, *HDST* high-dose dexamethasone suppression test. Adapted from Lindsay and Nieman, Endocrinol Metab Clin N Am. 2006;25:1–20

ACTH-independent primary adrenal causes of Cushing's syndrome. However, as ACTH concentrations were not suppressed in around half of individuals with primary adrenal disorders in one series in pregnancy, perhaps because of stimulation by the feto-placental unit, the application of standard criteria may lead to diagnostic inaccuracy [19, 27]. However, if ACTH concentrations are suppressed, further biochemical testing may not be required and imaging of the adrenals can be conducted (Fig. 16.2). It is important to highlight that ACTH samples should be collected in prechilled ethylenediaminetetraacetic (EDTA) acid tubes with rapid refrigerated centrifugation and plasma separation to permit accurate interpretation [46].

High-Dose Dexamethasone Suppression Testing

In nonpregnant individuals, the 8-mg overnight dexamethasone suppression test distinguishes Cushing's disease from ectopic ACTH secretion, using a cut-off point of serum cortisol suppression above 80%, with a sensitivity ranging from 60 to 80% and a specificity of more than 80% [62]. In pregnancy, the efficacy of the 8 mg dexamethasone suppression test is unknown due to the limited number of reported ectopic cases [19]. However, the high dose test appears to have utility in distinguishing adrenal from pituitary causes of Cushing's syndrome in pregnancy [19]. In one series, primary adrenal cases of Cushing's syndrome failed to suppress serum cortisol using criteria outlined above, whereas a majority of cases with pituitary ACTH-dependent Cushing's syndrome responded [27]. Therefore, high dose testing may help discriminate adrenal cases from Cushing's disease, which is helpful, given the difficulties in interpretation of plasma ACTH and the increased prevalence of adrenal disorders in pregnancy.

CRH Stimulation Testing

Patients with Cushing's disease retain responsiveness to CRH stimulation, in contrast to those with ectopic or adrenal causes [63, 64]. While no adverse effects were observed in a small number of cases during gestation, ovine CRH should only be considered for use in pregnancy when there is persistent diagnostic uncertainty after high-dose dexamethasone suppression and ACTH testing, as it is an FDA category C drug [47, 53, 64]. As third trimester plasma ACTH responses to human CRH are reduced in normal gestation, the interpretation of testing using standard criteria is more challenging in late pregnancy [65].

Imaging

Pituitary MRI should be considered in cases with suspected Cushing's disease. Noncontrast enhanced pituitary MRI is generally considered safe after 32 weeks gestation but should be avoided during the first trimester due to potentially unknown adverse effects on the fetus [19]. During the second and early third trimesters the risks and potential benefits of MRI need to be considered taking into account the potential for false-positive diagnoses, as normal pituitary doubles in size by the third trimester and also considering a reduced sensitivity of pituitary MRI without gadolinium contrast enhancement [66]. The prevalence of pituitary macroadenomas in pregnancy in earlier series was higher than expected [64, 67, 68].

In cases with suppressed plasma ACTH concentrations and failure to suppress serum cortisol following high-dose dexamethasone testing, adrenal imaging is recommended. Adrenal ultrasound imaging is safe and effective but has limited sensitivity for smaller tumor sizes [19, 69, 70]. MRI is preferred to CT during pregnancy due to the risks associated with ionizing radiation [52, 70, 71].

Inferior Petrosal Sinus Sampling

Inferior petrosal sinus sampling (IPSS) should only be considered when biochemical testing and pituitary imaging are discordant in view of the potential risks of ionizing radiation [64, 72]. Special precautions including the use of additional lead barrier protection and a direct jugular approach for catheter insertion are necessary to limit radiation exposure. Furthermore, it is not clear whether the usual criteria for interpretation will definitely exclude patients with adrenal disease as this has not been systematically studied. Therefore, we would generally recommend that patients with a pituitary adenoma ≥6 mm and consistent responses to high-dose dexamethasone suppression testing be considered for transsphenoidal surgery without proceeding to IPSS [19].

Therapeutic Options

It is assumed that the adverse maternal and fetal outcomes associated with Cushing's syndrome and pregnancy may be reduced or prevented by reducing UFC excretion to the upper part of the range observed in normal pregnancy [19, 58]. However, treatment for pregnant patients with Cushing's syndrome tends to have been implemented sporadically, generally late in the course of the pregnancy. A review of 136 pregnancies showed a higher rate of live births when treatment was implemented during the second trimester compared with no intervention [27].

Definitive surgical treatment of Cushing's syndrome in pregnancy is recommended where possible. Although transsphenoidal surgery has been used in a limited number of patients with pituitary ACTH-dependent hypercortisolism, this approach appears safe when performed by an experienced surgeon [27]. Adrenalectomy has usually been undertaken for patients with adrenal adenomas during the second trimester, and generally appears beneficial [29, 30, 73]. The live birth rate after unilateral or bilateral adrenalectomy is approximately 87% [19, 27]. Due to high rates of maternal and fetal morbidity, supportive treatment alone is usually not recommended, except perhaps late in the third trimester.

Medical therapy may be required if surgery is not feasible, or as an adjunct for severe adverse effects of hypercortisolism. As most of the available agents used for investigation and treatment of hypercortisolism are untested in pregnancy, the majority of these agents are classed as FDA category C (see Table 16.1). Metyrapone has been the most commonly used medical therapy [70, 73]. While its use has been associated with fetal hypoadrenalism and the potential for exacerbation of hypertension and progression to pre-eclampsia, it has generally been well tolerated [35, 70]. Other options such as ketoconazole or cyproheptadine have been attempted. Potential safety concerns with ketoconazole limits is use in pregnancy and has usually only considered in patients intolerant of metyrapone and in need of emergency medical therapy [19]. Cyproheptadine appears may be safe but is not effective and would not usually be considered [74, 75]. Mitotane is not recommended in pregnancy as it has potential teratogenic effects [68].

Conclusions

Cushing's syndrome is a rare occurrence in pregnancy, but is associated with significant morbidity. There is a need for development of criteria for interpretation of diagnostic tests and for increased consideration of Cushing's syndrome in pregnancy. It is likely that earlier recognition and treatment would improve outcomes for the fetus and mother. Surgery is the treatment of choice for Cushing's syndrome in pregnancy, except perhaps late in the third trimester, with medical treatment being an alternative option or for those awaiting surgery. While surgery or medical therapy is potentially an effective treatment for Cushing's syndrome in pregnancy, the prognosis for the

Table 16.1 FDA Classification for drugs used to treat hypercortisolism in pregnancy

Category	Drug	Interpretation	Summary
A		Controlled studies show no risk	Adequate and well-controlled studies have failed to demonstrate a risk to the fetus in the first trimester of pregnancy (and there is no evidence of risk in later trimesters).
B	Cyproheptadine	No evidence of risk in humans	Animal reproduction studies have failed to demonstrate a risk to the fetus and there are no adequate and well-controlled studies in pregnant women.
C	Dexamethasone Ovine CRH Metyrapone Ketoconazole Mitotane	Risk cannot be ruled out	Human studies are lacking and animal studies are either positive for fetal risk or lacking as well. However, potential benefits may justify the potential risk.
D		Positive evidence of risk	There is positive evidence of human fetal risk based on adverse reaction data from investigational or marketing experience or studies in humans, but potential benefits may warrant use of the drug in pregnant women despite potential risks.
X		Contraindicated in pregnancy	Studies in animals or humans have demonstrated fetal abnormalities and/or there is positive evidence of human fetal risk based on adverse reaction data from investigational or marketing experience, and the risks involved in use of the drug in pregnant women clearly outweigh potential benefits.

fetus remains guarded in the setting of persistent hypercortisolism. An increased suspicion for diagnosis of this rare disease may facilitate early treatment and improved outcomes for both mother and fetus.

References

1. Carr BR, Parker Jr CR, Madden JD, et al. Maternal plasma adrenocorticotropin and cortisol relationships throughout human pregnancy. Am J Obstet Gynecol. 1981;139(4):416–22.
2. Cousins L, Rigg L, Hollingsworth D, et al. Qualitative and quantitative assessment of the circadian rhythm of cortisol in pregnancy. Am J Obstet Gynecol. 1983;145(4):411–6.
3. Nolten WE, Lindheimer MD, Rueckert PA, et al. Diurnal patterns and regulation of cortisol secretion in pregnancy. J Clin Endocrinol Metab. 1980;51(3):466–72.
4. Patrick J, Challis J, Natale R, et al. Circadian rhythms in maternal plasma cortisol, estrone, estradiol, and estriol at 34 to 35 weeks' gestation. Am J Obstet Gynecol. 1979;135(6):791–8.
5. Martin JD, Mills IH. The effects of pregnancy on adrenal steroid metabolism. Clin Sci (Lond). 1958;17(1):137–46.

6. Scott EM, McGarrigle HH, Lachelin GC. The increase in plasma and saliva cortisol levels in pregnancy is not due to the increase in corticosteroid-binding globulin levels. J Clin Endocrinol Metab. 1990;71(3):639–44.
7. Hillhouse EW, Grammatopoulos DK. Role of stress peptides during human pregnancy and labour. Reproduction. 2002;124(3):323–9.
8. Sorem KA, Smikle CB, Spencer DK, et al. Circulating maternal corticotropin-releasing hormone and gonadotropin-releasing hormone in normal and abnormal pregnancies. Am J Obstet Gynecol. 1996;175(4 Pt 1):912–6.
9. Goland RS, Wardlaw SL, Blum M, et al. Biologically active corticotropin-releasing hormone in maternal and fetal plasma during pregnancy. Am J Obstet Gynecol. 1988;159(4):884–90.
10. Sasaki A, Liotta AS, Luckey MM, et al. Immunoreactive corticotropin-releasing factor is present in human maternal plasma during the third trimester of pregnancy. J Clin Endocrinol Metab. 1984;59(4):812–4.
11. Sasaki A, Shinkawa O, Yoshinaga K. Immunoreactive corticotropin-releasing hormone in amniotic fluid. Am J Obstet Gynecol. 1990;162(1):194–8.
12. Sasaki A, Tempst P, Liotta AS, et al. Isolation and characterization of a corticotropin-releasing hormone-like peptide from human placenta. J Clin Endocrinol Metab. 1988;67(4):768–73.
13. Potter E, Behan DP, Fischer WH, et al. Cloning and characterization of the cDNAs for human and rat corticotropin releasing factor-binding proteins. Nature. 1991;349(6308):423–6.
14. Linton EA, Perkins AV, Woods RJ, et al. Corticotropin releasing hormone-binding protein [CRH-BP]: plasma levels decrease during the third trimester of normal human pregnancy. J Clin Endocrinol Metab. 1993;76(1):260–2.
15. McLean M, Bisits A, Davies J, et al. A placental clock controlling the length of human pregnancy. Nat Med. 1995;1(5):460–3.
16. Wadhwa PD, Porto M, Garite TJ, et al. Maternal corticotropin-releasing hormone levels in the early third trimester predict length of gestation in human pregnancy. Am J Obstet Gynecol. 1998;179(4):1079–85.
17. Allolio B, Hoffmann J, Linton EA, et al. Diurnal salivary cortisol patterns during pregnancy and after delivery: relationship to plasma corticotrophin-releasing-hormone. Clin Endocrinol (Oxf). 1990;33(2):279–89.
18. Mukherjee K, Swyer GI. Plasma cortisol and adrenocorticotrophic hormone in normal men and non-pregnant women, normal pregnant women and women with pre-eclampsia. J Obstet Gynaecol Br Commonw. 1972;79(6):504–12.
19. Lindsay JR, Nieman LK. The hypothalamic-pituitary-adrenal axis in pregnancy: challenges in disease detection and treatment. Endocr Rev. 2005;26(6):775–99.
20. Demey-Ponsart E, Foidart JM, Sulon J, et al. Serum CBG, free and total cortisol and circadian patterns of adrenal function in normal pregnancy. J Steroid Biochem. 1982;16(2):165–9.
21. Odagiri E, Ishiwatari N, Abe Y, et al. Hypercortisolism and the resistance to dexamethasone suppression during gestation. Endocrinol Jpn. 1988;35(5):685–90.
22. Elliott CL, Read GF, Wallace EM. The pharmacokinetics of oral and intramuscular administration of dexamethasone in late pregnancy. Acta Obstet Gynecol Scand. 1996;75(3):213–6.
23. Seckl JR, Cleasby M, Nyirenda MJ. Glucocorticoids, 11beta-hydroxysteroid dehydrogenase, and fetal programming. Kidney Int. 2000;57(4):1412–7.
24. Murphy BE. Conversion of cortisol to cortisone by the human uterus and its reversal in pregnancy. J Clin Endocrinol Metab. 1977;44(6):1214–7.
25. Greenwood J, Parker G. The dexamethasone suppression test in the puerperium. Aust N Z J Psychiatry. 1984;18(3):282–4.
26. Owens PC, Smith R, Brinsmead MW, et al. Postnatal disappearance of the pregnancy-associated reduced sensitivity of plasma cortisol to feedback inhibition. Life Sci. 1987;41(14):1745–50.
27. Lindsay JR, Jonklaas J, Oldfield EH, et al. Cushing's syndrome during pregnancy: personal experience and review of the literature. J Clin Endocrinol Metab. 2005;90(5):3077–83.
28. Hunt AB, McConahey CW. Pregnancy associated with diseases of the adrenal glands. Am J Obstet Gynecol. 1953;66:970–87.

29. Buescher MA, McClamrock HD, Adashi EY. Cushing syndrome in pregnancy. Obstet Gynecol. 1992;79(1):130–7.
30. Aron DC, Schnall AM, Sheeler LR. Cushing's syndrome and pregnancy. Am J Obstet Gynecol. 1990;162(1):244–52.
31. Koerten JM, Morales WJ, Washington 3rd SR, et al. Cushing's syndrome in pregnancy: a case report and literature review. Am J Obstet Gynecol. 1986;154(3):626–8.
32. Sheeler LR. Cushing's syndrome and pregnancy. Endocrinol Metab Clin North Am. 1994;23(3):619–27.
33. Tajika T, Shinozaki T, Watanabe H, et al. Case report of a Cushing's syndrome patient with multiple pathologic fractures during pregnancy. J Orthop Sci. 2002;7(4):498–500.
34. Cabezon C, Bruno OD, Cohen M, et al. Twin pregnancy in a patient with Cushing's disease. Fertil Steril. 1999;72:371–2.
35. Connell JM, Cordiner J, Davies DL, et al. Pregnancy complicated by Cushing's syndrome: potential hazard of metyrapone therapy. Case report. Br J Obstet Gynaecol. 1985;92(11):1192–5.
36. Klibanski A, Stephen AE, Greene MF, et al. Case records of the Massachusetts General Hospital. Case 36–2006. A 35-year-old pregnant woman with new hypertension. N Engl J Med. 2006;355(21):2237–45.
37. Guilhaume B, Sanson ML, Billaud L, et al. Cushing's syndrome and pregnancy: aetiologies and prognosis in twenty-two patients. Eur J Med. 1992;1(2):83–9.
38. Pickard J, Jochen AL, Sadur CN, et al. Cushing's syndrome in pregnancy. Obstet Gynecol Surv. 1990;45(2):87–93.
39. Casson IF, Davis JC, Jeffreys RV, et al. Successful management of Cushing's disease during pregnancy by transsphenoidal adenectomy. Clin Endocrinol (Oxf). 1987;27(4):423–8.
40. Oh HC, Koh JM, Kim MS, et al. A case of ACTH-producing pheochromocytoma associated with pregnancy. Endocr J. 2003;50(6):739–44.
41. Wallace C, Toth EL, Lewanczuk RZ, et al. Pregnancy-induced Cushing's syndrome in multiple pregnancies. J Clin Endocrinol Metab. 1996;81(1):15–21.
42. Hána V, Dokoupilová M, Marek J, et al. Recurrent ACTH independent Cushing's syndrome in multiple pregnancies and its treatment with metyrapone. Clin Endocrinol (Oxf). 2001;54:277–81.
43. Carlson HE. Human adrenal cortex hyperfunction due to LH/hCG. Mol Cell Endocrinol. 2007;269:46–50.
44. Rask E, Schvarcz E, Hellman P, et al. Adrenocorticotropin-independent Cushing's syndrome in pregnancy related to overexpression of adrenal luteinizing hormone/human chorioic gonadotropin receptors. J Endocinol Invest. 2009;32:313–6.
45. Lacroix A, Hamet P, Boutin JM. Leuprolide acetate therapy in luteinizing hormone-dependent Cushing's syndrome. N Engl J Med. 1999;341(21):1577–81.
46. Lindsay JR, Nieman LK. Adrenal disorders in pregnancy. Endocrinol Metab Clin N Am. 2006;35:1–20.
47. Ross RJ, Chew SL, Perry L, et al. Diagnosis and selective cure of Cushing's disease during pregnancy by transsphenoidal surgery. Eur J Endocrinol. 1995;132(6):722–6.
48. Nakada T, Koike H, Katayama T. Uneventful delivery following series of successive treatments for virilized Cushing syndrome due to adrenocortical carcinoma. Urology. 1990;36(4):359–63.
49. Bevan JS, Gough MH, Gillmer MD, et al. Cushing's syndrome in pregnancy: the timing of definitive treatment. Clin Endocrinol (Oxf). 1987;27:225–33.
50. Avril-Ducarne C, Leclerc P, Thobois B, et al. Adrenal adenoma disclosing after delivery. Rev Med Interne. 1990;11:245–7.
51. Blumsohn D, Munyadziwa EH, Dajie SK, et al. Cushing's syndrome and pregnancy: a case report. S Afr Med. 1978;53:338–40.
52. Doshi S, Bhat A, Lim KB. Cushing's syndrome in pregnancy. J Obstet Gynaecol. 2003;23(5):568–9.
53. Mellor A, Harvey RD, Pobereskin LH, et al. Cushing's disease treated by trans-sphenoidal selective adenomectomy in mid-pregnancy. Br J Anaesth. 1998;80(6):850–2.

54. Newell-Price J, Trainer P, Perry L, et al. A single sleeping midnight cortisol has 100% sensitivity for the diagnosis of Cushing's syndrome. Clin Endocrinol (Oxf). 1995;43:545–50.
55. Evans PJ, Peters JR, Dyas J, et al. Salivary cortisol levels in true and apparent hypercortisolism. Clin Endocrinol. 1984;20:709–15.
56. Viardot A, Huber P, Puder JJ, et al. Reproducibility of nighttime salivary cortisol and its use in the diagnosis of hypercortisolism compared with urinary free cortisol and overnight dexamethasone suppression test. J Clin Endocrinol Metab. 2005;90:5730–6.
57. Billaud L, Sanson ML, Guilhaume B, et al. Cushing's syndrome during pregnancy. New diagnostic methods used in 3 cases of adrenal cortex carcinoma. Presse Med. 1992;21:2041–5.
58. Boscaro M, Arnaldi G. Approach to the patient with Cushing's syndrome. J Clin Endocrinol Metab. 2009;94:3121–31.
59. Newell-Price J, Trainer P, Besser GM, et al. The diagnosis and differential diagnosis of Cushing's syndrome and pseudo-Cushing's states. Endocr Rev. 1998;19:647–72.
60. Newell-Price J, Bertagna X, Grossman AB, et al. Cushing's syndrome. Lancet. 2006;367:1605–17.
61. Vilar L, Freitas M, Lima L, et al. Cushing's syndrome in pregnancy: an overview. Arq Bras Endocrinol Metab. 2007;51:1293–302.
62. Aron DC, Raff H, Findling JW. Effectiveness versus efficacy: the limited value in clinical practice of high dose dexamethasone suppression testing in the differential diagnosis of adrenocorticotropin-dependent Cushing's syndrome. J Clin Endocrinol Metab. 1997;82:1780–5.
63. Nieman LK, Chrousos GP, Oldfield EH, et al. The ovine corticotropin-releasing hormone stimulation test and the dexamethasone suppression test in the differential diagnosis of Cushing's syndrome. Ann Intern Med. 1986;105(6):862–7.
64. Pinette MG, Pan YQ, Oppenheim D, et al. Bilateral inferior petrosal sinus corticotropin sampling with corticotropin-releasing hormone stimulation in a pregnant patient with Cushing's syndrome. Am J Obstet Gynecol. 1994;171(2):563–4.
65. Schulte HM, Weisner D, Allolio B. The corticotrophin releasing hormone test in late pregnancy: lack of adrenocorticotrophin and cortisol response. Clin Endocrinol (Oxf). 1990;33(1):99–106.
66. Tabarin A, Laurent F, Catargi B, et al. Comparative evaluation of conventional and dynamic magnetic resonance imaging of the pituitary gland for the diagnosis of Cushing's disease. Clin Endocrinol (Oxf). 1998;49(3):293–300.
67. Mampalam TJ, Tyrrell JB, Wilson CB. Transsphenoidal microsurgery for Cushing disease. A report of 216 cases. Ann Intern Med. 1988;109(6):487–93.
68. Leiba S, Weinstein R, Shindel B, et al. The protracted effect of o, p'-DDD in Cushing's disease and its impact on adrenal morphogenesis of young human embryo. Ann Endocrinol (Paris). 1989;50(1):49–53.
69. Martin RW, Lucas JA, Martin JN, et al. Conservative management of Cushing's syndrome in pregnancy. A case report. J Reprod Med. 1989;34(7):493–5.
70. Shaw JA, Pearson DW, Krukowski ZH, et al. Cushing's syndrome during pregnancy: curative adrenalectomy at 31 weeks gestation. Eur J Obstet Gynecol Reprod Biol. 2002;105(2):189–91.
71. Finkenstedt G, Gasser RW, Hofle G, et al. Pheochromocytoma and sub-clinical Cushing's syndrome during pregnancy: diagnosis, medical pre-treatment and cure by laparoscopic unilateral adrenalectomy. J Endocrinol Invest. 1999;22(7):551–7.
72. Oldfield EH, Doppman JL, Nieman LK, et al. Petrosal sinus sampling with and without corticotropin-releasing hormone for the differential diagnosis of Cushing's syndrome. N Engl J Med. 1991;325(13):897–905.
73. Close CF, Mann MC, Watts JF, et al. ACTH-independent Cushing's syndrome in pregnancy with spontaneous resolution after delivery: control of the hypercortisolism with metyrapone. Clin Endocrinol (Oxf). 1993;39(3):375–9.
74. Khir AS, How J, Bewsher PD. Successful pregnancy after cyproheptadine treatment for Cushing's disease. Eur J Obstet Gynecol Reprod Biol. 1982;13:343–7.
75. Kasperlik-Zaluska A, Migdalska B, Hartwig W, et al. Two pregnancies in a woman with Cushing's syndrome treated with cyproheptadine. Case report. Br J Obstet Gynaecol. 1980;87:1171–3.

Chapter 17
Nelson's Syndrome: Corticotroph Tumor Progression After Bilateral Adrenalectomy in Cushing's Disease

Guillaume Assie, Laurence Guignat, Jérôme Bertherat, and Xavier Bertagna

Abstract Since Don Nelson's first description in 1958 of a pituitary macroadenoma occurring after adrenalectomy in a patient with Cushing's disease, the "Nelson's syndrome" has long been feared. However, major advances including pituitary MRI imaging, transsphenoidal surgery, and improvements in radiotherapy have changed the way Corticotroph Tumor Progression (CTP) can be monitored and treated. This chapter reviews the incidence, diagnosis, and management strategies for Corticotroph Tumor Progression.

Keywords Corticotroph tumor progression • Macroadenoma • Adrenalectomy • Adrenocorticotropic hormone • Transsphenoidal surgery • Radiotherapy

Introduction

Since Don Nelson's first description in 1958 of a pituitary macroadenoma occurring after adrenalectomy in a patient with Cushing's disease, the "Nelson's syndrome" has long been feared. However, major advances including pituitary MRI imaging, transsphenoidal surgery, and improvements in radiotherapy have changed the way Corticotroph Tumor Progression (CTP) can be monitored and treated. Rather than wait for the late occurrence of Nelson's syndrome, as defined originally by the complications associated with invasive macroadenomas, we can now detect the development of CTP long before the classical features of Nelson's syndrome have occurred.

X. Bertagna (✉)
Service des Maladies Endocriniennes et Métaboliques, Centre de Référence des Maladies Rares de la Surrénale, INSERM U-567, Institut Cochin, Hôpital Cochin,
Faculté de Médecine Paris Descartes, Université Paris 5, Paris, France

Department of Endocrinology, Hôpital Cochin, 27, rue Fg St Jacques, 75014 Paris, France
e-mail: xavier.bertagna@cch.aphp.fr

In a recent study of 53 patients followed by MRI after bilateral adrenalectomy, we showed that 3 years after adrenalectomy, the proportion of patients showing evidence of CTP reached 39%; this number plateaued at 47% after 7 years. Thus, about 50% of the patients showed no evidence of CTP during this time period. Factors that were found to be significantly associated with a higher risk of developing CTP were duration of Cushing's disease, baseline ACTH plasma level in the year following adrenalectomy, and the rate of increase in ACTH plasma levels after adrenalectomy. CTP does not seem to accelerate during pregnancy.

There is no question that pituitary surgery remains the first line treatment in most patients with Cushing's disease. However, when complete removal of a corticotroph tumor is not possible, total bilateral adrenalectomy can be considered among the various therapeutic options in Cushing's disease. CTP does not occur in all patients and is manageable in most cases. After bilateral adrenalectomy, if necessary, pituitary surgery and/or radiotherapy can control the CTP in a majority of situations. New pharmacologic agents directed against corticotroph tumors may prove beneficial in CTP as well.

Historical Perspective

In 1958, Don Nelson et al. [1] first reported the occurrence of a pituitary macroadenoma secreting high amounts of ACTH after total bilateral adrenalectomy for Cushing's syndrome: "a 33 year old woman who developed marked skin hyperpigmentation, and evidence of pituitary tumor (enlarged sella on skull x-ray and visual field defects), 3 years after she had been subjected to bilateral adrenalectomy for Cushing's syndrome. ACTH plasma levels were high enough to be measured by a bioassay in the hypophysectomized dog..." Other authors independently reported similar cases [2–5], demonstrating the existence of ACTH-secreting pituitary adenomas, as had been previously surmised by Harvey Cushing [6]. These observations came as an illuminating clue for the pathogenesis of Cushing's disease. They also raised the fear that adrenalectomy in Cushing's disease could induce the occurrence or trigger the growth of a pituitary adenoma, with the risk of subsequent complications related to the tumor burden. In 1960, Nelson et al. published the first series of patients [7] and "Nelson's syndrome" was born, which, 50 years later, still remains an ill-defined condition.

Nelson's Syndrome: Is There a Definition?

About 50 series [8, 9] have reported on Nelson's syndrome (NS), grossly defined by the association of an expanding pituitary tumor and increased ACTH secretion after adrenalectomy in Cushing's disease. The diagnostic criteria have varied over the years, including (1) the presence of a pituitary macroadenoma either diagnosed on x-ray or sellar tomography, or on the occurrence of associated visual defects and

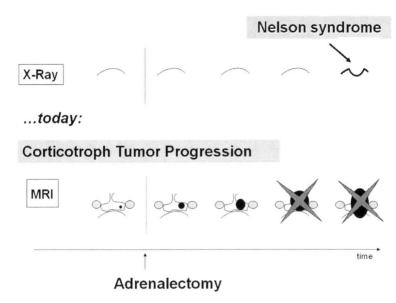

Fig. 17.1 Nelson's syndrome…or Corticotroph tumor progression? Late diagnosis of Nelson's syndrome when the diagnostic techniques lacked sensitivity (*upper part*). Close follow-up of possible corticotroph tumor progression, with modern tools such as pituitary MRI (*lower part*)

(2) the diagnosis of high plasma ACTH levels based either on qualitative assessment of cutaneous pigmentation, or on various baseline plasma ACTH cut-offs. In addition, the cohorts of patients to which the term has been applied have received heterogeneous treatments, including some directly interfering with potential tumor growth such as pituitary irradiation. Moreover, major advances in therapy and radiographic monitoring, such as transsphenoidal surgery or pituitary MRI, were developed during the inclusion period.

With these various and heterogeneous definitions, the prevalence of NS ranged from 8 to 29% in the largest series, with a time interval between adrenalectomy and the diagnosis of NS ranging from 0.5 to 24 years [8].

Corticotroph Tumor Progression

Today we know that the corticotroph adenoma is indeed the cause of Cushing's disease, and we can use highly sensitive imaging and biological means to visualize it and assess its function through pituitary MRI and ACTH measurements with immunoassays. In cases where bilateral adrenalectomy is eventually performed, these modern approaches are now routinely used for the follow-up of patients with Cushing's disease.

Rather than awaiting the late occurrence of NS, as originally defined (Fig. 17.1, upper), we can now detect, early on and with precision, the possible occurrence of CTP, long before the classical features of NS have developed (Fig. 17.1, lower).

Because progression of corticotroph adenomas can now be recognized prior to the development of hyperpigmentation and symptoms of mass effect, the term CTP is preferable.

After our initial paper of 2004 suggested that the definition of NS be revisited [8], a subsequent manuscript retrospectively analyzed the historical perspectives and current concepts in Nelson's syndrome [10]. Acknowledging the need to reassess this condition, these authors eventually wrote "…the authors believe this disease must be reevaluated in the contemporary era and a modern paradigm adapted." Among the authors of this paper was Don Nelson himself!

Assessing Corticotroph Tumor Progression

Is CTP Inevitable?

We recently studied [9] the rate of occurrence of CTP in a cohort of 53 patients with Cushing's disease who were carefully followed in a single center after bilateral adrenalectomy, using repeat MRI, for a median duration of follow-up after adrenalectomy of 4.6 years (range 0.5–13.5). None had received pituitary radiotherapy. CTP was defined either by the occurrence of an adenoma on MRI, or the growth of a pre-existing adenoma on pituitary MRI [9].

The Kaplan–Meyer representation evaluates that CTP will be detected in approximately one third of patients at 3 years, and one half at 7 years (Fig. 17.2). Thus, about 50% of the patients showed no evidence of CTP during this time interval. Among the ten patients who developed CTP, a single neurologic complication was observed where spontaneous tumor necrosis induced a transient ocular nerve palsy. Four patients were subsequently treated with conventional pituitary radiotherapy.

The Early Detection of CTP

There is a definite need to improve the accuracy of assessing pituitary tumor growth by imaging. Pituitary MRI has revolutionized the field [11–13], yet few data are available that provide us with clear tools to evaluate subtle morphological changes. They will be useful not only to follow CTP after adrenalectomy in Cushing's disease, but also in other circumstances, when other types of adenomas are subjected to direct – medical or radiotherapeutic – treatments, or, when patients with acromegaly are treated with GH antagonists. We have thoroughly evaluated the performance of pituitary MRI to specifically assess pituitary ACTH secreting adenomas [14].

CTP can indeed be easily detected by repeat pituitary MRI. It is recommended that it be performed before and 6 months after adrenalectomy, then every year,

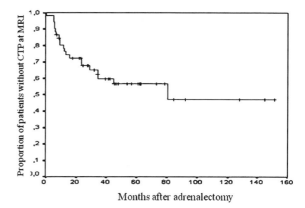

Fig. 17.2 Survival without evidence of CTP on MRI after total bilateral adrenalectomy in a cohort of 53 patients with Cushing's disease not subjected to pituitary irradiation

at least for the next 5–6 years. In the absence of CTP after this period, it seems reasonable to increase the time intervals of MRI surveillance thereafter.

Repeat determinations of ACTH plasma levels also add valuable information [9]. There is, however, no definitive threshold or accepted protocol (e.g., baseline, before or after the morning glucocorticoid administration, stimulated, suppressed, etc.) that has proven to be a valid and sensitive biochemical detector of early CTP. In general, higher ACTH plasma levels are associated with visible adenomas, but there is no definite threshold which differentiates those patients with visible from non-visible adenomas.

Can We Predict CTP?

In the past, studies [9] have attempted to identify predictive factors for classical NS with varying results, including young age at adrenalectomy, lack of pituitary irradiation prior to adrenalectomy, the surgical or morphological documentation of a pituitary adenoma before adrenalectomy, the existence of an adrenal remnant after adrenalectomy, duration of the Cushing's disease, and urinary cortisol excretion before adrenalectomy. For most of these variables, some studies indicated a correlation with the risk of developing NS, whereas others showed no significant association. Finally, some factors have never been demonstrated to be predictive, including gender, basal ACTH in the morning before adrenalectomy, the level of glucocorticoid substitution after adrenalectomy, and pregnancy.

Eventually many studies agreed that a high baseline ACTH plasma value in the year following adrenalectomy was the best validated predictive factor [9].

In our recent study [9], factors that were found to be significantly associated with a higher risk to develop CTP were a short duration of Cushing's disease, a high baseline ACTH plasma level in the year following adrenalectomy, and the rate of increase in ACTH plasma levels after adrenalectomy. Some of our patients had been treated by O,p'DDD at some point in the course of their disease; we showed that increases in plasma ACTH concentration during O,p'DDD-induced cortisol deprivation tended to predict CTP after adrenalectomy, but this relationship did not reach significance ($p=0.08$).

In those patients treated by pituitary surgery prior to adrenalectomy, pathological studies of the tissue thus far have not revealed predictors of CTP. In our recent study [9], neither the presence of mitoses nor a high percentage of Ki67-immunopositive nuclei in the adenoma was predictive of CTP.

Does Pregnancy Accelerate CTP?

Because Cushing's disease often occurs in young female patients, the desire for pregnancy is frequently an issue that must be considered when selecting a therapeutic option after failed pituitary surgery. We have thoroughly examined the hypothesis that pregnancy could stimulate CTP.

A retrospective cohort study was performed on patients who became pregnant after bilateral adrenalectomy, followed in a single center (Cochin Hospital, Paris). There were 20 pregnancies in 11 patients. None had had pituitary irradiation. CTP was assessed by pituitary MRI. Plasma ACTH levels and corticotroph tumor volume variations before, during, and after pregnancy were monitored and compared using paired Wilcoxon rank test. Data on maternal and neonatal outcomes were recorded by phone and obstetrical correspondence. CTP occurred in 8 out of 17 pregnancies, and ACTH increased in 8 out of 10 pregnancies. However, when compared to data obtained prior to pregnancy, neither the corticotroph tumor volume variation, nor the ACTH variation, increased during or after pregnancy. We concluded that pregnancy does not accelerate CTP after bilateral adrenalectomy. Pregnancy in these conditions is manageable, provided the patients can be followed closely [15].

Managing Corticotroph Tumor Progression

Can We Prevent or Treat CTP?

The historical cases of Nelson's syndrome were characterized by large invasive pituitary macroadenomas and presented a major therapeutic challenge. Today, with pituitary MRI, the tumor can be detected much earlier at a smaller size, and treated more effectively.

After adrenalectomy, the goal is to manage CTP so that no complication related to the tumor burden occurs. Regular MRI follow-up is necessary for an early CTP diagnosis. Some cases may be carefully followed with serial MR imaging if no progression is evident. If there is progression, the tumor may be removed transsphenoidally

17 Nelson's Syndrome: Corticotroph Tumor Progression...

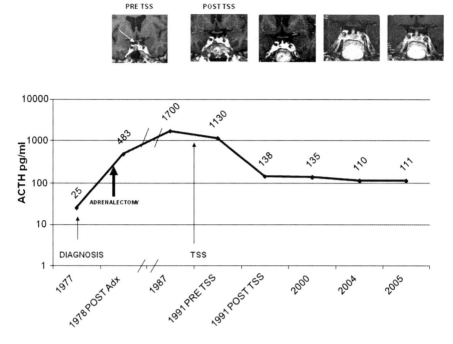

Fig. 17.3 Successful removal of a pituitary corticotroph adenoma that had appeared on MRI years after total bilateral adrenalectomy

if accessible (Fig. 17.3), or radiated if not. Some, but not all, studies have shown a protective effect of radiotherapy performed immediately following bilateral adrenalectomy [9].

The identification of clinical and molecular factors which could predict aggressive CTP is needed. With such factors, we could modify the pituitary MRI surveillance schedule, propose early pituitary irradiation in high risk patients, and better choose the appropriate time for pituitary surgery in the face of a growing pituitary adenoma. It is clear that further, prospective studies will be necessary to answer these questions; a goal that is difficult to achieve in such a rare disease.

Is There a Role for Bilateral Adrenalectomy in Cushing's Disease?

Bilateral adrenalectomy is by no means the ideal treatment of Cushing's disease. Pituitary surgery, usually by the transsphenoidal route, is indeed the first line treatment. In cases of failure or recurrence, the choice is generally between pituitary irradiation (with inconstant and delayed success and the risk of pituitary insufficiency) and adrenal directed therapy, either pharmacological (usually ketoconazole or O,p'DDD with their inconstant efficacy and frequent side effects, and precluding pregnancy) or adrenalectomy (immediate success, but adrenal failure…and the risk of NS).

We know that CTP is not inevitable, and close follow up with repeat MRI allows us to treat it before the classical NS develops. Under these conditions, adrenalectomy is an effective therapeutic modality in difficult cases of CD, particularly in young women who wish to become pregnant.

The Need for Medical Treatments for Cushing's Disease

The corticotroph adenoma is an "orphan pituitary tumor." In contrast with other secreting adenomas such as PRL, GH, or TSH adenomas, there are, at this time, no pharmacological agents that have clearly and consistently shown to be of therapeutic benefit on ACTH-secreting pituitary tumors.

Ongoing studies show promise: dopaminergic and/or somatostatinergic drugs, such as cabergoline and the preferential SST5 ligand SOM-230, are actively being studied, and clinical trials in patients with Cushing's disease are underway [16, 17]. PPAR gamma agonists have not proved as to be as useful in humans as was suggested by experimental studies [18], while animal studies with retinoic acid may show some benefit [19]. Yet, one should remain cautious until clear safety and efficacy are demonstrated.

Summary and Recommendations

Rather than awaiting the development of Nelson's syndrome, one should closely monitor for the possible occurrence of CTP. A baseline pituitary MRI should be obtained prior to adrenalectomy (within 6 months). There is no fully accepted predictor of CTP prior to adrenalectomy. A high ACTH plasma level in the year following adrenalectomy, and high absolute increases thereafter, may be predictive parameters.

Repeat pituitary MRI and ACTH plasma level determinations are mandatory and should be first performed at 3–6 months after adrenalectomy and yearly thereafter. Continued surveillance is recommended. In the absence of CTP after 6 years, it might be safe to decrease imaging frequency, perhaps to every 2 years.

There is no proven medical treatment for CTP. Early detection may permit curative transsphenoidal surgery. Alternatively, an invasive adenoma might require radiotherapy. There is no need for prophylactic radiotherapy after adrenalectomy.

Acknowledgments The authors are indebted to Stéphan Gaillard (Neurosurgery Department, Hôpital Foch), Hélène Bahurel, Marie Bienvenue, Paul Legmann (Radiology Department, Hôpital Cochin), Bertrand Dousset (Endocrine Surgery, Hôpital Cochin), and Michèle Kujas (Pathology Department, Hôpital La Pitié).

References

1. Nelson DH, Meakin JW, Dealy Jr JB, Matson DD, Emerson Jr K, Thorn GW. ACTH-producing tumor of the pituitary gland. N Engl J Med. 1958;259(4):161–4.
2. Salassa RM, Kearns TP, Kernohan JW, Sprague RG, Maccarty CS. Pituitary tumors in patients with Cushing's syndrome. J Clin Endocrinol Metab. 1959;19:1523–39.
3. Montgomery DA, Welbourn RB, McCaughey WT, Gleadhill CA. Pituitary tumours manifested after adrenalectomy for Cushing's syndrome. Lancet. 1959;2:707–10.
4. Glenn F, Karl RC, Horwith M. The surgical treatment of Cushing's syndrome. Ann Surg. 1958;148(3):365–74.
5. Rees JR, Zilva JF. Diabetes insipidus complicating total adrenalectomy. J Clin Pathol. 1959;12:530–4.
6. Cushing H. The basophil adenomas of the pituitary body and their clinical manifestations (pituitary basophilism). Bull John Hopkins Hosp. 1932;50:137–95.
7. Nelson DH, Meakin JW, Thorn GW. ACTH-producing pituitary tumors following adrenalectomy for Cushing's syndrome. Ann Intern Med. 1960;52:560–9.
8. Assié G, Bahurel H, Bertherat J, Kujas M, Legmann P, Bertagna X. The Nelson's syndrome… revisited. Pituitary. 2004;7(4):209–15. Review.
9. Assié G, Bahurel H, Coste J, Silvera S, Kujas M, Dugué MA, et al. Corticotroph tumor progression after adrenalectomy in Cushing's Disease: a reappraisal of Nelson's syndrome. J Clin Endocrinol Metab. 2007;92(1):172–9. Epub 2006 Oct 24.
10. Hornyak M, Weiss MH, Nelson DH, Couldwell WT. Nelson syndrome: historical perspectives and current concepts. Neurosurg Focus. 2007;23(3):E12.
11. Juliani G, Avataneo T, Potenzoni F, Sorrentino T. CT and MR compared in the study of hypophysis. Radiol Med (Torino). 1989;77(1–2):51–64.
12. Johnson MR, Hoare RD, Cox T, et al. The evaluation of patients with a suspected pituitary microadenoma: computer tomography compared to magnetic resonance imaging. Clin Endocrinol (Oxf). 1992;36(4):335–8.
13. Vest-Courtalon C, Ravel A, Perez N, et al. Pituitary gland MRI and Cushing disease: report of 14 operated patients. J Radiol. 2000;81(7):781–6.
14. Bahurel-Barrera H, Assie G, Silvera S, Bertagna X, Coste J, Legmann P. Inter- and intra-observer variability in detection and progression assessment with MRI of microadenoma in Cushing's disease patients followed up after bilateral adrenalectomy. Pituitary. 2008;11(3):263–9.
15. Jornayvaz FR, Assie G, Bienvenu-Perrard M, Coste J, Guignat L, Bertherat J, Silvera S, Bertagna X, Legmann P. Pregnancy does not accelerate corticotroph tumor progression in Nelson's syndrome. J Clin Endocrinol Metab. 2011;96(4):E658–62. Epub 2011 Feb 2.
16. Pivonello R, De Martino MC, Cappabianca P, De Leo M, Faggiano A, Lombardi G, et al. The medical treatment of Cushing's disease: effectiveness of chronic treatment with the dopamine agonist cabergoline in patients unsuccessfully treated by surgery. J Clin Endocrinol Metab. 2009;94(1):223–30. Epub 2008 Oct 28.
17. Boscaro M, Ludlam WH, Atkinson B, Glusman JE, Petersenn S, Reincke M, et al. Treatment of pituitary-dependent Cushing's disease with the multireceptor ligand somatostatin analog pasireotide (SOM230): a multicenter, phase II trial. J Clin Endocrinol Metab. 2009;94(1):115–22. Epub 2008 Oct 28.
18. Heaney AP, Fernando M, Yong WH, Melmed S. Functional PPAR-gamma receptor is a novel therapeutic target for ACTH-secreting pituitary adenomas. Nat Med. 2002;8(11):1281–7. Epub 2002 Oct 15.
19. Paez-Pereda M, Kovalovsky D, Hopfner U, Theodoropoulou M, Pagotto U, Uhl E, et al. Retinoic acid prevents experimental Cushing syndrome. J Clin Invest. 2001;108(8):1123–31.

Chapter 18
Psychosocial Aspects of Cushing's Disease

Nicoletta Sonino

Abstract In recent years, there has been a conceptual shift from a merely biomedical approach in disease treatment to a psychosomatic consideration of the entire person and his/her quality of life; with the goal of more effective patient management. The term "psychosomatic" refers to the assumption that mind and body are inseparably linked, and that the person invariably functions and reacts as an integrated mind–body unit. The application of psychosomatic research tools is providing new insight in the setting of endocrine disorders, as it has in other fields of medicine. This chapter reviews the psychosocial aspects in Cushing's syndrome, characterized by an array of debilitating symptoms and clinical features, in which psychological manifestations play a prominent part, and which may persist despite correction of the underlying biochemical disorder.

Keywords Cushing's disease • Life events • Depression • Anxiety • Quality of life • Cognitive impairment

N. Sonino (✉)
Department of Statistical Sciences, University of Padova,
Via Battisti 241, 35121 Padova, Italy

Department of Mental Health, Padova City Hospital,
35100 Padova, Italy

Department of Psychiatry, State University of New York
at Buffalo, Buffalo, NY, USA
e-mail: nicoletta.sonino@unipd.it

Introduction

In recent years, there has been a conceptual shift from a merely biomedical approach in disease treatment to a psychosomatic consideration of the entire person and his/her quality of life; with the goal of more effective patient management. The term "psychosomatic" refers to the assumption that mind and body are inseparably linked, and that the person invariably functions and reacts as an integrated mind–body unit [1, 2]. The application of psychosomatic research tools is providing new insight in the setting of endocrine disorders, as it has in other fields of medicine [3]. As the issues of psychological well-being, functional capacity, and social and interpersonal components of medical illness are being developed in endocrinology, there is increasing understanding of the importance of psychosocial aspects in Cushing's syndrome, characterized by an array of debilitating symptoms and clinical features [4], in which psychological manifestations play a prominent part.

Pituitary-dependent Cushing's disease, the most common form of endogenous hypercortisolism, presents with distinctive features and extremely complex issues to assess and manage. In spite of ongoing progress in both diagnostic and therapeutic procedures, it remains a challenge for the clinician and burdensome for the patient [5–9]. Psychosocial aspects extend from the role of life stress as a potential pathogenic factor to the association with affective disorders and the presence of residual symptoms long after adequate treatment (Table 18.1).

Role of Life Events

A life event is defined as a discrete change in the subject's social or personal environment [10]. The event should represent a change as opposed to a persisting state, and should be externally verifiable rather than psychological. The use of standardized methods of life events assessment and of controlled and prospective research designs has suggested that recent life events may, in some cases, play a substantial role in exposing individual vulnerability to a particular physical or psychiatric illness [10]. The notion that meaningful events and situations in a person's life that elicit emotional distress may be followed by physical illness is an old clinical observation. Harvey Cushing himself postulated that "psychic traumas" may play an important role in the pathogenesis of pituitary disease [11]. Trethowan and Cobb [12] found "psychological stress" (such as divorce, loss of a child, etc.) to be a possible pathogenetic factor in some of their cases. Gifford and Gunderson [13] reported "emotional losses," usually involving separation or death in a close relationship, in eight of their selected ten patients. Cohen [14] found a "disturbing" life event in 6 of 29 consecutive patients. These psychosomatic papers, however, had considerable shortcomings, as they lacked structured methods of data collection and control groups. We decided to further study this issue, based on both the previous demonstration of a role for recent life events in nonendocrine major depression and the

Table 18.1 Psychosocial aspects during the course of Cushing's disease

Prodromal phase
Life events
Mood disorders

Active phase
Mood disorders
Cognitive disturbances
Impaired quality of life

Post-treatment phase
Residual symptoms
Mood disorders
Cognitive disturbances
Impaired quality of life

high prevalence of major depression in Cushing's syndrome. We investigated the occurrence of life events in the year before the first signs of disease onset in 66 patients with Cushing's syndrome [15], by means of Paykel's Interview for Recent Life Events [10]. This cohort was compared to a control group of 66 healthy subjects matched for sociodemographic variables. Patients with Cushing's syndrome reported significantly more losses, undesirable and uncontrolled events than controls. The results did not depend on the well-known relationship between life events and major depression, since there were no differences between patients with and without depression within the Cushing's syndrome group. Of great interest is that a subdivision between patients with pituitary-dependent (Cushing's disease) and pituitary-independent (primary adrenal hyperfunction or ectopic ACTH production) forms, compared with their matched controls, indicated a causal role for stressful life events exclusively in Cushing's disease [15]. The results in Cushing's disease are remarkably similar to those obtained by comparing depressed patients to the general population, and, in particular, to those of a study performed with the same methods in the same geographic area [16]. In view of the methods used (careful estimate of the onset of symptoms, rigorous event definition, delay of the interview until hormone abnormalities were corrected, blind rating of independence and objective negative impact), and within a multifactorial frame of reference, a causal relationship of stressful life events was suggested in Cushing's disease.

In the still controversial pathogenesis of this condition, data on life events would support the hypothesis of limbic–hypothalamic involvement. A disturbance of the regulatory mechanisms of the limbic structures and, particularly, of the hypothalamus (where changes in the balance of biogenic amines may affect hormone release) can trigger complex biochemical reactions. This would particularly apply to the cases of Cushing's disease where a pituitary tumor cannot be found [17, 18]. However, even in the case of a clonal pituitary tumor, implying a local genetic defect, serotonin may play a permissive role in the clonal expansion of a mutated pituitary cell [19]. Stress has been associated with activation of the hypothalamic–pituitary–adrenal (HPA) axis and CRH hypersecretion in a model that is more linked to acute than chronic situations. Chronic stress, however, particularly if associated with anxiety and irritability, may also result in enhanced 5HT2 receptor function and hence in overactivity of the HPA axis [20, 21], with possible consequences that depend on the preexisting conditions. Life events might be relevant in increasing individual vulnerability to both onset and relapse of Cushing's disease, as it seemed to be the case in some of the patients in our study population (unpublished observations).

Affective Disorders

Several psychiatric and psychological disturbances may be associated with Cushing's syndrome, regardless of tumor location [22, 23]. Depression is the most common psychiatric manifestation, occurring in more than half of the patients, as reported by studies that used a standardized assessment (Table 18.2). Haskett [24] obtained a longitudinal psychiatric history from 30 patients with Cushing's syndrome. He found that 24 (80%) met the criteria for a major depressive disorder (MDD); in about 80% of such cases depression reached melancholic proportions. Eight of the 24 patients had a bipolar affective disorder, i.e., history of mania or hypomania and depression [24]. Schizophrenic symptoms were not evident. Major psychiatric disturbances other than mood and anxiety disorders are infrequent in Cushing's syndrome and, if psychotic symptoms occur, they are likely to be a complication of mania or severe depression. Hudson et al. [25] also found a high lifetime incidence of mood disorder (56%) in 16 patients with Cushing's disease. The rate of familial mood disorder among these patients was significantly lower than that found among patients with major depression not associated with physical conditions. Loosen et al. [26], however, obtained similar rates of depression in family members of patients with Cushing's disease and nonendocrine major depression. They found a MDD to be present in 68% of their patients and to be frequently associated with an anxiety disorder, suggesting a syndrome of anxious depression to be characteristic of the illness. Sonino et al. [15] found major depression to occur in 62% of 66 patients with Cushing's syndrome. There were no significant differences in depression between patients with pituitary-dependent and pituitary-independent forms of the illness (see above), a finding later confirmed by an independent investigation [27]. Depression appeared in the prodromal phase in about a quarter of patients [26, 27]. In a study including an expanded sample of 162 patients with pituitary-dependent Cushing's disease [28], Sonino et al. found DSM-IV major depression in 88 (54%) of their 162 patients. In these patients, a subsequent analysis showed that major depression was significantly associated with older age, female sex, higher pretreatment urinary cortisol levels, relatively more severe clinical condition, and absence of pituitary adenoma [29]. Patients with Cushing's disease and depression appeared to suffer from a more severe form of illness, both in terms of cortisol production and clinical presentation, compared to those who were not depressed. Kelly [27] also examined a large sample of patients with Cushing's syndrome ($n=209$) and found depression to occur in 120 (57%) of them. In all these investigations that used diagnostic criteria such as the DSM, the similarities between

Table 18.2 Prevalence of major depressive disorder (MDD) in patients with Cushing's syndrome

Author	References	Patients	Patients with MDD (%)	Diagnosis
Haskett	[24]	30	24 (80%)	All forms
Hudson	[25]	16	9 (56%)	Cushing's disease
Loosen	[26]	20	13 (68%)	Cushing's disease
Dorn	[30]	33	17 (52%)[a]	All forms
Kelly	[27]	209	120 (57%)	All forms
Sonino	[28]	162	88 (54%)	Cushing's disease
		470	271 (58%)	

[a]Defined as "atypical depression"

depression occurring in the setting of Cushing's syndrome and depression not associated with endocrine disease were emphasized. At variance with these findings, Dorn et al. [30] reported a high prevalence of atypical depressive features in their sample of 33 patients with Cushing's syndrome (Table 18.2). The definition of atypical depression referred to the presence of increased appetite, fatigue, and excessive sleep, not associated with melancholic features. There could be, however, confusion between symptoms that may be present in Cushing's syndrome regardless of depression (such as increased appetite, weight, and fatigue) and specific manifestations of a mood disorder.

Bipolar disorder and manic and hypomanic episodes may also occur in Cushing's syndrome. They were reported in about 30% of patients of Haskett [24] and of Hudson et al. [25]. Subthreshold fluctuations of mood are, however, common in the course of illness. Manic and hypomanic symptoms were described among the early manifestations [24, 31]. Conversely, the onset of Cushing's disease superimposed on a long-standing seasonal bipolar disorder rendered the underlying psychiatric condition refractory to treatment until a pituitary tumor was removed [32].

It is difficult to establish whether anxiety disorders are a consequence of depression, since they are usually present in about half of patients with nonendocrine major depression [1, 2]. Loosen et al. [26] included anxiety disorders in their assessment and found that 70% of their patients with Cushing's disease met the criteria for generalized anxiety (a percentage higher than that of major depression) and 53% met the criteria for panic disorder. Symptoms of anxiety may persist independently after resolution of depression with remission [23, 31, 33].

While psychiatric symptoms may be obvious in some patients, the absence of psychopathology as defined by psychiatric diagnostic criteria cannot be equated with well-being. To assess subclinical symptoms (demoralization, irritable mood, somatization) that are subtle but pervasive manifestations of distress, we used the Diagnostic Criteria for Psychosomatic Research (DCPR) and their specific interview [3, 33]. We also employed the Psychosocial Index (PSI), a simple self-rated instrument designed to evaluate stress, psychological distress, abnormal illness behavior, and psychological well-being [3, 33]. In Cushing's disease, the PSI documented that conditions of stress and lack of well-being persisted over 9–36 months of follow-up with remission after treatment [33].

Cognitive Disturbances

Neuropsychological testing has indicated that about two thirds of patients suffering from Cushing's syndrome have varying degrees of diffuse bilateral cerebral dysfunction, with impairment in nonverbal, visual-ideational, visual-memory, and spatial-constructional abilities, and that there are several correlations between affective symptoms and cognitive impairment [23, 34–36]. Difficulties with concentration, reasoning ability, comprehension, and processing of new information have also been reported. Patients complain of forgetfulness (appointments made, names of people, location of objects, important dates in their personal or medical histories, and trouble with previously familiar tasks). Deficits in cognition have been shown in a controlled study in 19 patients (11 with pituitary-dependent Cushing's disease and 8 with ACTH-independent Cushing's syndrome; mean estimated duration of disease from symptom onset to diagnosis confirmation 42.7 ± 26.9 months, range 15–120 months) [37]. A general decline in most cognitive domains after chronic exposure to elevated glucocorticoid levels may be related to the wide distribution of glucocorticoid receptors throughout the cerebral cortex, in addition to the hippocampus. Hook et al. [38] examined cognitive function in 27 patients with Cushing's disease at baseline and at 3 follow-up periods up to 18 months after successful surgery and found that younger patients improved more quickly than older participants. Neurocognitive effects of hypercortisolism, however, may not be fully reversible [35, 38–41]. Cognitive dysfunctions usually occur together with loss of brain volume and other related abnormalities, including decreased volume of the hippocampus and amygdala and enlargement of the third ventricle [35, 38–40] on imaging studies (CT and MRI). Brain abnormalities were also found in children and adolescents [42, 43] in whom a significant decline in cognitive function was recorded 1 year after correction of hypercortisolism, in spite of a rapid reversibility of cerebral atrophy by imaging [42].

Quality of Life

The domain of quality of life includes functional capacity (the ability to perform activities of daily life, social adjustment, intellectual and psychological functions, and economic status), perceptions (levels of well-being and satisfaction with life), and impact of disease symptoms (with resultant impairment) [1–3]. There are many questionnaires available to assess quality of life [1]. A disease-specific questionnaire has been recently proposed to evaluate health-related quality of life in Cushing's syndrome [44]. Depressive mood and cognitive impairments, adding to other disabling symptoms, may markedly influence how the pathological process is experienced [22, 23]. The impact of depression on quality of life, particularly as to well-being and social functioning, is indeed remarkable, as it is repeatedly emphasized in patients' accounts [45, 46] and in the newsletters of patients' associations (e.g., the Cushing's Support and Research Foundation and the Pituitary Network Association in the USA).

Although progressive improvement of psychological distress and cognitive deficits is usually observed after successful control of hypercortisolism, a considerable degree of symptomatology may persist [22, 23]. While most patients experience dramatic recovery in the year after remission, psychiatric symptoms may not resolve in some patients even with proper endocrine treatment [22, 23, 31, 33, 47, 48]. Using specific criteria for psychiatric improvement [47], it was found that about 70% of patients fully recovered from their depression after successful treatment of Cushing's syndrome, while others remained the same or even worsened. Dorn et al. [31] observed a slight increase in the frequency of suicidal ideation and panic after correction of hypercortisolism.

The quality of life in Cushing's syndrome is generally impaired even over the long term, with little difference among etiologies and type of treatment [31, 33, 44, 47–54]. In the study of van Aken et al. [52], with a mean duration of remission of 13.4 ± 6.7 years, the general perceived well-being of patients with Cushing's disease was significantly reduced compared to controls, especially in the presence of hypopituitarism. Heald et al. [53] found that patients treated for Cushing's disease perceived themselves as being more depressed, anxious, fatigued, and with poorer physical health, environmental and social adjustment, than patients with other pituitary tumors. Similar results were obtained recently by Santos et al. [49]. In a population of 40 children and adolescents with Cushing's syndrome, 34 of whom had Cushing's disease, quality of life was impaired 1 year after cure and younger children scored worse in cognitive function [55].

Since personality traits may increase neuroendocrine vulnerability to stressful life situations and mood changes and may influence quality of life, controlled investigations have been carried out in Cushing's syndrome [56]. There were no significant differences in personality variables between patients and controls, and therefore did not seem to play a role in the quality of life of patients with Cushing's syndrome. Personality characteristics might be expected to be more relevant in the hypothalamic–pituitary forms. However, separate analyses on Cushing's disease patients compared to their matched controls did not yield statistical significance in this preliminary study [56]. Based on the scant data available, no conclusion can be drawn at present.

Treatment

Treatment primarily directed to the underlying physical condition is usually more effective than psychotropic drugs in organic affective syndromes associated with endocrine disease. Depression may improve in Cushing's syndrome upon achievement of normal cortisol levels [22, 23, 31, 47, 48, 51–54]. In the study by Dorn et al. [31], in which 67% of patients with Cushing's syndrome had significant psychopathology before cure, overall psychiatric symptoms decreased to 54% at 3 months, 36% at

6 months, and 24% at 12 months. There was a parallel recovery of the HPA axis and an inverse correlation between psychological improvement and baseline morning cortisol [31]. Endocrinologists may thus tend to overestimate the reversibility of psychiatric symptoms by adequate specific treatment. However, for some patients correction of hypercortisolism alone is not sufficient to treat depression and, in addition to normalization of cortisol levels, antidepressant agents are required. In our experience [47], a few individual patients actually deteriorated, and in those cases appropriate psychiatric intervention was valuable. Interestingly, one of them responded to an antidepressant drug that had been ineffective when she was hypercortisolemic. Treatment may encompass both psychotropic agents (use of antidepressant drugs such as tricyclic agents and selective serotonin uptake inhibitors) and psychotherapeutic strategies (particularly cognitive behavioral therapies used in affective disorders). In case of marked anxiety, benzodiazepines may also be beneficial. Adding to psychological and cognitive impairments (as outlined above), long-standing hypercortisolism may be associated with underlying organic pathological processes [57, 58]. Nonetheless, when surgery is performed, i.e., pituitary surgery in Cushing's disease [6–9, 28, 33, 38, 49, 52, 53, 59, 60], the patient is likely to have expectations of a quick recovery to his/her former condition. Unrealistic hopes of "cure" may foster discouragement and apathy.

The subset of patients with persistent psychiatric issues or impaired quality of life despite biochemical remission may need new types of clinical intervention. We have recently conceptualized this as rehabilitation of endocrine patients [61, 62], envisioning above all the demanding connotations of Cushing's disease. Rehabilitation units, with contributions from physical therapy and psychological care, might be suitable to address the multifaceted problems that these patients manifest, particularly in the post-treatment phase. Additional factors that may impair the quality of life and the speed of recovery involve maintenance medication and hormone replacement requirements, addressing any intervening pituitary hormone deficiency [59, 63, 64]. In particular, a recent publication highlights the need for evaluation and treatment of GH deficiency in adults with controlled Cushing's disease [65]. Treatment should be carefully individualized.

Clinical Implications

Addressing the psychosocial aspects of Cushing's disease will greatly support the patient and his/her family in the "fight against the psychic incapacitations of the malady," as Harvey Cushing said [11]. Mood disorders were present in about 58% of our large population of patients with Cushing's syndrome [66], and were among the eight main features we incorporated into a clinical index [67] for assessing the response to treatment. Mood disorders were present in 70% of cases in a subsequent survey of the literature [68], and in 55% of cases reported from a single center [69]. The presence of depression was associated with the severity of the clinical presentation and is of prognostic value [28]. Treatment with common antidepressant drugs seldom results in clinical improvement while the patient is hypercortisolemic.

If definitive treatment for the disease is delayed, temporary therapy with inhibitors of steroid production should be provided [70]. These pharmacological tools are generally successful in improving both psychological and physical symptoms. Of great research interest are the findings that, in nonendocrine major depression, normalization of the HPA axis is required for a favorable outcome, and inhibitors of steroid production were beneficial in cases refractory to antidepressant treatment alone [23]. The similarities between the psychological aspects of Cushing's disease and nonendocrine major depression, therefore, start with the potential pathogenetic role of recent life events and continue with the response to pharmacological manipulation and remission/recurrence [22, 23, 29].

Long after successful treatment, when the patient is apparently doing well from an endocrine viewpoint, the quality of life may still be seriously compromised from residual psychological and neurocognitive deficits, as well as persistent physical effects [22, 23, 38–41, 44, 45, 50–53, 56, 57]. Other factors that may influence the speed of recovery include the type and dosage of hormone replacement and the patient's behavior and attitude toward his/her illness. Since psychological impairment often persists in the remission phase, patients may be less likely to resume their usual activities. However, the avoidance of situations that induce undue anxiety may lead to its continuation. Specialized help should be provided when psychological symptoms persist or increase in the few months after surgery. In case of residual depression after hypercortisolism is corrected, the use of antidepressant drugs may be highly successful.

On the basis of these clinical research findings, psychiatric/psychological care has been proposed as part of a new interdisciplinary approach in clinical medicine [1, 2, 71, 72], and in the field of endocrinology in particular [3, 61, 62, 73]. It is mandatory in the management of Cushing's disease.

Conclusions

Despite ongoing progress in diagnosis and treatment modalities, Cushing's disease still represents a challenge for both treating physician and patient. Psychosocial aspects are of paramount importance throughout all illness phases and should not be overlooked. They include the possible pathogenetic role of life stress, in the form of recent life events, and the occurrence of psychiatric/psychological symptoms, which may be prodromal or persist in the post-treatment and remission phases. As a result of long-standing hypercortisolism, there are cognitive deficits that may be very slowly (and only partially) reversible. They contribute to the impairment of quality of life that negatively impacts both the patient and his/her environment. Addressing psychosocial issues may alleviate the burden of the disease and improve the quality of management, in which replacement of pituitary hormone deficiency on an individualized basis is important. An effective approach should be interdisciplinary with rehabilitation measures, including psychological interventions and the judicious use of psychotropic agents.

References

1. Fava GA, Sonino N. Psychosomatic medicine. Int J Clin Pract. 2010;64:1155–61.
2. Fava GA, Sonino N. Psychosomatic assessment. Psychother Psychosom. 2009;78:333–41.
3. Sonino N, Tomba E, Fava GA. Psychosocial approach to endocrine disease. In: Porcelli P, Sonino N, editors. Psychosocial factors affecting medical conditions: a new classification for DSM-V, Advances in Psychosomatic Medicine, vol. 28. Basel: Karger; 2007. p. 21–33.
4. Nieman LK, Biller BMK, Findling JW. The diagnosis of Cushing's syndrome: an endocrine society clinical practice guideline. J Clin Endocrinol Metab. 2008;93:1526–40.
5. Pecori Giraldi F. Recent challenges in the diagnosis of Cushing's syndrome. Horm Res. 2009;71(Supp 1):123–7.
6. Mullan KR, Atkinson B. Endocrine clinical update: where are we in the therapeutic management of pituitary-dependent hypercortisolism? Clin Endocrinol. 2008;68:327–37.
7. Aghi MK. Management of recurrent and refractory Cushing's disease. Nat Clin Pract Endocrinol Metab. 2008;4:560–8.
8. Boscaro M, Ludlam WH, Atkinson B, et al. Treatment of pituitary-dependent Cushing's disease with the multireceptor ligand somatostatin analog pasireotide (SOM230): a multicenter, phase II trial. J Clin Endocrinol Metab. 2009;94:115–22.
9. Wagenmakers MAEM, Netea-Maier RT, van Lindert EJ, et al. Repeated transsfenoidal pituitary surgery (TS) via the endoscopic technique: a good therapeutic option for recurrent or persistent Cushing's disease (CD). Clin Endocrinol. 2009;70:274–80.
10. Paykel ES. The interview for recent life events. Psychol Med. 1997;27:301–10.
11. Cushing H. Psychic disturbances associated with disorders of the ductless glands. Am J Insanity. 1913;69:965–90.
12. Trethowan WH, Cobb S. Neuropsychiatric aspects of Cushing's syndrome. AMA Arch Neurol Psychiat. 1952;67:283–309.
13. Gifford S, Gunderson JG. Cushing's disease as a psychosomatic disorder. Medicine. 1970;49:397–409.
14. Cohen SI. Cushing's syndrome. A psychiatric study of 29 patients. Br J Psychiatry. 1980;136:120–4.
15. Sonino N, Fava GA, Boscaro M. A role for life events in the pathogenesis of Cushing's disease. Clin Endocrinol. 1993;38:261–4.
16. Fava GA, Munari F, Pavan L, et al. Life events and depression. J Affect Disord. 1981;3:159–65.
17. Krystallenia IA, Kaltsas GA, Isidori AM, et al. The prevalence and characteristic features of cyclicity and variability in Cushing's disease. Eur J Endocrinol. 2009;160:1011–8.
18. Boscaro M, Rampazzo A, Paoletta A, et al. Patterns of ACTH response to oCRH in Cushing's disease: correlation with histological/immunocytochemical findings. Neuroendocrinology. 1994;60:237–42.
19. Dahia PLM, Grossman AB. The molecular pathogenesis of corticotroph tumors. Endocr Rev. 1999;20:136–55.
20. Chrousos GP. Stress and disorders of the stress system. Nat Rev Endocrinol. 2009;5:374–81.
21. McEwen BS. Central effects of stress hormones in health and disease: understanding the protective and damaging effects of stress and stress mediators. Eur J Pharmacol. 2008;583:174–85.
22. Sonino N, Fava GA. Psychosomatic aspects of Cushing's disease. Psychother Psychosom. 1998;67:140–6.
23. Sonino N, Fava GA. Psychiatric disorders associated with Cushing's syndrome. CNS Drugs. 2001;15:361–73.
24. Haskett RF. Diagnostic categorization of psychiatric disturbance in Cushing's syndrome. Am J Psychiatry. 1985;142:911–6.
25. Hudson JI, Hudson MS, Griffing GT, et al. Phenomenology and family history of affective disorder in Cushing's disease. Am J Psychiatry. 1987;144:951–3.

26. Loosen PT, Chambliss B, de Bold CR, et al. Psychiatric phenomenology in Cushing's disease. Pharmacopsychiatry. 1992;25:192–8.
27. Kelly WF. Psychiatric aspects of Cushing's syndrome. Q J Med. 1996;89:543–51.
28. Sonino N, Zielezny M, Fava GA, et al. Risk factors and long-term outcome in pituitary-dependent Cushing's disease. J Clin Endocrinol Metab. 1996;81:2647–52.
29. Sonino N, Fava GA, Raffi AR, et al. Clinical correlates of major depression in Cushing's disease. Psychopathology. 1998;31:302–6.
30. Dorn LD, Burgess ES, Dubbert B, et al. Psychopathology in patients with endogenous Cushing's syndrome: atypical or melancholic features. Clin Endocrinol. 1995;43:433–42.
31. Dorn LD, Burgess ES, Friedman TC, et al. The longitudinal course of psychopathology in Cushing's syndrome after correction of hypercortisolism. J Clin Endocrinol Metab. 1997;82:912–9.
32. Ghadirian AM, Marcovitz S, Pearson Murphy BE. A case of seasonal bipolar disorder exacerbated by Cushing's disease. Compr Psychiatry. 2005;46:155–8.
33. Sonino N, Ruini C, Navarrini C, et al. Psychosocial impairment in patients treated for pituitary disease: a controlled study. Clin Endocrinol. 2007;67:719–26.
34. Starkman MN, Giordani B, Berent S, et al. Elevated cortisol levels in Cushing's disease are associated with cognitive decrements. Psychosom Med. 2001;63:985–93.
35. Sherwood Brown E, Rush AJ, McEwen BS. Hippocampal remodeling and damage by corticosteroids: implications for mood disorders. Neuropsychopharmacology. 1999;21:474–84.
36. Tooze A, Gittoes NJ, Jones CA, et al. Neurocognitive consequences of surgery and radiotherapy for tumours of the pituitary. Clin Endocrinol. 2009;70:503–11.
37. Forget H, Lacroix A, Somma M, et al. Cognitive decline in patients with Cushing's syndrome. J Int Neuropsychol Soc. 2000;6:20–9.
38. Hook JN, Giordani B, Schteingart DE, et al. Patterns of cognitive change over time and relationship to age following successful treatment of Cushing's disease. J Int Neuropsychol Soc. 2007;13:21–9.
39. Forget H, Lacroix A, Cohen H. Persistent cognitive impairment following surgical treatment of Cushing's syndrome. Psychoneuroendocrinology. 2002;27:367–83.
40. Bourdeau I, Bard C, Forget H, et al. Cognitive function and cerebral assessment in patients who have Cushing's syndrome. Endocrinol Metab Clin N Am. 2005;34:357–69.
41. Dorn LD, Cerrone P. Cognitive function in patients with Cushing's syndrome. A longitudinal perspective. Clin Nurs Res. 2000;9:420–40.
42. Merke DP, Giedd JN, Keil MF, et al. Children experience cognitive decline despite reversal of brain atrophy one year after resolution of Cushing's syndrome. J Clin Endocrinol Metab. 2005;90:2531–6.
43. Mahen FS, Mazzone L, Merke DP, et al. Altered amygdala and hippocampus function in adolescents with hypercortisolemia: A functional magnetic resonance imaging study of Cushing's syndrome. Dev Psychopathol. 2008;20:1177–89.
44. Webb SM, Badia X, Barahona MJ, et al. Evaluation of health-related quality of life in patients with Cushing's syndrome with a new questionnaire. Eur J Endocrinol. 2008;158: 623–30.
45. Armstrong A, Fachnie JD. The phenomenology of Cushing's syndrome: one patient account. Henry Ford Hosp Med J. 1991;39:8–9.
46. Gotch PM. Cushing's syndrome from the patient perspective. Endocrinol Metab Clin N Am. 1994;23:607–17.
47. Sonino N, Fava GA, Belluardo P, et al. Course of depression in Cushing's syndrome: response to treatment and comparison with Graves' disease. Horm Res. 1993;39:202–6.
48. Kelly WF, Kelly MJ, Faragher B. A prospective study of psychiatric and psychological aspects of Cushing's syndrome. Clin Endocrinol. 1996;45:715–20.
49. Santos A, Resmini E, Martinez MA, et al. Quality of life in patients with pituitary tumors. Curr Opin Endocrinol Diabetes Obes. 2009;16:299–303.
50. Smith PW, Turza KC, Carter CO, et al. Bilateral adrenalectomy for refractory Cushing's disease: a safe and definitive therapy. J Am Coll Surg. 2009;208:1059–64.

51. Lindsay JR, Nansel T, Baid S, et al. Long term impaired quality of life in Cushing's syndrome despite initial improvement after surgical remission. J Clin Endocrinol Metab. 2006;91:447–53.
52. van Aken MO, Pereira AM, Biermasz NR, et al. Quality of life in patients after long-term biochemical cure of Cushing's disease. J Clin Endocrinol Metab. 2005;90:3279–86.
53. Heald AH, Ghosh S, Bray S, et al. Long-term negative impact on quality of life in patients with successfully treated Cushing's disease. Clin Endocrinol. 2004;61:458–65.
54. Pikkarainen L, Sane T, Reunanen A. The survival and well-being of patients treated for Cushing's syndrome. J Int Med. 1999;245:463–8.
55. Keil MF, Merke DP, Gandhi R, et al. Quality of life in children and adolescents 1-year after cure of Cushing's syndrome: a prospective study. Clin Endocrinol. 2009;71:326–33.
56. Sonino N, Bonnini S, Fallo F, et al. Personality characteristics and quality of life in patients treated for Cushing's syndrome. Clin Endocrinol. 2006;64:314–8.
57. Barahona MJ, Sucunza N, Resmini E, et al. Persistent body fat mass and inflammatory marker increases after long-term cure of Cushing's syndrome. J Clin Endocrinol Metabol. 2009;94:3365–71.
58. Pivonello R, De Martino MC, De Leo M, et al. Cushing's syndrome: aftermath of the cure. Arq Bras Endocrinol Metab. 2007;51:1381–91.
59. Biller BMK, Grossman AB, Stewart PM, et al. Treatment of adrenocorticotropin-dependent Cushing's syndrome: a consensus statement. J Clin Endocrinol Metab. 2008;53:2454–62.
60. Prevedello DM, Pouratian N, Sherman J, et al. Management of Cushing's disease: outcome in patients with microadenoma detected on pituitary magnetic imaging. J Neurosurg. 2008;109:751–9.
61. Sonino N, Fava GA. Rehabilitation in endocrine patients: a novel psychosomatic approach. Psychother Psychosom. 2007;76:319–24.
62. Sonino N. The need for rehabilitation teams in endocrinology. Expert Rev Endocrinol Metab. 2008;3:291–3.
63. Danilovicz K, Bruno OD, Manavela M, et al. Correction of cortisol overreplacement ameliorates morbidity in patients with hypopituitarism: a pilot study. Pituitary. 2008;11:279–85.
64. Johannsson G, Stibrant Sunnerhagen K, Svensson J. Baseline characteristics and the effects of two years of growth hormone replacement therapy in adults with growth hormone deficiency previously treated for Cushing's disease. Clin Endocrinol. 2004;60:550–9.
65. Hoyby C, Ragnarsson O, Jonsson PJ, et al. Clinical features of GH deficiency and effects of GH replacement in adults with controlled Cushing's disease. Eur J Endocrinol. 2010;162:677–84.
66. Boscaro M, Barzon L, Fallo F, et al. Cushing's syndrome. Lancet. 2001;357:783–91.
67. Sonino N, Boscaro M, Fallo F, et al. A clinical index for rating severity in Cushing's syndrome. Psychother Psychosom. 2000;69:216–20.
68. Newell-Price J, Bertagna X, Grossman AB, et al. Cushing's syndrome. Lancet. 2006;367:1605–17.
69. Boscaro M, Arnaldi G. Approach to the patient with possible Cushing's syndrome. J Clin Endocrinol Metab. 2009;94:3121–31.
70. Sonino N, Boscaro M. Medical therapy for Cushing's disease. Endocrinol Metab Clin N Am. 1999;28:211–22.
71. Porcelli P, Sonino N. Psychological factor affecting medical conditions: a new classification for DSM-V. Basel: Karger; 2007.
72. Fava GA, Sonino N. The biopsychosocial model thirty years later. Psychother Psychosom. 2008;77:1–2.
73. Sonino N, Peruzzi P. A psychoneuroendocrinology service. Psychother Psychosom. 2009;78:346–51.

Index

A
ACTH. *See* Adrenocorticotropic hormone; Adrenocorticotropin
Adiposogenital syndrome, 9
Adrenocorticotropic hormone (ACTH), 121
  CRH, 86
  Cushing's syndrome algorithm, 100–101
  dependent Cushing's syndrome
    biochemical testing, 90–91
    clinical features, 89–90
    corticotroph adenomas, 91
    IPS (*see* Inferior petrosal sinus)
    pituitary microsurgery, 89
    secreting pituitary adenomas, 91
  dependent *vs.* independent Cushing's syndrome
    contralateral adrenal gland, 89
    CRH simulation test, 87–88
    nodular adrenal disease, 89
    plasma, 87
  ectopic ACTH syndrome, 95–96
  etiologic considerations, 86–87
  independent Cushing's syndrome
    adrenocortical carcinoma, 98
    exogenous, 96–97
    macronodular adrenal hyperplasia, 98
    McCune–Albright syndrome, 99
    PPNAD, 98–99
    solitary adrenal adenomas, 97–98
    subclinical Cushing's syndrome, 99–100
  pathologic endogenous hypercortisolism, 86
Adrenocorticotropin
  H&E, 33
  hypothalamic–pituitary–endocrine axis, 33
  immunohistochemistry, 34
  intraoperative consultation, 40–41
  PAS, 34
  POMC, 34
  producing pituitary carcinomas, 39
  producing pituitary tumors
    ACTH hypersecretion, 35
    ACTH immunoreactivity, 35, 36
    corticotroph cells, 34
    Crooke's cell adenomas, 35
    glucocorticoid syndrome, 34
    LH, 35
    Nelson's syndrome, 35
    producing adenomas, 34
    prognosis and predictive factors, 39–40
    RER, 35
    silent ACTH-producing adenomas, 38

B
11β-hydroxysteroid dehydrogenase (11β-HSD), 63
Bilateral adrenalectomy, 191–192
Bilateral inferior petrosal sinus sampling (BIPSS), 73
Biomedical research, 15

C
Carney complex (CNC), 12
Cerebrospinal fluid rhinorrhea, 133
Computed tomography (CT)
  coronal precontrast, 110
  microadenomas, 110
  multidetector CT (MDCT) technology, 110
  paranasal sinus mucosal inflammatory changes, 108, 109
  pituitary microadenomas, 108

Computed tomography (CT) *(cont.)*
  protocols, 108, 109
  vascular structure and sellar contents, 108
Corticotroph adenomas, 27–28
Corticotroph tumor progression (CTP)
  assessment
    early detection, 240–241
    inevitable, 240
    prediction, 241–242
    pregnancy acceleration, 242
  Cushing's disease, 237
    bilateral adrenalectomy role, 243–244
    medical treatment, 244
  description, 237
  historical perspective
    ACTH plasma levels, 238
    diagnostic criteria, 238–239
    diagnostic techniques, 239–240
    Nelson's syndrome, definition, 238–239
  pituitary surgery, 238
  prevention/treatment, 242–243
Corticotropin-releasing hormone (CRH), 86
Crooke's cell adenomas, 35
Cushing, Harvey
  ACTH, 9
  adiposogenital dystrophy, 6
  adiposogenital syndrome, 9
  adrenal glands, 4
  adrenal lesions, 9
  Frohlich's syndrome, 7
  Galenic concept, 5
  glandulae renibus incumbentes, 4–5
  hyperadrenalism, 9
  hypercortisolism, 7, 8
  intracranial pressure symptoms, 8
  neurosurgeon, 6–7
  pituitary gland, 5–6
  polyglandular syndrome, 7, 9
Cushing's disease
  biochemical screening tests
    corticotrope cells, 53
    dehydroepiandrosterone, 53–54
    dexamethasone suppression test (DST), 51–52
    diagnosis, guideline, 48, 49
    IPSS, 54
    salivary cortisol assays, 50–51
    second line tests, 52–53
    urine cortisol excretion, 49–50
  biochemical testing, 47–48
  clinical entity
    clinical observation and comparison, 3
    Fuller Albright and hyperadrenocorticism, 9–11

  Harvey Cushing (*see* Cushing, Harvey)
  hypercortisolism, 4
  clinical epidemiology and healthcare delivery, 12–14
  clinical features, 46–47
  cortisol adrenal production, 46
  endocrinology, 2
  glucocorticoid, 46
  hormone characterization, 2
  history, 2
  NIH roadmap, 3
  pathophysiology and clinical features, 11–12
  radioimmunoassay, 3
Cyclic Cushing's disease
  biochemical indices, 71
  BIPSS, 73
  clinical/biochemical disease activity, 80
  clinical features and laboratory findings, 75–76
  definition and prevalence, 72–73
  diagnostic approach
    cortisol and synthetic glucocorticoids, 79
    cyclic hypercortisolism, 77, 78
    endogenous hypercortisolism, 78
    exogenous glucocorticoid, 79
    factitious hypercortisolism, 79
    pseudo-Cushing's, 77–78
  glucocorticoid hormonogenesis, 72
  hypercortisolism, 73, 74
  low-dose dexamethasone, 79
  medical therapy, 80
  pathophysiology, 76–77
  pituitary microsurgery, 79
  salivary cortisol profile, 73, 74
  transsphenoidal exploration, 73
  transsphenoidal surgery, 80
  weight gain, 73

D
Direct endonasal approach, 123–124
Drugs, FDA classification, 232

E
Ectopic ACTH syndrome, 11
Endocrine neoplasms, 39
Endoscopic approach, 124–125
Epidermal growth factor (EGF), 27
External beam radiation therapy (EBRT), 152–153

Index

F
^{18}Fluoro-deoxy-glucose (^{18}FDG), 116
Fractionated stereotactic radiotherapy (FSRT), 155
Frohlich's syndrome, 7
Fuller Albright and hyperadrenocorticism, 9–11

G
Galenic concept, 5
Gamma knife (GK), 153–154
Glucocorticoid receptor (GR), 26
    abnormalities, 63
    antagonists, 176–177

H
Hematoxylin and eosin (H&E), 33
Hyperadrenalism, 9
Hypercortisolism, 7, 8
Hypothalamic–pituitary–adrenal (HPA) axis, 59, 223

I
Inferior petrosal sinus (IPS)
    anomalous venous drainage, 92
    anterior pituitary hormone, 92
    cavernous sinus sampling, 94–95
    desmopressin uses, 93
    dexamethasone/peripheral CRH testing, 94
    normocortisolemia, 93
Inferior petrosal sinus sampling (IPSS), 54, 230
Insulin tolerance test (ITT), 66–67
Intraoperative ultrasound (IOUS), 108

L
Laparoscopic adrenalectomy (LA), 14
Luteinizing hormones (LH), 35

M
Magnetic resonance imaging (MRI)
    ACTH-producing pituitary tumors, 115
    contrast-enhanced 3 T, 113
    intrasellar and suprasellar pathology, 110
    microadenomas, 111, 113–114
    pituitary carcinomas secrete ACTH, 115
    pituitary gland, 111, 112
    pituitary hyperplasia, 115
    protocol, 111
    sellar and parasellar structures, 110–111
Major depressive disorder (MDD), 250

McCune–Albright syndrome, 99
Medical management
    adrenal-directed therapy
        antiseizure medication, aminoglutethimide, 171
        ketoconazole, 170–171
        metyrapone, 169–170
        mitotane, 171
        non-opioid anesthetic etomidate, 171–172
    current approaches, 168–169
    drug therapy, efficacy and safety, 168
    glucocorticoid receptor antagonists, 176–177
    morbidity and mortality, 167
    pituitary-directed therapy
        cabergoline, 173
        dopamine agonists, 172–173
        octreotide, efficacy and treatment, 174–175
        pasireotide, 175–176
        PPARγ, 172
        quinagolide, 173
        somatostatin, preferential affinitie, 175
        somatostatin receptor, 173–174
        sst2 glucocorticoids downregulation, 174
        treatment, 175
        UFC normalization, 176
        urinary glucocorticoid assessment, 173
Metabolic syndrome, 62
Methionine, 116
Molecular biology
    hormonal and growth factor signals, 21
    molecular pathogenesis (*see* Molecular pathogenesis)
    pituitary corticotroph adenomas, 20
    pituitary POMC-cell tumors, 22–23
    spontaneous disorders mimicking, 23
    transgenic mice models, 21
    transgenic oncogene overexpression, 20–21
Molecular pathogenesis
    corticotroph tumor, 23–24
    endocrinopathies, 23
    microRNA expression, 27–28
    neuroendocrine hormones and regulatory factors
        corticotroph adenoma cells, 25
        corticotroph hyperplasia and hypercortisolism, 25
        corticotroph proliferation and ACTH secretion, 25
        CRH, 25
        EGF, 27
        GR, 26

Molecular pathogenesis *(cont.)*
    melanocortin 2 receptor, 26
    pituitary Nelson's tumors, 26–27
    POMC, 26
    tumor suppressor gene and cell cycle
        regulators, 24–25

N
Nelson's syndrome, 35. *See also* Corticotroph
    tumor progression (CTP)

P
Pediatric Cushing's disease
    children, diagnosis and treatment, 198
    classification, 198
    clinical features
        growth and auxological
            parameters, 200–201
        pubertal development, 201–202
        salient feature, 200
    epidemiology, 198–200
    investigation
        BIPSS for ACTH, 204–205
        confirmation, 203–204
        imaging studies, 204
        obese children, 202
        syndrome, confirmation/exclusion,
            202–203
    symptoms and signs, 197
    treatment
        childhood, 205
        metyrapone/ketoconazole, 206
        options, 205
        pituitary radiotherapy, 206
        postcure growth and development,
            207–208
        transsphenoidal surgery, 206
Periodic acid Schiff (PAS), 34
Peroxisome proliferator-activated receptor≈
    (PPAR≈), 172
Pharmacological therapy, 218–219
Pituitary radiotherapy, 206
Polycystic ovary syndrome (PCOS), 62
Polyglandular syndrome, 7, 9
Positron emission tomography, 10
Postoperative management
        and assessment
    classical postoperative management, 147
    continued glucocorticoid replacement,
        148–149
    cortisol production, 144
    ideal situation, 147–148

influencing factor
    pituitary tissue amount, 145
    postoperative steroid replacement,
        144–145
    preoperative adenoma sixe, 144
pituitary adenoma, 143
remission, Cushing's disease
    ACTH cells, 146
    biochemical criteria, 145
    HPA function, 145–146
    UFC concentration, 146–147
symptoms, 144
Pregnancy
    diagnostic strategies
        CRH stimulation testing, 230
        differential diagnosis test, 228–229
        high-dose dexamethasone suppression
            testing, 229
        imaging, 230
        IPSS, 230
        screening and diagnosis, 227–228
    normal HPA axis
        clinical presentation, 225–226
        CRH concentrations, 224
        etiology, 226–227
        fetal morbidity and mortality, 226
        hypothalamic–pituitary
            responsiveness, 225
        maternal morbidity and mortality, 226
        placental clock, 224
        plasma ACTH concentration, 224
        plasma concentration, 225
    therapeutic options, 231
Primary pigmented nodular adrenocortical
        disease (PPNAD), 12, 98–99
Pro-opiomelanocortin (POMC), 34
Proton therapy, 155–156
Pseudo-Cushing's syndrome (PCS)
    alcohol intake, 63
    chronic diseases, 61
    cortisol production, 58
    depression, 60
    drug induced, 62–63
    emotional stress, 60
    endocrine testing, 58
    factitious glucocorticoid administration, 62
    glucocorticoid receptor abnormalities, 64
    growth hormone deficiency, 62
    HPA, 59
    hypercortisolism, 58–29
    laboratory confirmation and test
        confirm hypercortisolism, 64
        desmopressin test, 66
        dexamethasone-CRH test, 65–66

diagnostic accuracy, 67
ITT, 67
low-dose dexamethasone suppression tests, 65
midnight serum/salivary cortisol, 65
morning serum total and free cortisol levels, 64–65
nutrition (morbid obesity, anorexia), 61–62
peripheral cortisol metabolism, 63
physical stresses (aerobic exercise), 59–60
psychiatric disorders and alcoholism, 59
severe illnesses, 60–61
treatment, 67
Psychosocial aspects
affective disorders
anxiety disorders, 251
anxious depression, 250
manic and hypomanic episodes, 251
MDD patients, 250, 251
mood disorder, 250
psychiatric and psychological disturbances, 250
psychopathology, 251
clinical implications, 254–255
cognitive disturbances, 252
Cushing's disease, 249
life event
chronics stress, 249–250
Cushing's disease, 249
definition, 248
emotional losses, 248
pathogenesis, 249
psychic traumas, 248
quality of life, 252–253
treatment, 253–254

R
Radiation therapy
dose, 157
fractionated EBRT vs. SRS
CTH-producing adenomas, 156–157
FSRT, 155
interstitial brachytherapy, 156
proton therapy, 155–156
gamma knife, 153–154
late effects, after
cerebrovascular accidents, 163
hypopituitarism, 162
radionecrosis, 163
secondary tumors, 163
visual deficits, 162
latency period, 161
linear accelerator-based stereotactic radiosurgery, 154
pituitary irradiation, 151–152
remission after
fractionated EBRT, 160
heavy-charged particles, 160–161
series, 157–159
stereotactic radiosurgery, 160
schedules and technology
EBRT, 152–153
stereotactic radiosurgery, 153
Radiologic imaging techniques
IOUS, 108
pituitary imaging
CT (*see* Computed tomography)
MRI (*see* Magnetic resonance imaging)
positron emission tomography, 10
ultrasound, 9–10
Radionecrosis, 163
Radiotherapy, 189–190, 217
Recurrent Cushing's disease
adjuvant therapies
bilateral adrenalectomy, 191–192
medical treatment, 190
radiotherapy, 189–190
definition, 184
patients surveillance, 184
transsphenoidal surgical treatment
adenoma resection, 185
cavernous sinus, 186
conventional microscope technique, 185
CTH-secreting adenomas, 188
diagnosis, 186
Dickerman and Oldfield's series, 187
extracapsular dissection, 187
hemihypophysectomy, 188
Hofmann's series, 187
MRI, 185
Nakane's series, 187
persistent, after failed, 186
pituitary adenomas, surgical management, 187–188
postoperative CSF, 188–189
reoperation, 188
safe and effective access, 187
soft tissue, adhesions, 186
Remission, Cushing's disease
ACTH cells, 146
biochemical criteria, 145
HPA function, 145–146
UFC concentration, 146–147
Rough endoplasmic reticulum (RER), 35

S

Salivary cortisol assays, 50–51
Silent corticotroph adenomas (SCAs)
    classification, 212
    clinical features
        haemorrhage, 215
        headaches, 215
        patients clinical characteristics, 214, 215
        secondary hypogonadism and hypothyroidism, 215
        visual deficit, 215
    nonfunctioning pituitary tumors, 211–212
    nonsurgical management
        pharmacological therapy, 218–219
        radiotherapy, 217
    post-operative recurrence, 215–216
    "silence", reasons of, 212–213
Stereotactic radiosurgery, 153, 160

T

Transsphenoidal surgery, 206
    adrenocorticotropic hormone, 121
    Cushingoid signs, 122
    indications for, 122–123
    postoperative complications
        comorbid medical risk, 131
        CSF rhinorrhea, 133
        epistaxis, 134
        hormone insufficiency, 131–133
        infection, 134
        neurologic, 133
        venous thrombosis, 133
    recurrent disease, 127, 134–135
    surgical remission and long-term outcome
        determination of remission, 128, 129
        HPA axis, 128–131
        hypophysectomy/adenomectomy, 127
        hypopituitarism, 127
        persistent hypercortisolemia, 126
        persistent/recurrent disease, 125, 127
        unweighted average rates, 125, 126
        withdrawal of replacement, 128–131
    surgical techniques
        direct endonasal approach, 123–124
        endoscopic approach, 124–125
        oxymetazoline hydrochloride, 123
        pituitary microadenoma, 123

U

Ultrasound imaging, 9–10
Urine cortisol excretion, 49–50

V

Venous thrombosis, 133